Testis Cancer

Guest Editor

TIMOTHY GILLIGAN, MD

HEMATOLOGY/ONCOLOGY CLINICS OF NORTH AMERICA

www.hemonc.theclinics.com

Consulting Editors
GEORGE P. CANELLOS, MD
NANCY BERLINER, MD

June 2011 • Volume 25 • Number 3

SAUNDERS an imprint of ELSEVIER, Inc.

W.B. SAUNDERS COMPANY
A Division of Elsevier Inc.

1600 John F. Kennedy Blvd. ● Suite 1800 ● Philadelphia, PA 19103-2899

http://www.theclinics.com

HEMATOLOGY/ONCOLOGY CLINICS OF NORTH AMERICA Volume 25, Number 3
June 2011 ISSN 0889-8588, ISBN 13: 978-1-4557-1038-6

Editor: Patrick Manley

Photocopying
Single photocopies of single articles may be made for personal use as allowed by national copyright laws. Permission of the Publisher and payment of a fee is required for all other photocopying, including multiple or systematic copying, copying for advertising or promotional purposes, resale, and all forms of document delivery. Special rates are available for educational institutions that wish to make photocopies for non-profit educational classroom use. For information on how to seek permission visit www.elsevier.com/permissions or call: (+44) 1865 843830 (UK)/(+1) 215 239 3804 (USA).

Derivative Works
Subscribers may reproduce tables of contents or prepare lists of articles including abstracts for internal circulation within their institutions. Permission of the Publisher is required for resale or distribution outside the institution. Permission of the Publisher is required for all other derivative works, including compilations and translations (please consult www.elsevier.com/permissions).

Electronic Storage or Usage
Permission of the Publisher is required to store or use electronically any material contained in this journal, including any article or part of an article (please consult www.elsevier.com/permissions). Except as outlined above, no part of this publication may be reproduced, stored in a retrieval system or transmitted in any form or by any means, electronic, mechanical, photocopying, recording or otherwise, without prior written permission of the Publisher.

Notice
No responsibility is assumed by the Publisher for any injury and/or damage to persons or property as a matter of products liability, negligence or otherwise, or from any use or operation of any methods, products, instructions or ideas contained in the material herein. Because of rapid advances in the medical sciences, in particular, independent verification of diagnoses and drug dosages should be made.

Although all advertising material is expected to conform to ethical (medical) standards, inclusion in this publication does not constitute a guarantee or endorsement of the quality or value of such product or of the claims made of it by its manufacturer.

Hematology/Oncology Clinics (ISSN 0889-8588) is published bimonthly by Elsevier Inc., 360 Park Avenue South, New York, NY 10010-1710. Months of issue are February, April, June, August, October, and December. Business and Editorial Offices: 1600 John F. Kennedy Blvd., Ste. 1800, Philadelphia, PA 19103–2899. Customer Service Office: 3251 Riverport Lane, Maryland Heights, MO 63043. Periodicals postage paid at New York, NY and at additional mailing offices. Subscription prices are $327.00 per year (domestic individuals), $541.00 per year (domestic institutions), $160.00 per year (domestic students/residents), $371.00 per year (Canadian individuals), $662.00 per year (Canadian institutions) $442.00 per year (international individuals), $662.00 per year (international institutions), and $216.00 per year (international and Canadian students/residents). International air speed delivery is included in all *Clinics* subscription prices. All prices are subject to change without notice. **POSTMASTER:** Send address changes to *Hematology/Oncology Clinics of North America*, Elsevier Health Sciences Division, Subscription Customer Service, 3251 Riverport Lane, Maryland Heights, MO 63043. Customer Service (orders, claims, online, change of address): Elsevier Health Sciences Division, Subscription Customer Service, 3251 Riverport Lane, Maryland Heights, MO 63043. Tel: 1-800-654-2452 (U.S. and Canada); 314-447-8871 (outside U.S. and Canada). Fax: 314-447-8029. E-mail: journalscustomerservice-usa@elsevier.com (for print support); journalsonlinesupport-usa@elsevier.com (for online support).

Reprints. For copies of 100 or more, of articles in this publication, please contact the Commercial Reprints Department, Elsevier Inc., 360 Park Avenue South, New York, New York 10010-1710; Tel.: 212-633-3813, Fax: 212-462-1935, E-mail: reprints@elsevier.com.

Hematology/Oncology Clinics of North America is covered in *MEDLINE/PubMed (Index Medicus)*, *EMBASE/ Excerpta Medica*, and *BIOSIS*.

Printed and bound by CPI Group (UK) Ltd, Croydon, CR0 4YY
Transferred to Digital Print 2011

Contributors

CONSULTING EDITORS

GEORGE P. CANELLOS, MD
William Rosenberg Professor of Medicine, Department of Medical Oncology, Dana-Farber
Cancer Institute, Boston, Massachusetts

NANCY BERLINER, MD
Chief, Division of Hematology, Brigham and Women's Hospital; Professor of Medicine,
Harvard Medical School, Boston, Massachusetts

GUEST EDITOR

TIMOTHY GILLIGAN, MD
Director, Late Effects Clinic, Taussig Cancer Institute; Program Director, Hematology/
Oncology Fellowship; Deputy Editor, Cleveland Clinic Journal of Medicine, Cleveland
Clinic, Cleveland, Ohio

AUTHORS

PHILIPPE BEDARD, MD, FRCPC
Staff Physician, Department of Medical Oncology/Haematology, Princess Margaret
Hospital; Assistant Professor, Department of Medicine, University of Toronto, Toronto,
Ontario, Canada

CARSTEN BOKEMEYER, MD
Professor of Medicine; Director, Department of Oncology/Hematology/Bone Marrow
Transplantation/Pneumology, University Medical Center Eppendorf, Hamburg, Germany

GEORGE J. BOSL, MD
Genitourinary Oncology Service, Department of Medicine, Memorial Sloan-Kettering
Cancer Center, New York, New York

PETER W.M. CHUNG, MBChB, FRCPC
Staff Physician, Radiation Medicine Program, Princess Margaret Hospital; Assistant
Professor, Department of Radiation Oncology, University of Toronto, Toronto, Ontario,
Canada

G. COOK, FRCP, FRCR
Department of Nuclear Medicine, Royal Marsden Hospital, Sutton, Surrey, England,
United Kingdom

MICHAEL H. CULLEN, MD
The Cancer Centre, University Hospital Birmingham NHS Foundation Trust, Birmingham,
United Kingdom

DARREN R. FELDMAN, MD
Genitourinary Oncology Service, Department of Medicine, Memorial Sloan-Kettering Cancer Center, New York, New York

SOPHIE D. FOSSÅ, MD, PhD
Department of Clinical Cancer Research, The Norwegian Radium Hospital; University of Oslo, Oslo, Norway

TIMOTHY GILLIGAN, MD
Director, Late Effects Clinic, Taussig Cancer Institute; Program Director, Hematology/Oncology Fellowship; Deputy Editor, Cleveland Clinic Journal of Medicine, Cleveland Clinic, Cleveland, Ohio

SYED A. HUSSAIN, MD
The Cancer Centre, University Hospital Birmingham NHS Foundation Trust; Cancer Research UK, Institute for Cancer Studies, School of Cancer Sciences, University of Birmingham, Birmingham, United Kingdom

DOW-MU KOH, MRCP, FRCR
Department of Diagnostic Radiology, Royal Marsden Hospital, Sutton, Surrey, England, United Kingdom

CHRISTIAN KOLLMANNSBERGER, MD
Clinical Associate Professor of Medicine, Division of Medical Oncology, British Columbia Cancer Agency-Vancouver Cancer Centre, University of British Columbia, Vancouver, British Columbia, Canada

OLIVER KUSS, PhD
Institut für Medizinische Epidemiologie, Biometrie und Informatik, Medizinische Fakultät, Martin-Luther-Universität Halle-Wittenberg, Halle (Saale), Germany

ANJA LORCH, MD
Department of Oncology, Marburg University Clinic, Marburg, Germany

YUK TING MA, MD, PhD
The Cancer Centre, University Hospital Birmingham NHS Foundation Trust, Birmingham, United Kingdom

GARY MOK, MD, FRCPC
Clinical Fellow, Radiation Medicine Program, Princess Margaret Hospital, Toronto, Ontario, Canada

ROBERT J. MOTZER, MD
Genitourinary Oncology Service, Department of Medicine, Memorial Sloan-Kettering Cancer Center, New York, New York

CRAIG NICHOLS, MD
Director of the Multidisciplinary Testicular Cancer Clinic, Division of Medical Oncology, Virginia Mason Medical Center, Seattle, Washington

CARVELL T. NGUYEN, MD, PhD
Glickman Urological and Kidney Institute, Cleveland Clinic, Cleveland, Ohio

KARIN OECHSLE, MD
Department of Oncology/Hematology/Bone Marrow Transplantation/Pneumology, University Medical Center Eppendorf, Hamburg, Germany

JAN OLDENBURG, MD, PhD
Department of Oncology, The Norwegian Radium Hospital, Oslo; Buskerud University College, Institute of Health, Drammen, Norway

THOMAS POWLES, MRCP, MD
Senior Lecturer in Medical Oncology, St Bartholomew's Hospital, Barts and the London NHS Trust, London, United Kingdom

S.A. SOHAIB, MRCP, FRCR
Department of Diagnostic Radiology, Royal Marsden Hospital, Sutton, Surrey, England, United Kingdom

ANDREAS STANG, MD, MPH
Institut für Klinische Epidemiologie, Medizinische Fakultät, Martin-Luther-Universität Halle-Wittenberg, Halle (Saale), Germany

ANDREW J. STEPHENSON, MD
Director, Center for Urological Oncology, Glickman Urological and Kidney Institute, Cleveland Clinic, Cleveland, Ohio

DAVID J. VAUGHN, MD
Professor of Medicine, Division of Hematology/Oncology, University of Pennsylvania, Philadelphia, Pennsylvania

CHRISTINE M. VEENSTRA, MD
Chief Fellow, Division of Hematology/Oncology, University of Pennsylvania, Philadelphia, Pennsylvania

MARTIN H. VOSS, MD
Department of Medicine, Memorial Sloan-Kettering Cancer Center, New York, New York

PADRAIG WARDE, MB, FRCPC
Professor, Department of Radiation Oncology, University of Toronto; Radiation Medicine Program, Princess Margaret Hospital, Toronto, Ontario, Canada

Contents

Preface xiii

Timothy Gilligan

Biology of Germ Cell Tumors 457

Yuk Ting Ma, Michael H. Cullen, and Syed A. Hussain

> Testicular cancer has been a model for a curable malignancy. The existence of an array of potential new therapies is the result of a prodigious effort in the researching and defining of the molecular components of the cancer phenotype and the subsequent rational design of agents to target candidate pathways. A better understanding of the molecular biology of cancer may also aid in guiding the most appropriate use of existing therapies, such as conventional chemotherapy.

Etiologic Differences Between Seminoma and Nonseminoma of the Testis: A Systematic Review of Epidemiologic Studies 473

Andreas Stang and Oliver Kuss

> Descriptive epidemiologic features of testicular cancer suggest that the etiologies of seminoma and nonseminoma of the testis differ. To address this, the authors conducted a systematic review of 150 case-control and cohort studies of the etiology of testicular cancer including 1,148 relative risk estimates, stratified by histologic subgroup, reflecting 631 exposures. Their results do not support the hypothesis that seminoma and nonseminoma have different etiologies among adolescents and young men. To date, only descriptive epidemiologic features, including incidence age patterns and incidence time trends of seminoma and nonseminoma, provide evidence suggesting different etiologies, especially among newborns, infants, and elderly men.

Imaging Studies for Germ Cell Tumors 487

S.A. Sohaib, G. Cook, and Dow-Mu Koh

> Imaging plays an important role in the management of patients with testicular germ cell tumors. This article reviews the role of imaging in the diagnosis, staging, and posttreatment restaging of these patients. CT remains the main radiologic technique used, although ultrasound, MRI, and positron emission tomography also have specific roles in the clinical management of these patients.

Management of Stage I Testicular Seminoma 503

Gary Mok and Padraig Warde

> Adjuvant treatment options for stage I seminoma include surveillance, radiation, and hemotherapy. Despite excellent results for both adjuvant chemotherapy and radiotherapy, many concerns have been raised in regards to the potential long-term toxicities of these treatments. To

minimize the burden of treatment, there has been a shift away from adjuvant treatments for stage I testicular seminomas toward surveillance protocols for seminoma survivors. This article reviews the evidence for all adjuvant treatment options for stage I testicular seminomas with a particular focus on surveillance.

Stage I Nonseminomatous Germ Cell Tumor of the Testis: More Questions than Answers?   517

Thomas Powles

The outcome of patients with stage I nonseminomatous germ cell tumors (NSGCTs) is excellent, with 99% overall 5-year survival. If treated with orchiectomy alone, approximately 30% of patients relapse with metastatic disease. Therefore adjuvant therapy with either chemotherapy or retroperitoneal lymph node dissection (RPLND) is often recommended, despite impressive results with active surveillance alone. This article addresses the risks and benefits of each approach.

Stage II Seminomas and Nonseminomas   529

Peter W.M. Chung and Philippe Bedard

Although a rare presentation for testicular germ cell tumors, the optimal management for stage II disease generates considerable debate, which is, in large part, because of the potential curative role of single-modality treatment in many patients and overall excellent survival in those who require salvage treatment. Individualizing the treatment of each patient to ensure cure with minimal toxicity is challenging, given the rudimentary tools available for predicting disease relapse after initial therapy. Long-term toxicity and patient choice should be taken into account when selecting the management options.

First-Line Chemotherapy of Disseminated Germ Cell Tumors   543

Craig Nichols and Christian Kollmannsberger

The development of effective chemotherapy has been the defining event in the history of testicular cancer treatment. The discovery of cisplatin-based chemotherapy created a massive inflection that sharply defined the relatively grim precisplatin era from the astonishing postcisplatin era. The ripple effects of this discovery continue today with the rewriting of management of early-stage germ cell tumors to surveillance-based programs. This article reviews the discovery, development, and delivery of cisplatin-based chemotherapy; expected outcomes of chemotherapy treatment; remaining controversies in primary chemotherapy treatment of disseminated disease; and practical management tips for delivery of bleomycin, etoposide, and cisplatin and after chemotherapy treatment.

A Review of Second-line Chemotherapy and Prognostic Models for Disseminated Germ Cell Tumors   557

Martin H. Voss, Darren R. Feldman, George J. Bosl, and Robert J. Motzer

Despite an excellent prognosis even for patients with disseminated disease, about 20% to 30% of men with advanced germ cell tumors are refractory to first-line chemotherapy or experience disease recurrence after an initial remission with such treatment. Many of these are cured with conventional dose cisplatin/ifosfamide-based regimen or high-dose chemotherapy with stem cell rescue. Controversy exists regarding the optimal choice between these 2 second-line approaches, and available data for each is reviewed here. Clinical factors can help prognosticate patients, and recently an international effort developed a prognostic model for the second-line setting that can be universally applied in future studies.

Third-Line Chemotherapy and Novel Agents for Metastatic Germ Cell Tumors   577

Christine M. Veenstra and David J. Vaughn

Although germ cell tumors (GCT) are among the most curable solid tumors, a subset of patients with GCT experience relapse or progression despite appropriate cisplatin-based therapy or first-line salvage therapy. This article describes the molecular mechanisms of cisplatin resistance, outlines single-agent chemotherapy and combination chemotherapy regimens that are active against GCT in the third-line or later setting, discusses the use of drug therapy for treating growing teratoma syndrome and teratoma with malignant transformation, outlines novel agents used to treat GCT, and highlights ongoing clinical trials and future directions in the treatment of refractory GCT.

Role of Postchemotherapy Retroperitoneal Lymph Node Dissection in Advanced Germ Cell Tumors   593

Carvell T. Nguyen and Andrew J. Stephenson

Advanced germ cell tumors (GCTs) are curable with the appropriate integration of cisplatin-based chemotherapy and postchemotherapy surgical resection of residual masses. For men with retroperitoneal metastases, postchemotherapy retroperitoneal lymph node dissection (PC-RPLND) is a vital component of this treatment algorithm. The rationale for PC-RPLND is based on the consistent 10% to 20% and 35% to 55% incidence of viable malignancy and teratoma, respectively. Prognostic factors and nomograms cannot predict the presence of necrosis with sufficient accuracy to obviate the need for PC-RPLND. This article reviews the indications, technique, and outcomes of PC-RPLND in the management of advanced GCT.

Treatment of Brain Metastases from Germ Cell Tumors   605

Karin Oechsle and Carsten Bokemeyer

Brain metastases occur in approximately 10% of patients with advanced metastatic germ cell tumors. Patients with nonseminomatous histology, lung metastases, and high β-human chorionic gonadotropin levels are at higher risk for synchronous brain metastases at first diagnosis and for relapsing with brain metastases after successful cisplatin-based chemotherapy. Patients with brain metastases should undergo multimodal treatment strategies, including cisplatin-based combination chemotherapy plus radiotherapy or surgery. However, the optimal combination and sequence of these strategies remain unclear and may differ between subgroups. But in all cases, chemotherapy must be part of treatment, even in patients with isolated cerebral relapse without systemic disease.

Late Relapse of Germ Cell Tumors   615

Jan Oldenburg, Anja Lorch, and Sophie D. Fosså

> This article highlights relevant aspects of the rare late relapses of malig-
> nant germ cell tumors (MGCTs), which by definition occur at least 2 years
> after successful treatment. In most reports, 1% to 6% of patients with
> MGCT experience a late relapse. Surgery is the most important part in
> the treatment of late relapses. Viable MGCT or teratoma with malignant
> transformation may require multimodal treatment with chemotherapy,
> radiotherapy, and/or surgery. Salvage chemotherapy should be based
> on a representative biopsy. Referring patients with late relapse to high-
> volume institutions ensures the best chances of cure and enables multi-
> modal treatment.

Testicular Cancer Survivorship   627

Timothy Gilligan

> Because of a rising incidence of, and declining mortality from, testicular
> cancer, there are an increasing number of survivors of testicular cancer.
> Given their young age at diagnosis, the survivors have many years of life
> ahead of them during which they may experience adverse consequences
> from cancer and its treatment. Over the past few decades and particularly
> in this century, research into the short- and long-term effects of treatments
> of testicular cancer has grown rapidly, and now there exist a much greater
> body of data to help us counsel patients about the risks and side effects of
> these treatments.

Index   641

FORTHCOMING ISSUES

August 2011
Renal Cell Carcinoma
Toni K. Choueri, MD,
Guest Editor

October 2011
Acute Leukemia
Martin Tallman, MD,
Guest Editor

RECENT ISSUES

April 2011
Hematologic Disorders in Pregnancy
Jean M. Connors, MD,
Guest Editor

February 2011
Immunodeficiency, Infection, and Stem Cell Transplantation
Nancy Berliner, MD,
Guest Editor

December 2010
Thalassemia
Bernard G. Forget, MD,
Guest Editor

THE CLINICS ARE NOW AVAILABLE ONLINE!

Access your subscription at:
www.theclinics.com

Preface

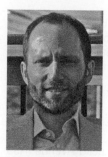

Timothy Gilligan, MD
Guest Editor

The development of effective treatment for testicular germ cell tumors represents one of the great success stories of modern medicine. A cancer that was once almost universally and rapidly fatal unless caught at an early stage is now curable even for most patients with distant metastatic disease. Most patients with testicular cancer are in their 20s, 30s, or 40s, and therefore, the development of successful therapies has resulted in decades of extra life for these men. However, this means that any complications or side effects from treatment may affect their health and quality of life for many years. The stakes are thus very high with regard to getting the treatment right. Mistakes in management that result in failure to cure can result in the loss of many years of life, while unnecessarily aggressive treatment can result in many years of disability or diminished quality of life.

For reasons that remain unclear, the incidence of testicular germ cell tumors is increasing, while, as a result of more effective treatments and the diagnosis of a higher proportion of men with early stage disease, the mortality rate is declining. The treatment of men with early-stage disease remains an area of significant controversy. The development of highly effective chemotherapy for metastatic disease has made postorchiectomy surveillance a widely accepted management strategy for men with stage I cancers because those who relapse can be successfully salvaged. The role of chemotherapy, retroperitoneal lymph node dissection (for nonseminomas), and radiation therapy (for seminomas) for clinical stage I disease is now the subject of frequent debates in the medical literature and at oncology meetings. The treatment of advanced stage disease, in contrast, is much more standardized as a result of a long series of randomized controlled trials.

The major themes of testis cancer research at this time are developing effective treatment for the small number of men with cancers refractory to currently available chemotherapy and the prevention of late effects in men with curable cancers by avoiding overtreatment and unnecessary exposure to radiation due to imaging studies. With regard to the former challenge, it is hoped that our increasing understanding of the biology of germ cell tumors will result in new and more effective treatments for those cancers that are currently incurable. Investigations into the experiences and medical problems of testis cancer survivors are also receiving increasing attention as it has

Hematol Oncol Clin N Am 25 (2011) xiii–xiv
doi:10.1016/j.hoc.2011.04.001

become clear that men with a history of testis cancer who have received radiation therapy and/or chemotherapy have an increased risk of death from cardiovascular disease, secondary malignancies, and several other causes.

This issue of *Hematology/Oncology Clinics of North America* brings together an internationally renowned group of thought leaders, many of whom played central roles in the development of our current treatment paradigms. Together, their articles provide a comprehensive review of the management of this important disease.

Timothy Gilligan, MD
Late Effects Clinic
Taussig Cancer Institute
Cleveland Clinic
9500 Euclid Avenue, R35
Cleveland, OH 44195, USA

E-mail address:
gilligt@ccf.org

Biology of Germ Cell Tumors

Yuk Ting Ma, MD, PhD[a], Michael H. Cullen, MD[a],
Syed A. Hussain, MD[a,b],*

KEYWORDS

• Testicular • Germ cell tumors • Biology • Cisplatin resistance

Germ cell tumors are derived from cells belonging to the germ cell lineage. They occur primarily in the gonads, and less than 10% arise in specific extragonadal sites along the midline of the body. This pattern of distribution is thought to reflect the migration route of the primordial germ cells (PGCs) during embryogenesis—from the yolk sac to the genital ridges.[1]

Germ cell tumors of the testis (TGCTs) account for more than 95% of all testicular tumors, and they are the most common solid malignancies to affect young white men.[1] Histologically, TGCTs comprise 2 major subgroups: seminomas and nonseminomatous germ cell tumors (NSGCTs). Seminomas are composed of uniform tumor cells that resemble PGCs/gonocytes. In contrast, NSGCTs may contain one or more histologic subtypes that represent different differentiation lineages and stages of embryonic development—embryonal carcinoma, choriocarcinoma, yolk sac carcinoma, and teratoma.[1] Ten percent of TGCTs comprise elements of both seminomas and NSGCTs.

TGCTs are characterized by extreme sensitivity to chemotherapy. Despite this, approximately 20% of patients with metastatic TGCTs fail to achieve a complete response or relapse from complete remission; this is due to intrinsic cisplatin resistance or acquired resistance after an initial response. Understanding the molecular biology of TGCTs may thus allow the development of new therapies for the small subset of patients with a poor prognosis.

PREINVASIVE DISEASE

Despite the clinical and histologic differences between seminomas and NSGCTs, all TGCTs are thought to arise from a common precursor lesion, carcinoma in situ, first

The authors have nothing to disclose.
[a] The Cancer Centre, University Hospital Birmingham NHS Foundation Trust, Edgbaston, Birmingham B15 2TH, UK
[b] Cancer Research UK, Institute for Cancer Studies, School of Cancer Sciences, University of Birmingham, Edgbaston, Birmingham B15 2TT, UK
* Corresponding author. Cancer Research UK, Institute for Cancer Studies, School of Cancer Sciences, University of Birmingham, Edgbaston, Birmingham B15 2TT, UK.
E-mail address: s.a.hussain@bham.ac.uk

Hematol Oncol Clin N Am 25 (2011) 457–471
doi:10.1016/j.hoc.2011.03.004
0889-8588/11/$ – see front matter © 2011 Elsevier Inc. All rights reserved.

described by Skakkebaek in 1972.[2] This hypothesis is supported by the frequent observation of carcinoma in situ in the testicular tissue adjacent to TGCTs as well as the development of TGCTs in patients previously diagnosed with carcinoma in situ.[3,4] Due to the absence of epithelial differentiation in these precursors, the term, *intratubular germ cell neoplasia, unclassified (ITGCNU)*, is now more commonly used. Spontaneous regression of ITGCNU does not seem to occur and eventually all ITGCNUs progress to TGCTs. The median time to the development of invasive disease is 5 years.[5]

ITGCNUs are thought to be derived from transformation of a PGC or gonocyte during fetal development.[6] Evidence supporting this includes the morphologic similarities and the presence of overlapping developmental immunohistochemical markers (PLAP, KIT, and OCT3/4) between ITGCNUs and PGCs and early gonocytes.[6–12] In addition, biallelic expression of the imprinted genes, *H19* and *IGF2*, has been reported in TGCTs, indicating again that these tumors may have arisen from PGCs, where genomic imprinting is temporarily erased.[13] More recently, gene expression profiling studies have revealed a substantial overlap between the expression profile of ITGC-NUs and that of embryonic stem cells, providing further evidence of the fetal origin of ITGCNUs.[14,15]

The precise molecular events underlying the initiation of malignant transformation from gonocyte to ITGCNU remains poorly understood; 2 theories have been put forward. Skakkebaek and colleagues[6] proposed that the origins of ITGCNU are fetal gonocytes that are unable to develop into normal spermatogonia.[16] These arrested germ cells are thought to be susceptible to postnatal or pubertal gonadotrophin stimulation, which may lead to further malignant progression later in development.[16,17] This model is supported by extensive data suggesting ITGCNU cells are transformed gonocytes. In the second model, Chaganti and Houldsworth postulated that transformation occurs after the onset of spermatogenesis, involving the zygotene-pachytene spermatocyte.[18] These cells contain replicated DNA, express wild-type p53 temporarily, and seem to be associated with a recombination checkpoint. Furthermore, aberrant chromatid exchange events associated with crossing-over during this stage may lead to increased copy number of the short arm of chromosome 12 (12p), consequential cyclin D2 (*CCND2*) overexpression, and aberrant reinitiation of the cell cycle. This model cannot explain, however, the development of ITGCNU in the gonads of children with sexual differentiation disorders.

Two models have also been proposed to explain the subsequent progression of ITGCNU into seminomas and NSGCTs.[19] In the linear progression model, TGCTs progress along a single pathway, from ITGCNU through seminomas to NSGCTs. Alternatively, the independent progression model postulates that ITGCNU progresses along independent pathways to produce both seminomas and NSGCTs.[19] Considerable evidence exists to support both models and it is likely that both pathways exist.

GENETIC CHANGES

TGCTs are characterized by the invariable gain of material from chromosome 12p.[20–24] In the majority of cases, this is due to an isochromosome of 12p, i(12p), first reported by Atkin and Baker in 1982.[20] This abnormal chromosome comprises 2 fused short arms of chromosome 12 and is common to both seminomas and NSGCTs. The remaining i(12p)-negative TGCTs have also been shown to contain gain of chromosome 12p sequences, either as tandem duplications located in situ or transposed elsewhere in the genome.[21,22]

In addition to gain of the complete 12p, amplification of subregions of chromosome 12p (12p11.2-p12.1 and 12p12 ~ 13) has also been reported in some TGCTs.[23–29] The 12p11.2-p12.1 amplification was first identified in a patient with metastatic seminoma and occurs almost exclusively in i(12p)-negative TGCTs.[23–27] It is associated with a younger age at first presentation compared with seminomas with gain of the complete 12p but does not predict clinical outcome.[27]

Because all TGCTs show gain of chromosome 12p sequences, many investigators have attempted to identify overexpressed genes on 12p, which may be important in the pathogenesis of TGCTs.[30–35] The growing list of candidate genes can be divided into 2 broad groups: those that confer the tumor cells with a growth advantage (eg, CCND2; K-RAS; DAD-R, a novel gene associated with decreased apoptosis in TGCTs; and ethanolamine kinase 1 [EKI1], which may protect cells from apoptotic cell death) and those that help to establish or maintain the stem cell phenotype (eg, the stem cell genes NANOG, STELLA, and GDF3).[30–35]

Gain of 12p is also thought to be associated with malignant progression of ITGCNU into invasive TGCTs. Using high-resolution comparative genomic hybridization, Ottesen and colleagues[36] analyzed the microdissected cells from 7 cases of ITGCNU adjacent to TGCTs and from 2 cases of ITGCNU without invasive elements. Gain of 12p was detected in 6 of 7 cases of ITGCNU adjacent to TGCTs but not in the 2 cases of ITGCNU without invasive disease.[36] Nevertheless, gain of 12p is not thought to be the initiating genetic event, because acquisition of i(12p) has been shown to be preceded by polyploidization.[37]

A nonrandom pattern of over-representation and under-representation of other chromosomal regions has also been reported, although at a lower frequency than the gain of 12p. These changes are common to both seminomas and NSGCTs, supporting the hypothesis of a common origin for all histologic subtypes of TGCTs.

Differential chromosomal gains and losses have also been reported between seminomas and NSGCTs. Gain of chromosomes 7, 15, 19, and 22 and loss of chromosome 17 have been associated with seminomas, whereas gain of chromosomes 5q, 6q, 13q, and 17q and loss of chromosomes 10q, 19, and 22 were detected in NSGCTs, suggesting these regions may be important in the differentiation of TGCTs.[28,38] Several recent studies have attempted to identify differentially expressed genes corresponding to such regions of chromosomal gains and losses.[39–41] Despite this, few of the identified genes have been shown to contribute to the development or progression of TGCTs.

EPIGENETIC CHANGES

Epigenetic silencing of tumor suppressor genes is known to play a significant role in carcinogenesis. The epigenetic regulation of gene expression involves DNA methylation, post-translational modifications of the histone proteins, or both.[42] Aberrant DNA methylation in the proximal promoter region of tumor suppressor genes has been reported in virtually every tumor type and is frequently associated with silencing of gene expression, although the genes inactivated by methylation varies with tumor type.[42]

Despite their genetic similarities, seminomas and NSGCTs are characterized by distinct epigenetic phenotypes.[43–46] Using restriction landmark genomic scanning, Smiraglia and colleagues[43] analyzed 16 TGCT samples and observed virtually no CpG island methylation in the seminomas, whereas CpG island methylation in NSGCTs was similar to that previously identified in other solid malignancies (mean 0.08% vs 1.11%, $P = .003$). Seminomas were also characterized by a higher level of global hypomethylation compared with NSGCTs.[43] This pattern was also demonstrated in several candidate gene studies: methylation of one or more gene promoters was frequently detected in NSGCTs (eg, *MGMT, RASSF1A, APC*, and *FHIT*) whereas minimal methylation was found in seminomas.[44–46] Consistent with these findings, Almstrup and colleagues[47] demonstrated upregulation of DNA methyltransferase 3B (DNMT3B) in NSGCTs but not in seminomas compared with ITGCNU. DNMT3B is predominantly involved in establishing de novo methylation patterns.[42]

Furthermore, aberrant promoter methylation was associated with absent or down-regulated gene expression in most of the methylated genes, and reactivation of gene expression was frequently observed, in vitro, after treatment with the demethylating agent, 5-aza-2'deoxycytidine.[44]

Recently, the distinct methylation profiles have been correlated with differentiation.[48,49] Using immunohistochemical staining against 5-methylcytosine to assess global methylation patterns, hypomethylation was observed in ITGCNU and seminomas, whereas the more differentiated nonseminomas (eg, yolk sac tumors, choriocarcinomas, and teratomas) were all consistently hypermethylated.[48,49] This was also observed using a candidate gene approach. Using microdissected cells, the upstream region of *OCT3/4* (a transcription factor involved in the maintenance of pluripotency in embryonic stem cells) was found hypomethylated in seminomas and in the undifferentiated nonseminomatous embryonal carcinoma, whereas this region was hypermethylated in the differentiated nonseminomatous components.[50] Distinguishing methylation changes that reflect normal development from those contributing to TGCT pathogenesis presents an important challenge.

GENE EXPRESSION PROFILING

Using gene expression profiling, distinct molecular signatures have also been observed between seminomas and the different histologic components of NSGCTs, providing further insight into germ cell tumorigenesis.[47,51–55] Port and colleagues[51] analyzed 11 TGCTs (5 seminomas and 6 NSGCTs) and revealed almost opposing gene expression profiles between seminomas and NSGCTs. The majority of the differentially expressed genes fell into 5 functional groups: cell cycle, intracellular transducer, apoptosis, DNA synthesis and repair, and transcription, irrespective of the histologic subtype.[51] Korkola and colleagues[53] performed gene expression profiling on 84 NSGCTs (42 pure and 42 mixed) and identified differentially expressed genes predictive of each subset of NSGCTs. Using hierarchical clustering, Hofer and colleagues[55] identified a new subgroup of seminomas with an expression profile similar to the embryonal carcinoma component of NSGCTs. The 2 subgroups of seminomas distinguished were otherwise histologically similar. Whether this allows identification of a subgroup of patients with a poorer prognosis remains unknown but is worthy of investigation.

Gene expression profiling studies have also been used to predict clinical outcome in patients with TGCTs. Sugimura and colleagues[56] performed gene expression microarray analysis on 17 metastatic NSGCTs and identified 11 differentially expressed genes that could distinguish early-relapse NSGCTs from late-relapse NSGCTs. More recently, Korkola and colleagues[57] performed gene expression profiling on 108 NSGCT patients treated with cisplatin-based chemotherapy and identified a gene expression signature that could predict overall survival.

BIOLOGY OF CHEMOSENSITIVITY

The exquisite sensitivity of TGCTs to cisplatin-based chemotherapy is thought to be related to their embryonal origin. Embryonic stem cells retain the potential to produce any cell type in the body, and these cells therefore have a high sensitivity to DNA damage to maintain genomic integrity.[58,59] The high sensitivity of TGCTs to chemotherapy in vivo is also maintained in vitro with many studies demonstrating that TGCT cells are 2-fold to 4-fold more sensitive to cytotoxic agents or irradiation compared with other types of tumor cells.[60–64] Thus, TGCT provides an ideal model in which to study the mechanisms of chemotherapy sensitivity.

In general, 4 factors determine the sensitivity of a cell to chemotherapeutic agents: transport of the drug across the cell membrane, drug metabolism, accessibility of the drug to DNA, and the cell's response to DNA damage.[65] The molecular basis for the extreme chemosensitivity of TGCTs remains poorly understood but is thought to be predominantly related to the DNA damage response pathways.[65]

Expression of p53

It was initially proposed that the absence of p53 mutations and the expression of high levels of wild-type p53 in TGCTs might account for the chemosensitivity of these tumors.[66–68] More than 30% of TGCTs, however, show no p53 staining using immunohistochemistry.[68] Furthermore, in clinical samples, a high level of p53 expression did not relate to treatment sensitivity of the TGCTs; p53 was detected in 59% of the treatment-sensitive tumors compared with 89% of the treatment-resistant TGCTs.[68] Thus, the expression of wild-type p53 alone is insufficient to account for the chemosensitivity of TGCTs.

Apoptosis

Studies investigating the role of apoptosis in TGCTs have reported conflicting data. An initial study reported relatively high levels of expression of the proapoptotic protein Bax in 3 TGCT cell lines and no expression of the antiapoptotic protein Bcl-2, and this high Bax:Bcl-2 ratio was hypothesized to contribute to the 15-fold higher sensitivity to etoposide-induced apoptosis observed in the TGCT cell lines compared with 3 bladder cancer cell lines.[69] Subsequent transfection of one of these TGCT cell lines (833K) with Bcl-2 resulted in a surprising increase in sensitivity to drug-induced apoptosis, and the observed reciprocal down-regulation of the Bcl-2 homolog, Bcl-X_L was proposed as the mechanism by which Bcl-2 transfection resulted in activation of apoptosis.[70] A separate study, however, using 4 different TGCT cell lines observed no correlation between the expression of Bax, Bcl-2, and cisplatin-induced apoptosis.[71] Furthermore, although a high Bax:Bcl-2 ratio was also detected in the invasive components of 46 TGCT samples derived from patients with both chemosensitive and chemotherapy-refractory disease, this was not associated with treatment outcome.[72]

Seladin-1 is a multifunctional protein involved in apoptosis. Recently, an inverse relationship between the expression levels of seladin-1 in TGCT cell lines and sensitivity to cisplatin was demonstrated, and the antiapoptotic effect was mediated through inhibition of caspase-3 activation.[73]

DNA Repair Pathways

In mammalian cells, nucleotide excision repair (NER) is the main mechanism by which cisplatin-induced intrastrand DNA cross-links are removed.[74,75] In 1988, Bedford and colleagues[76] provided the first evidence that NER was defective in TGCTs: using atomic absorption spectroscopy and alkaline elution, TGCT cell lines demonstrated a reduced ability to remove platinum-DNA adducts from the genome compared with a bladder cancer cell line. The reduced capacity for NER in TGCT cell lines has been attributed to low levels of the core NER proteins, xeroderma pigmentosum group

A protein, and the ERCC1-XPF endonuclease.[77,78] Clinical data correlating low NER protein levels to adverse clinical outcome, however, are currently lacking.

Interstrand DNA cross-links (ICLs) account for less than 5% of all cisplatin lesions and these are repaired by ICL repair. Recently, it has been demonstrated that TGCT cell lines are also deficient in ICL repair, due to low level expression of ERCC1-XPF, and that this accounts, at least in part, to the sensitivity to cisplatin.[79]

High-mobility group domain proteins have also been investigated. These proteins specifically recognize and bind to the main cisplatin-induced intrastrand cross-link, 1,2 d(GpG) adduct and block these lesions from NER.[80–82] In TGCT cell lines, the human testis-determining factor, SRY, and the murine testis-specific high-mobility group domain protein have been shown to bind to the cisplatin-DNA adducts with high affinity.[83–85] Again, however, clinical data are lacking.

BIOLOGY OF CHEMOTHERAPY RESISTANCE

Many mechanisms associated with resistance to chemotherapy have been identified, predominantly from studies using drug-resistant cell lines. Cisplatin resistance has been the most widely studied.

Transport of Cisplatin Across Cell Membrane

One potential mechanism for resistance is to reduce the intracellular concentration of cisplatin that is available to target DNA, either by preventing drug influx or by exporting the drug out of the cell. Transporters involved in the maintenance of copper homeostasis have been found to be important in the transport of platinum agents.[86,87] Decreased expression of CTR1, the major influx transporter, and overexpression of ATP7A and ATP7B, the efflux transporters, have been associated with cisplatin resistance in vitro.[88–91] In ovarian and gastric carcinomas that were refractory to cisplatin, overexpression of ATP7B has also been reported.[92,93] The expression of these transporters in TGCT in vivo, however, has yet to be reported.

Overexpression of the ABC transporters has also been investigated but not been shown to contribute significantly to chemotherapy resistance. No significant difference in the levels of 4 ABC transporters (Pgp, MRP1, MRP2, and BRCP) or the major vault protein, LRP, were detected between TGCT samples taken from patients with responsive and those with resistant disease, although individual samples from chemotherapy-resistant cases showed high expression of MRP2.[72]

Drug Metabolism

Elevated levels of the detoxifying agents, glutathione and metallothionein, can also decrease the intracellular levels of active drug. Conflicting data, however, have been published from different studies,[72,94–96] suggesting that drug detoxification does not contribute significantly to cisplatin resistance in TGCTs.

Cell's Response to DNA Damage

Mismatch repair pathway

The mismatch repair (MMR) pathway contributes to acquired cisplatin resistance. Platinum complexes interfere with normal MMR activity and prevent a complete repair of DNA damage. When the MMR pathway is intact, this leads to the initiation of apoptosis. When MMR is deficient, cells can continue to proliferate in spite of DNA damage caused by cisplatin. Studies in several human tumor cell lines have shown that loss of DNA mismatch repair due to lack of expression of hMSH2 or hMLH1 results in low-level resistance to cisplatin.[97,98] In addition, in a xenograft model, this low-level resistance (<2-fold) was sufficient to impair clinical response to cisplatin in vivo.[99]

There is increasing evidence that deficiency of MMR also contributes to chemotherapy resistance in TGCTs.[100–104] Mayer and colleagues[100] detected microsatellite instability, a determinant of deficiency of the MMR pathway, in 5 of 11 refractory TGCTs tested compared with 6 of 100 unselected TGCTs examined (45% vs 6%, P = .001). Furthermore, in a series of 162 TGCTs, Velasco and colleagues[102,103] demonstrated that decreased immunohistochemical staining for MMR proteins and/ or increased frequency of microsatellite instability was associated with a shorter time to tumor recurrence and death. Confirmation of these findings in a prospective study would be useful. Recently, a significantly higher incidence of the *BRAF* V600E mutation was detected in chemotherapy-resistant TGCTs compared with control TGCTs, and this was highly correlated with microsatellite instability.[104] Because multikinase inhibitors targeting BRAF are available (eg, sorafenib), it will be important to evaluate these agents in patients with chemotherapy-resistant TGCTs.

Apoptosis

p53 Mutations were initially thought to contribute to cisplatin resistance. Houldsworth and colleagues[105] detected p53 mutations in 4 of 23 patients with either primary resistant or chemotherapy-relapsed TGCTs. All the mutations, however, were identified in TGCTs with a teratomatous histology, which are known to be intrinsically resistant to chemotherapy. A subsequent study identified p53 mutations in only 1 of 17 treatment-sensitive TGCT and in 0 of 18 treatment-resistant TGCTs, and expression of p53 was not lower in the refractory tumors compared with the responsive group.[68] This second study contained a lower number of mature teratoma samples. Thus, p53 mutations are unlikely to account for cisplatin resistance in most patients with TGCTs.

Preclinical data have also shown that p53 mutations do not contribute significantly to cisplatin resistance: the susceptibility of 6 TGCT cell lines to induction of apoptosis was not associated with their p53 status.[106] Furthermore, inactivation of wild-type p53 function by transfecting cells with the HPV16 E6 gene did not affect cisplatin-induced or gamma irradiation–induced apoptosis.[106] Thus, wild-type p53 expression is not required for the efficient induction of apoptosis in TGCT cell lines. Cisplatin has been shown to mediate p53-independent apoptosis via activation of the Fas/CD95 or the MEK-ERK signaling pathways, and inactivation of these pathways has been associated with resistance to cisplatin-induced apoptosis in vitro.[106–108]

The caspase family of proteases also has been investigated. Inhibition of caspase-9 in TGCT cell lines almost completely blocked apoptosis and induced cisplatin resistance.[109] This effect was independent of the expression of p53, Fas receptor, Fas ligand, or the Bcl-2 family proteins.[109]

NER

Although reduced NER has been shown to contribute significantly to the chemosensitivity of TGCTs, enhanced NER has not emerged as a major contributor to cisplatin resistance. No difference in the DNA repair capacity was detected in 2 sublines with acquired cisplatin resistance, compared with the cisplatin-sensitive parental cell lines.[110]

Genome-wide Studies

Genome-wide studies have also been conducted to identify the genetic mechanisms underlying cisplatin resistance. Using comparative genomic hybridization, high-level amplification in 8 regions were observed in 5 of 17 chemotherapy-resistant

TGCTs: 1q31–32, 2p23–24, 7q21, 7q31, 9q22, 9q32–34, 15q23–24, and 20q11.2–12.[111] Further studies are needed, however, to identify potential candidate genes residing in these regions. Wilson and colleagues[112] performed comparative expressed sequence hybridization, a technique for gene expression profiling along chromosomes, on 3 pairs of TGCT cell lines, and revealed a striking overexpression of 16q in all 3 cisplatin-resistant cell lines compared with their cisplatin-sensitive parental cell lines. This suggests that a gene or group of genes from 16q plays an important role in cisplatin resistance in TGCTs, although, again, the relevant genes remain to be identified. More recently, gene expression profiling has been performed on these 3 pairs of TGCT cell lines and revealed only a few differentially expressed genes when comparing the parental cells with the resistant cells.[113] The most significantly differentially expressed gene was found to be CCND1, and in a series of 25 clinical samples (13 resistant and 12 sensitive), significantly higher levels of CCND1 expression were detected in the resistant cases compared with the sensitive samples.[113] Furthermore, CCND1 overexpression was detected in most of the resistant samples, suggesting that CCND1 overexpression may be a common mechanism of cisplatin resistance in TGCTs.

Epigenetics and Cisplatin Resistance

Two recent studies have demonstrated in vitro that chemical demethylation using 5-azacytidine or 5-aza-2'-deoxycytidine can resensitize cisplatin-resistant cells to cisplatin-mediated toxicity.[49,114] Further in vitro and in vivo studies are needed to assess if these agents may provide an additional therapeutic modality for patients with resistant TGCTs.

SUMMARY

Testicular cancer has been a model for a curable malignancy. The existence of an array of potential new therapies is the result of a prodigious effort in the researching and defining of the molecular components of the cancer phenotype and the subsequent rational design of agents to target candidate pathways. A better understanding of the molecular biology of cancer may also aid in guiding the most appropriate use of existing therapies, such as conventional chemotherapy. This knowledge will facilitate the rational selection of drug combinations and/or sequencing based on their mechanisms of action at a molecular level. There has been considerable progress in understanding the molecular biology of TGCTs. These heterogeneous tumors originate from a common precursor lesion, ITGCNU, reflected in the broadly similar genetic profile of seminomas and NSGCTs, whereas the distinct epigenetic profiles are thought to explain their phenotypic differences. Although the majority of patients with TGCTs are cured, understanding the molecular mechanisms underlying cisplatin resistance is important and will enable the development of new approaches for those with resistant disease. A key goal for the molecular technologies described in this article is to improve risk stratification for patients with stage I disease so that adjuvant therapy can be recommended more rationally. In terms of metastatic disease, although the majority of patients with metatstatic disease can be cured by combination cisplatin-based chemotherapy, some patients are not cured. Currently, clinical parameters can identify a small group of high-risk patients, more than 50% of whom are still cured by standard chemotherapy regimens. Thus, it would be desirable to identify the 50% of high-risk patients not cured by conventional therapy so that they may be selected for clinical trials of novel therapies and novel approaches. The key is to define the patient population most likely to benefit from these agents through identification of clinical and biologic markers indicating a sensitive tumor phenotype. The integration of small molecules, multikinase inhibitors, and a range of pipeline products being developed by pharmaceutical industries with existing therapies should be based on robust preclinical data indicating potentially beneficial additive or even synergistic interactions. The correct clinical management strategy can be guided by preclinical modeling but can only be validated by carefully designed clinical trials. These need to be conducted with correlative translational research elements to allow selecting the most appropriate treatment strategy for individual patients. An understanding of tumors at the molecular level and of the mechanisms of drug resistance may go a long way toward achieving that goal. The future for cancer therapy is promising, but it is important to be prepared for disappointment, because early success in animal models cannot guarantee a successful human therapy.

REFERENCES

1. Looijenga LH, Oosterhuis JW. Pathogenesis of testicular germ cell tumours. Rev Reprod 1999;4:90–100.
2. Skakkebaek NE. Possible carcinoma-in-situ of the testis. Lancet 1972;2:516–7.
3. Jacobsen GK, Henriksen OB, von der Maase H. Carcinoma in situ of testicular tissue adjacent to malignant germ cell tumors: a study of 105 cases. Cancer 1981;47:2660–2.
4. Skakkebaek NE. Carcinoma *in situ* of the testis: frequency and relationship to invasive germ cell tumours in infertile men. Histopathology 1978;2:157–70.
5. Von der Maase H, Rørth M, Walbom-Jørgensen S, et al. Carcinoma in situ of contralateral testis in patients with testicular germ cell cancer: study of 27 cases in 500 patients. Br Med J 1986;293:1398–401.
6. Skakkebaek NE, Berthelsen JG, Giwercman A, et al. Carcinoma-in-situ of the testis: possible origin from gonocytes and precursor of all types of germ cell tumours except spermatocytoma. Int J Androl 1987;10:19–28.
7. Nielsen H, Nielsen M, Skakkebaek NE. The fine structure of possible carcinoma-in-situ in the seminiferous tubules in the testes of four infertile men. Acta Pathol Microbiol Scand A 1974;82:235–48.
8. Rajpert-De Meyts E, Bartkova J, Samson M, et al. The emerging phenotype of the testicular carcinoma in situ germ cell. APMIS 2003;111:267–78.
9. Koide O, Iwai S, Baba K, et al. Identification of testicular atypical germ cells by an immunohistochemical technique for placental alkaline phosphatase. Cancer 1987;60:1325–30.
10. Giwercman A, Cantell L, Marks A. Placental-like alkaline phosphatase as a marker of carcinoma in situ of the testis. Comparison with monoclonal antibodies M2A and 43-9F. APMIS 1991;99:586–94.
11. Jorgensen N, Rajpert-De Meyts E, Graem N, et al. Expression of immunohistochemical markers for testicular carcinoma in situ by normal human fetal germ cells. Lab Invest 1995;72:223–31.
12. Rajpert-De Meyts E, Hanstein R, Jorgensen N, et al. Developmental expression of POU5F1 (OCT3/4) in normal and dysgenetic human gonads. Hum Reprod 2004;19:1338–44.
13. van Gurp RJ, Oosterhuis JW, Kalscheuer V, et al. Biallelic expression of the H19 and IGF2 genes in human testicular germ cell tumors. J Natl Cancer Inst 1994; 86:1070–5.
14. Almstrup K, Hoei-Hansen CE, Wirkner U, et al. Embryonic stem cell-like features of testicular carcinoma in situ revealed by genome-wide gene expression profiling. Cancer Res 2004;64:4736–43.

15. Skotheim RI, Lind GE, Monni O, et al. Differentiation of human embryonal carcinomas in vitro and in vivo reveals expression profiles relevant to normal development. Cancer Res 2005;65:5588–98.
16. Rajpert-De Meyts E, Jørgensen N, Brøndum-Nielsen K, et al. Developmental arrest of germ cells in the pathogenesis of germ cell neoplasia. APMIS 1998; 106:198–204.
17. Rajpert-De Meyts E, Skakkebaek NE. The possible role of sex hormones in the development of testicular cancer. Eur Urol 1993;23:54–9.
18. Chaganti RS, Houldsworth J. Genetics and biology of adult human male germ cell tumors. Cancer Res 2000;60:1475–82.
19. Dieckmann KP, Skakkebaek NE. Carcinoma in situ of the testis: review of biological and clinical features. Int J Cancer 1999;83:815–22.
20. Atkin NB, Baker MC. Specific chromosome change, i(12p), in testicular tumours? Lancet 1982;11:1349.
21. Suijkerbuijk RF, Sinke RJ, Meloni AM, et al. Overrepresentation of chromosome 12p sequences and karyotypic evolution in i(12p)-negative testicular germ-cell tumors revealed by fluorescence in situ hybridization. Cancer Genet Cytogenet 1993;70:85–93.
22. Rodriguez E, Houldsworth J, Reuter VE, et al. Molecular cytogenetic analysis of i(12p)-negative human male germ cell tumors. Genes Chromosomes Cancer 1993;8:230–6.
23. Mostert MM, van de Pol M, Olde Weghuis D, et al. Comparative genomic hybridization of germ cell tumors of the adult testis: confirmation of karyotypic findings and identification of a 12p amplicon. Cancer Genet Cytogenet 1996;89:146–52.
24. Korn MW, Olde Weghuis DE, Suijkerbuijk RF, et al. Detection of chromosomal DNA gains and losses in testicular germ cell tumors by comparative genomic hybridization. Genes Chromosomes Cancer 1996;17:78–87.
25. Suijkerbuijk RF, Sinke RJ, Olde Weghuis DE, et al. Amplification of chromosome subregion 12p11.2–12.1 in a metastasis of an i(12p)-negative seminoma: relationship to tumor progression? Cancer Genet Cytogenet 1994;78:145–52.
26. Mostert MC, Verkerk AJ, van de Pol M, et al. Identification of the critical region of 12p over-representation in testicular germ cell tumors of adolescents and adults. Oncogene 1998;16:2617–27.
27. Roelofs H, Mostert MC, Pompe K, et al. Restricted 12p amplification and RAS mutation in human germ cell tumors of the adult testis. Am J Pathol 2000;57: 1155–66.
28. Kraggerud SM, Skotheim RI, Szymanska J, et al. Genome profiles of familial/ bilateral and sporadic testicular germ cell tumors. Genes Chromosomes Cancer 2002;34:168–74.
29. Henegariu O, Heerema NA, Thurston V, et al. Characterization of gains, losses, and regional amplification in testicular germ cell tumor cell lines by comparative genomic hybridization. Cancer Genet Cytogenet 2004;148:14–20.
30. Houldsorth J, Reuter V, Bosl GJ, et al. Aberrant expression of cyclin D2 is an early event in human male germ cell tumorigenesis. Cell Growth Differ 1997;8:293–9.
31. Zafarana G, Gillis AJ, van Gurp RJ, et al. Coamplification of DAD-R, SOX5 and EKI1 in human testicular seminomas, with specific overexpression of DAD-R, correlates with reduced levels of apoptosis and earlier clinical manifestation. Cancer Res 2002;62:1822–31.
32. Rodriguez S, Jafer O, Goker H, et al. Expression profile of genes from 12p in testicular germ cell tumors of adolescents and adults associated with i(12p) and amplification at 12p1.2-p12.1. Oncogene 2003;22:1880–91.

33. Bourdon V, Naef F, Rao PH, et al. Genomic and expression analysis of the 12p11–p12 amplicon using EST arrays identifies two novel amplified and over-expressed genes. Cancer Res 2002;62:6218–23.

34. Ezeh UI, Turek PJ, Reijo RA, et al. Human embryonic stem cell genes OCT4, NANOG, STELLAR, and GDF3 are expressed in both seminoma and breast carcinoma. Cancer 2005;104:2255–65.

35. Korkola JE, Houldsworth J, Chadalavada RS, et al. Down-regulation of stem cell genes, including those in a 200-kb gene cluster at 12p13.31, is associated with in vivo differentiation of human male germ cell tumors. Cancer Res 2006;66:820–7.

36. Ottesen AM, Skakkebaek NE, Lundsteen C, et al. High-resolution comparative genomic hybridization detects extra chromosome arm 12p material in most cases of carcinoma in situ adjacent to overt germ cell tumors, but not before the invasive tumor development. Genes Chromosomes Cancer 2003;38: 117–25.

37. Geurts van Kessel A, van Drunen E, de Jong B, et al. Chromosome 12q hetero-zygosity is retained in i(12p)-positive testicular germ cell tumor cells. Cancer Genet Cytogenet 1989;40:129–34.

38. Summersgill B, Osin P, Lu YJ, et al. Chromosomal imbalances associated with carcinoma in situ and associated testicular germ cell tumours of adolescents and adults. Br J Cancer 2001;85:213–9.

39. Skotheim RI, Monni O, Mousses S, et al. New insights into testicular germ cell tumorigenesis from gene expression profiling. Cancer Res 2002;62: 2359–64.

40. McIntyre A, Summersgill B, Jafar O, et al. Defining minimum genomic regions of imbalance involved in testicular germ cell tumors of adolescents and adults through genome wide microarray analysis of cDNA clones. Oncogene 2004; 23:9142–7.

41. Skotheim RI, Autio R, Lind GE, et al. Novel genomic aberrations in testicular germ cell tumors by array-CGH, and associated gene expression change. Cell Oncol 2006;28:315–26.

42. Jones PA, Baylin SB. The fundamental role of epigenetic events in cancer. Nat Rev Genet 2002;3:415–28.

43. Smiraglia DJ, Szymanska J, Kraggerud SM, et al. Distinct epigenetic pheno-types in seminomatous and nonseminomatous testicular germ cell tumors. Oncogene 2002;21:3909–16.

44. Koul S, Houldsworth J, Mansukhani MM, et al. Characteristic promoter hyperme-thylation signatures in male germ cell tumors. Mol Cancer 2002;1:8.

45. Smith-Sørensen B, Lind GE, Skotheim RI, et al. Frequent promoter hypermethy-lation of the O6-Methylguanine-DNA Methyltransferase (MGMT) gene in testic-ular cancer. Oncogene 2002;21:8878–84.

46. Honorio S, Agathanggelou A, Wernet N, et al. Frequent epigenetic inactivation of the RASSF1A tumour suppressor gene in testicular tumours and distinct methyl-ation profiles of seminoma and nonseminoma germ cell tumours. Oncogene 2003;22:461–6.

47. Almstrup K, Hoei-Hansen CE, Nielsen JE, et al. Genome-wide gene expression profiling of testicular carcinoma in situ progression into overt tumours. Br J Cancer 2005;92:1934–41.

48. Netto GJ, Nakai Y, Nakayama M, et al. Global DNA hypomethylation in intratub-ular germ cell neoplasia and seminoma, but not in nonseminomatous male germ cell tumors. Mod Pathol 2008;21:1337–44.

49. Wermann H, Stoop H, Gillis AJ, et al. Global DNA methylation in fetal human germ cells and germ cell tumours: association with differentiation and cisplatin resistance. J Pathol 2010;221:433–43.

50. De Jong J, Weeda S, Gillis AJM, et al. Differential methylation of the OCT3/4 upstream region in primary human testicular germ cell tumors. Oncol Rep 2007;18:127–32.

51. Port M, Schmelz HU, Stockinger M, et al. Gene expression profiling in seminoma and nonseminoma. J Clin Oncol 2005;23:58–69.

52. Okada K, Katagiri T, Tsunoda T, et al. Analysis of gene-expression profiles in testicular seminomas using a genome-wide cDNA microarray. Int J Oncol 2003;23:1615–35.

53. Korkola JE, Houldsworth J, Dobrzynski D, et al. Gene expression-based classification of nonseminomatous male germ cell tumors. Oncogene 2005;24: 5101–7.

54. Juric D, Sale S, Hromas RA, et al. Gene expression profiling differentiates germ cell tumors from other cancers and defines subtype-specific signatures. Proc Natl Acad Sci U S A 2005;102:17763–8.

55. Hofer MD, Browne TJ, He L, et al. Identification of two molecular groups of seminomas by using expression and tissue microarrays. Clin Cancer Res 2005;11: 5722–9.

56. Sugimura J, Foster RS, Cummings OW, et al. Gene expression profiling of early- and late-relapse nonseminomatous germ cell tumor and primitive neuroectodermal tumor of the testis. Clin Cancer Res 2004;10:2368–78.

57. Korkola JE, Houldsworth J, Feldman DR, et al. Identification and validation of a gene expression signature that predicts outcome in adult men with germ cell tumors. J Clin Oncol 2009;27:5240–7.

58. Aladjem MI, Spike BT, Rodewald LW, et al. ES cells do not activate p53-dependent stress responses and undergo p53-independent apoptosis in response to DNA damage. Curr Biol 1998;8:145–55.

59. Hong Y, Stambrook PJ. Restoration of an absent G_1 arrest and protection from apoptosis in embryonic stem cells after ionizing radiation. Proc Natl Acad Sci U S A 2004;101:14443–8.

60. Oosterhuis JW, Andrews PW, Knowles BB, et al. Effects of cis-platinum on embryonal cancer cell lines in vitro. Int J Cancer 1984;34:133–9.

61. Walker MC, Parris CN, Masters JR. Differential sensitivities to chemotherapeutic drugs between testicular and bladder cancer cells. J Natl Cancer Inst 1987;79:213–6.

62. Fry AM, Chresta CM, Davies SM, et al. Relationship between topoisomerase II level and chemosensitivity in human tumor cell lines. Cancer Res 1991;51: 6592–5.

63. Masters JR, Osborne EJ, Walker MC, et al. Hypersensitivity of human testis-tumour cell lines to chemotherapeutic drugs. Int J Cancer 1993;53:340–6.

64. Parris CN, Arlett CF, Lehmann AR, et al. Differential sensitivities to gamma radiation of human bladder and testicular tumour cell lines. Int J Radiat Biol Relat Stud Phys Chem Med 1988;53:599–608.

65. Masters JR, Köberle B. Curing metastatic cancer: lessons from testicular germ-cell tumours. Nat Rev Cancer 2003;3:517–25.

66. Peng HQ, Hogg D, Malkin D, et al. Mutations of the p53 gene do not occur in testis cancer. Cancer Res 1993;53:3574–8.

67. Heimdal K, Lothe RA, Lystad S, et al. No germline TP53 mutations detected in familial and bilateral testicular cancer. Genes Chromosomes Cancer 1993;6:92–7.

68. Kersemaekers AM, Mayer F, Molier M, et al. Role of P53 and MDM2 in treatment response of human germ cell tumors. J Clin Oncol 2002;20:1551–61.
69. Chresta CM, Masters JR, Hickman JA. Hypersensitivity of human testicular tumors to etoposide-induced apoptosis is associated with functional p53 and a high Bax:Bcl-2 ratio. Cancer Res 1996;56:1834–41.
70. Arriola EL, Rodriguez-Lopez AM, Hickman JA, et al. Bcl-2 overexpression results in reciprocal downregulation of Bcl-X$_L$ and sensitises human testicular germ cell tumours to chemotherapy-induced apoptosis. Oncogene 1998;18: 1457–64.
71. Burger H, Nooter K, Boersma AW, et al. Expression of p53, Bcl-2 and Bax in cisplatin-induced apoptosis in testicular germ cell tumour cell lines. Br J Cancer 1998;77:1562–7.
72. Mayer F, Stoop H, Scheffer GL, et al. Molecular determinants of treatment response in human germ cell tumors. Clin Cancer Res 2003;9:767–73.
73. Nuti F, Luciani P, Marinari E, et al. Seladin-1 and testicular germ cell tumours: new insights into cisplatin responsiveness. J Pathol 2009;219:491–500.
74. Fichtinger-Schepman AM, van der Veer JL, den Hartog JH, et al. Adducts of the antitumor drug cis-diamminedichloroplatinum(II) with DNA: formation, identification, and quantitation. Biochemistry 1985;24:707–13.
75. Zamble DB, Mu D, Reardon JT, et al. Repair of cisplatin–DNA adducts by the mammalian excision nuclease. Biochemistry 1996;35:10004–13.
76. Bedford P, Fichtinger-Schepman AM, Shellard SA, et al. Differential repair of platinum-DNA adducts in human bladder and testicular tumor continuous cell lines. Cancer Res 1988;48:3019–24.
77. Köberle B, Masters JR, Hartley JA, et al. Defective repair of cisplatin-induced DNA damage caused by reduced XPA protein in testicular germ cell tumours. Curr Biol 1999;9:273–6.
78. Welsh C, Day R, McGurk C, et al. Reduced levels of XPA, ERRC1 and XPF DNA repair proteins in testis tumor cell lines. Int J Cancer 2004;110:352–61.
79. Usanova S, Piee-Staffa A, Sied U, et al. Cisplatin sensitivity of testis tumour cells is due to deficiency in interstrand-crosslink repair and low ERCC1-XPF expression. Mol Cancer 2010;9:248.
80. Ohndorf UM, Rould MA, He Q, et al. Basis for the recognition of cisplatin-modified DNA by high-mobility-group proteins. Nature 1999;399:708–12.
81. Billings PC, Engelsberg BN, Hughes EN. Proteins binding to cisplatin-damaged DNA in human cell lines. Cancer Invest 1994;12:597–604.
82. Huang JC, Zamble DB, Reardon JT, et al. HMG-domain proteins specifically inhibit the repair of the major DNA adduct of the anticancer drug cisplatin by human excision nuclease. Proc Natl Acad Sci U S A 1994;91:10394–8.
83. Zamble DB, Mikata Y, Eng CE, et al. Testis-specific HMG-domain protein alters the response of cells to cisplatin. J Inorg Biochem 2002;91:451–62.
84. Ohndorf UM, Whitehead JP, Raju NL, et al. Binding to tsHMG, a mouse testis-specific HMG-domain protein, to cisplatin-DNA adducts. Biochemistry 1997; 36:14807–15.
85. Trimer EE, Zamble DB, Lippard SJ, et al. Human testis-determining factor SRY binds to the major DNA adduct of cisplatin and a putative target sequence with comparable affinities. Biochemistry 1998;37:352–62.
86. Safaei R, Howell SB. Copper transporters regulate the cellular pharmacology and sensitivity to Pt drugs. Crit Rev Oncol Hematol 2005;53:13–23.
87. Kuo MT, Chen HH, Song IS, et al. The roles of copper transporters in cisplatin resistance. Cancer Metastasis Rev 2007;26:71–83.

88. Song IS, Savaraj N, Siddik ZH, et al. Role of human copper transporter Ctr1 in the transport of platinum-based antitumor agents in cisplatin-sensitive and cisplatin-resistant cells. Mol Cancer Ther 2004;3:1543–9.

89. Komatsu M, Sumizawa T, Mutoh M, et al. Copper-transporting P-type adenosine triphosphatase (ATP7B) is associated with cisplatin resistance. Cancer Res 2000;60:1312–6.

90. Samimi G, Safaei R, Katano K, et al. Increased expression of the copper efflux transporter ATP7A mediates resistance to cisplatin, carboplatin, and oxaliplatin in ovarian cancer cells. Clin Cancer Res 2004;10:4661–9.

91. Katano K, Safaei R, Samimi G, et al. The copper export pump ATP7B modulates the cellular pharmacology of carboplatin in ovarian carcinoma cells. Mol Pharmacol 2003;64:466–73.

92. Nakayama K, Kanzaki A, Terada K, et al. Prognostic value of the cu-transporting ATPase in ovarian carcinoma patients receiving cisplatin-based chemotherapy. Clin Cancer Res 2004;10:2804–11.

93. Ohbu M, Ogawa K, Konno S, et al. Copper-transporting P-type adenosine triphosphate (ATP7B) is expressed in human gastric carcinoma. Cancer Lett 2003;189:33–8.

94. Masters JR, Thomas R, Hall AG, et al. Sensitivity of testis tumour cells to chemotherapeutic drugs: role of detoxifying pathways. Eur J Cancer 1996;32A:1248–53.

95. Koropatnick J, Kloth DM, Kadhim S, et al. Metallothionein expression and resistance to cisplatin in a human germ cell tumor cell line. J Pharmacol Exp Ther 1995;275:1681–7.

96. Meijer C, Timmer A, De Vries EG, et al. Role of metallothionein in cisplatin sensitivity of germ cell tumours. Int J Cancer 2000;85:777–81.

97. Fink D, Nebel S, Aebi S, et al. The role of DNA mismatch repair in platinum drug resistance. Cancer Res 1990;56:4881–9.

98. Aebi S, Kurdi-Haidar B, Gordon R, et al. Loss of DNA mismatch repair in acquired resistance to cisplatin. Cancer Res 1996;56:3087–90.

99. Fink D, Zheng H, Nebel S, et al. In vitro and in vivo resistance to cisplatin in cells that have lost DNA mismatch repair. Cancer Res 1997;57:1841–5.

100. Mayer F, Gillis AJ, Dinjens W, et al. Microsatellite instability of germ cell tumors is associated with resistance to systemic treatment. Cancer Res 2002;62:2758–60.

101. Olasz J, Mándoky L, Géczi L, et al. Influence of hMLH1 methylation, mismatch repair deficiency and microsatellite instability on chemoresistance of testicular germ-cell tumours. Anticancer Res 2005;25:4319–24.

102. Velasco A, Riquelme E, Schultz M, et al. Microsatellite instability and loss of heterozygosity have distinct prognostic value for testicular germ cell tumor recurrence. Cancer Biol Ther 2004;3:1152–8.

103. Velasco A, Corvalan A, Wistuba II, et al. Mismatch repair expression in testicular cancer predicts recurrence and survival. Int J Cancer 2008;122:1774–7.

104. Honecker F, Wermann H, Mayer F, et al. Microsatellite instability, mismatch repair deficiency, and BRAF mutation in treatment-resistant germ cell tumors. J Clin Oncol 2009;27:2129–36.

105. Houldsworth J, Xiao H, Murty VV, et al. Human male germ cell tumor resistance to cisplatin is linked to TP53 gene mutation. Oncogene 1998;16:2345–9.

106. Burger H, Nooter K, Boersma AW, et al. Distinct p53-independent apoptotic cell death signalling pathways in testicular germ cell tumour cell lines. Int J Cancer 1999;81:620–8.

107. Spierings DC, de Vries EG, Vellenga E, et al. Loss of drug-induced activation of the CD95 apoptotic pathway in a cisplatin-resistant testicular germ cell tumour cell line. Cell Death Differ 2003;10:808–22.
108. Schweyer S, Soruri A, Meschter O, et al. Cisplatin-induced apoptosis in human malignant testicular germ cell lines depends on MEK/ERK activation. Br J Cancer 2004;91:589–98.
109. Mueller T, Vogt W, Simon H, et al. Failure of activation of caspase-9 induces a higher threshold for apoptosis and cisplatin resistance in testicular cancer. Cancer Res 2003;63:513–21.
110. Köberle B, Payne J, Grimaldi KA, et al. DNA repair in cisplatin-sensitive and resistant human cell lines measured in specific genes by quantitative polymerase chain reaction. Biochem Pharmacol 1996;52:1729–34.
111. Rao PH, Houldsworth J, Palanisamy N, et al. Chromosomal amplification is associated with cisplatin resistance of human germ cell tumors. Cancer Res 1998;58:4260–3.
112. Wilson C, Yang J, Streffod J, et al. Overexpression of genes on 16q associated with cisplatin resistance of testicular germ cell tumor cell lines. Genes Chromosomes Cancer 2005;43:211–6.
113. Noel EE, Yeste-Velasco M, Mao X, et al. The association of CCND1 overexpression and cisplatin resistance in testicular germ cell tumors and other cancers. Am J Pathol 2010;176:2607–15.
114. Beyrouthy MJ, Garner KM, Hever MP, et al. High DNA methyltransferase 3B expression mediates 5-azadeoxycytidine hypersensitivity in testicular germ cell tumors. Cancer Res 2009;69:9360–6.

Etiologic Differences Between Seminoma and Nonseminoma of the Testis: A Systematic Review of Epidemiologic Studies

Andreas Stang, MD, MPH[a],*, Oliver Kuss, PhD[b]

KEYWORDS

- Testicular neoplasms • Seminoma • Nonseminoma
- Epidemiology • Etiology • Systematic review

The vast majority of testicular cancers are germ cell cancers. The World Health Organization (WHO) classification of testicular germ cell cancers distinguishes between 3 types of germ cell cancers: teratomas and yolk-sac tumors in newborns and infants, seminomatous and nonseminomatous tumors in adolescents and young adults, and spermatocytic seminomas in the elderly.[1] The most well-established risk factors for testicular germ cell cancer are cryptorchidism, a previous germ cell tumor, and a family history of testicular cancer.[2]

The rapid increase in the incidence of testicular cancer over the past 40 years suggests that critical changes in environmental factors may contribute to the development of these tumors.[3] Opinion is divided between those who propose that testicular germ cell cancers represent a single disease with variable morphologic phenotypes (the so-called lumpers) and those who consider these morphologies to be separate diseases, with shared etiologic and clinical features (the so-called splitters). For example, from a developmental biology perspective it has been recently proposed "that the various types of germ cell cancers are in fact one disease, reflecting the

Disclosures: The authors have nothing to disclose.
[a] Institut für Klinische Epidemiologie, Medizinische Fakultät, Martin-Luther-Universität Halle-Wittenberg, Magdeburger Street 8, 06097 Halle (Saale), Germany
[b] Institut für Medizinische Epidemiologie, Biometrie und Informatik, Medizinische Fakultät, Martin-Luther-Universität Halle-Wittenberg, Magdeburger Strasse 8, 06097 Halle (Saale), Germany
* Corresponding author.
E-mail address: andreas.stang@medizin.uni-halle.de

Hematol Oncol Clin N Am 25 (2011) 473–486
doi:10.1016/j.hoc.2011.03.003
0889-8588/11/$ – see front matter © 2011 Elsevier Inc. All rights reserved.

developmental potential of germ cells in different stages of maturation."[4] In addition, based on incidence time trend analyses among men aged 15 to 54 years, it has been recently hypothesized that "similar temporal patterns in the cohort dimension imply that the etiologies of seminoma and non-seminoma are largely similar if not identical."[5,6] In contrast, incidence time trend analyses in Canada,[7] and other epidemiologic features,[8] suggest that seminoma and nonseminoma have different etiologies.[7] In a recent review of international trends in the incidence of testicular cancer, Chia and colleagues[9] concluded that "differences between seminoma and nonseminoma remain evident and suggest that some of the unknown causative factors of testicular cancer may partially or exclusively affect risk of a single histologic group."

Descriptive epidemiologic features, such as incidence age patterns and incidence time trends for testicular cancer, have provided several hints that the etiology of seminoma and nonseminoma may differ. First, age-specific incidence analyses have revealed that, among children aged 0 to 14 years, nonseminoma are virtually the only type of testicular germ cell cancer.[10–12] Thus, the etiologies of seminoma and nonseminoma must be different for young boys, otherwise nonseminoma germ cell cancers would not be predominant among young boys. In addition, the incidence rate of testicular cancer among boys aged 0 to 14 years has remained constant over time,[11,13] whereas incidence rates among adolescents and young men have increased[4,11,13] indicating that the etiology of testicular cancer among boys and young men differs. Furthermore, additional descriptive epidemiologic features that do not support the hypothesis of identical etiologies of germ cell cancers have been published recently.[14]

Here, we postulated that analytical epidemiologic studies, such as case-control and cohort studies, may provide evidence that the risk of germ cell cancers of the testis differs by histologic group. The aim of this study was to summarize the available evidence on etiologic differences among seminoma and nonseminoma based on a systematic review of published case-control and cohort studies, which present separate measures of effects for seminoma and nonseminoma.

MATERIAL AND METHODS

To identify epidemiologic studies that report separate measures of effects for the association between exposure (environmental or genetic) and the risk of testicular cancer, one of us (AS) used a detailed Medline search on September 29, 2010 and included all available calendar years. A professional librarian confirmed the appropriateness of the search algorithm. We restricted our literature search to case-control and cohort studies published in the English language. To increase the recall of our search, we included several similar medical subject headings. To increase the precision of the search, we also included several restrictions, such as "cancer (sb)" and restriction to relevant publication types. We refined our search algorithm after comparison of the output with a priori known relevant case-control and cohort studies (**Fig. 1**).

After downloading all 158 references retrieved by the search algorithm, one of us (AS) read all 158 full articles and checked if the study results were based on case-control or cohort studies. We did not contact the authors of the manuscripts. A list of all retrieved publications is available upon request. We excluded the following 8 publications from this study based on the following criteria: 2 studies were narrative reviews or meta-analyses,[15,16] 1 study was an ecological analysis,[17] 1 study was a re-analysis of previously published case-control study data,[18] 2 studies were case-only analyses,[19,20] 1 study was a prevalence study,[21] and 1 study analyzed

("case-control studies"[MESH] OR "cohort studies"[MESH]) AND ("Testicular
Neoplasms/etiology"[MAJR] OR "Testicular Neoplasms/epidemiology"[MAJR]) AND
("humans"[MeSH Terms] AND "male"[MeSH Terms]) AND (Meta-Analysis[ptyp] OR
Review[ptyp] OR Classical Article[ptyp] OR Comparative Study[ptyp] OR Journal
Article[ptyp] OR Multicenter Study[ptyp] OR Twin Study[ptyp]) AND English[lang]
AND cancer[sb]

Fig. 1. Medline search algorithm to identify relevant epidemiologic studies.

the association between date of birth and testicular cancer.[22] The remaining 150 publications included 110 case-control and 40 cohort studies. One of us (AS) checked whether these publications reported measures of effects by histologic subgroup. Overall, 61 case-control studies and 12 cohort studies reported histology-specific results (**Fig. 2**).

For each reference, we documented the study size (number of cases and controls, cohort size, and number of events), the age range of testicular cancer cases studied, the classification scheme used for germ cell cancers, and details about the exposures of interest. In addition, for each study, we extracted published relative risk (RR) estimates and their estimated 95% confidence intervals (CI) for seminoma and nonseminoma to the exposures of interest. We grouped exposures according to the following categories: (1) predisposing diseases, serologic findings, hormonal concentrations (index persons); (2) factors related to puberty, sex hormones, and fertility-related factors (index persons); (3) anthropometric measures (index persons); (4) lifestyle factors (index persons); (5) socioeconomic status and profession (both parents and

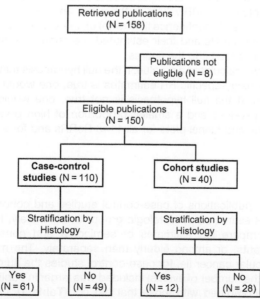

Fig. 2. Results of the literature search on case-control and cohort studies in the etiology of testicular cancer.

index persons); (6) pregnancy-related factors (mothers and index persons); (7) genetic factors (index persons); and (8) family history.

If several effect estimates for the same exposure with different degrees of adjustment were presented, we chose the most thoroughly adjusted RR estimates. If investigators distinguished between subtypes of nonseminoma, we used inverse-variance weighting to produce a single effect estimate for nonseminoma. When studies separately reported RR estimates for nonseminoma and for mixed germ cell cancers, we chose only the RR estimates for nonseminoma.

To quantify the etiologic heterogeneity of seminoma and nonseminoma, we calculated the ratio of RR estimates (RoRR). For example, estimated RRs for seminoma and nonseminoma associated with a history of cryptorchidism was 4.21 (95% CI: 2.48–7.14) and 3.55 (95% CI: 1.74–7.21), respectively, in a recent case-control study.[23] The ratio of RR estimates (seminoma/nonseminoma) thus equals 4.21/3.55 = 1.19. To estimate the 95% confidence interval for this ratio we estimated the variance (Var) of the difference between the βs (natural logarithms of the effect estimates) with S indicating seminoma and N indicating nonseminoma:

$Var(\beta_S - \beta_N) = Var(\beta_S) + Var(\beta_N) - 2 \, Cov(\beta_S, \beta_N)$ ([24] see page 184) and set the covariance $Cov(\beta_S, \beta_N)$ arbitrarily to zero, because this information cannot be extracted from the published reports included in this study. After calculation of the confidence interval for the difference between βs, we retranslated this confidence interval to the linear scale. We assumed that confidence intervals for the RR estimates in the published reports were based on Wald confidence intervals. RR estimates related to age were sometimes presented using a 1-year or 5-year increment. We recalculated these RR estimates to include 10-year increments.[25–27]

To study the distribution of RoRRs, we produced histograms, with Log(RoRR) on the x-axis and the relative frequency on the y-axis. In addition, we superimposed a kernel density estimate on the histograms through the use of a normal kernel function. The bandwidth of the kernel was estimated from the data. To investigate any pattern between the magnitude of the estimated RoRRs and the estimated precisions, we produced funnel plots with RoRR values on the y-axis and the estimated RoRR precision (the inverse of the 95% confidence limit ratio) on the x-axis. To better visualize the relationship between RoRRs and their estimated precisions, we fitted a parametric spline smoother and added it to the figures.

For each RoRR, we calculated a p-value. If the null hypothesis that no heterogeneity exists between histology-specific RR estimates is true, one would expect a uniform p-value distribution. If the null hypothesis is not true, one would expect a larger proportion of low p-values and a smaller proportion of high p-values. We plotted p-value distributions and funnel plots for all 1148 RoRRs and for separate groups of exposures.

RESULTS

Overall, 61 and 12 publications of case-control studies and cohort studies respectively, stratified RR estimates by histologic group. Unfortunately, not a single study enabled us to compare RR estimates of seminoma and nonseminoma among newborns and infants, or among elderly men separately. The median number of patients with testicular cancer (ie, for case-control studies the number of cases and for cohort studies the number of events) included was larger in publications that stratified by histology compared with those that did not (**Table 1**). Overall, 36% of all case-control studies and 58% of all cohort studies that provided histology-specific RR estimates were based on less than or equal to 200 patients with testicular germ

Table 1
Comparison of studies that stratified and did not stratify effect estimates by histology

	Reporting of Separate RR Estimates for Seminoma and Nonseminoma	
	No	Yes
Case-control studies		
Number of studies	49	61
Median number of case	243	289
Minimum-maximum	10–8498	58–6415
P25-P75	129–418	163–158
Cohort studies		
Number of studies	28	12
Median number of events	28	123
Minimum-maximum	2–5441	6–7035
P25-P75	7.5–283.0	29.0–2390.5

P25, 25% percentile; P75, 75% percentile.

cell cancer (either as cases in case-control studies or as events in cohort studies). Year of publication was positively associated with stratification by histologic subgroup (<1995: 18%; 1996–2000: 53%; 2001–2005: 45%; 2006–2010: 68%) and adjustment for study size did not alter this time trend.

We extracted a total of 1148 RR estimates (including RR estimates from disjoint indicator variables) from the 73 publications with histology-specific RR estimates, stratified by histologic subgroups, reflecting 631 exposures. Overall 30.9% of these 631 stratified analyses were related to lifestyle factors followed by pregnancy-related factors (20.9%), family history (12.7%), genetic factors (10.8%), and others (**Table 2**).

Ratios of RR estimates were symmetrically distributed with a peak at the reference value (RR = 1 or log[RR] = 0) (**Fig. 3**). The funnel plot indicates that the RoRR depends on the estimated precision; studies that provided more precise RoRR values tended to produce RoRR estimates closer to the null value (RoRR = 1) than studies with less precise RoRR estimates. The symmetry of the funnel plot suggests a lack of publication bias (**Fig. 4**). The corresponding p-value distribution is close to the expected distribution under the null hypothesis of no histologic heterogeneity of RR estimates (**Fig. 5**). Our sensitivity analyses according to predefined exposure groups revealed the same null results as our main analysis (data not shown).

DISCUSSION

Overall, 49% of the 150 published case-control and cohort studies on the etiology of testicular cancer identified in this study stratified effect estimates by histologic subgroups among adolescents and young adults. In total, we compared 1148 relative-risk estimates for seminoma and nonseminoma. Despite evidence based on descriptive epidemiologic features, which suggests that the etiology of seminoma and nonseminoma differs, our systematic review of case-control and cohort studies does not support the hypothesis that RR estimates for seminoma and nonseminoma differ. Publication bias is an unlikely explanation for this finding because the funnel plots and p-value distributions were not consistent with publication bias. Unfortunately, because we could not separately study histology-specific RR estimates for seminoma and nonseminoma among newborns, infants, and among elderly men, it

Table 2
Potential risk factors of case-control and cohort studies that stratified effect estimates by histologic subgroups

Exposures	N	%
Predisposing diseases, serologic findings, hormonal concentrations	44	7.0
CMV IgG positivity, VCA Ig positivity, EA-R/d IgG positivity[28]; IgG EBV, IgG CMV[29]; history of mumps, history of measles[30]; insulinlike growth factor, insulinlike growth factor binding protein[31]; HIV positivity[32]; history of STD[33]; parvovirus B19 positivity[34]; abnormal semen characteristics[35]; low sperm count[36]; undescended testis[23,33,37–40]; congenital defects[41]; atrophic testis[40]; inguinal hernia[33,38]; testis/groin injury[33,40]; Down syndrome[10,42]		
Puberty, sex hormone, and fertility-related factors	93	7.8
Age at first nocturnal emissions[33,43]; age when voice broke[33,43]; age when started to shave[43]; ever impregnated woman[36,44,45]; ever fathered child, number of children, relative fertility[44]; several sex hormone active chemicals[46–48]; pesticide use for gardening[41]		
Anthropometric measures (index persons)	9	1.4
BMI,[23,43,49] height,[23,46,50,51] weight[43]		
Lifestyle factors	195	30.9
Physical activity[33,40,52,53]; smoking,[40,49,54] passive smoking,[54] marijuana use[55]; dietary/nutritional factors[23,43,49,56–58]; immigration[59,60]; mobile phone use[37]; Vietnam military service[61]; urban/rural residence[40,41,62]; electric blanket use[63]		
Socioeconomic status, profession	54	8.6
Profession, job[23,40,62,64–67]; socioeconomic status[26,30,40,41,68]; years at school[23]; occupational exposure to magnetic fields[69]; occupational physical activity[40]; night work[40]		
Pregnancy-related factors	132	20.9
Maternal BMI before pregnancy[70]; history of previous fetal death[25]; previous miscarriages[30]; maternal health before pregnancy[10,71]; maternal age[10,25–27,41,72–77]; paternal age[25,73,76]; maternal parity[10,25,27,73,76]; placenta weight[27]; retained placenta[10,71]; bleeding/threatened miscarriages[30]; maternal smoking during pregnancy[39,78–80]; weight gain during pregnancy[70]; severe nausea during pregnancy[76,81]; hyperemesis gravidarum[10,76]; preeclampsia[27,76]; bleeding during pregnancy[40,76]; gestational hypertension[10,70,76]; proteinuria, anemia, glucosuria during pregnancy[70]; hormone use during pregnancy[39]; DHEAS level, androstenedione level[82] during pregnancy; any abnormality during pregnancy[40]; gestational age[10,25,27,76,83]; gestational duration[26,39]; birth date (compared with expected date)[72]; signs of prematurity[77]; dimension for gestational age[26]; presentation/delivery (breech, cesarean, head first)[76]; birth order[26,30,39,72–75,77,83]; born as twin[10,83]; singleton versus multiple births[76]; sibship size[30,74,75]; interval from son's birth to the previous delivery of the mother[73]; birth weight[10,25–27,40,41,72,76,77,83]; birth length[25,27,72,76]; neonatal jaundice[27,71,76]		

(continued on next page)

Table 2
(continued)

Exposures	N	%
Genetic factors (index persons)	68	10.8
SNPs of 8q24[84]; KITLG 12q22[85]; SPRY4 5q31.3[85]; SNPs in 6 genes (INHA, INHBA, INHBB, INHBC, INHBE, SMAD4)[86]; SNPs in 16 immune function genes[87]; SNPs in hormone-metabolizing genes[88]; several SNPs on chromosomes 1, 4, 5, 6, 12[89]; phenotype and genotype of glutathione S-transferase μ[90]		
Family history	80	12.7
Family history of several cancers,[23,40,91–94] ethnicity of parents[25]		
Total	631	100

Exposures that were modeled by disjoint indicator variables were counted only once in this table. That is, 1148 ratio estimates reflected 631 exposures.

Abbreviations: BMI, body mass index; CMV, cytomegalovirus; DHEAS, dehydroepiandrosterone sulfate; EA-R/d IgG positivity, EBV early antigen of restricted or diffuse type; EBV, Epstein-Barr virus; Ig, immunoglobulin; STD, sexually transmitted disease; VCA Ig positivity, EBV viral capsid antigen positivity.

remains unclear if our findings can be generalized to these other groups. However, descriptive epidemiologic features do not support such a generalization.

The fact that 51% of published case-control and cohort studies did not report histology-specific effect estimates may be caused by several factors, including a lack of sufficient numbers of testicular cancer events or cases. Furthermore, some studies were not able to distinguish between histologic testicular cancer subtypes for technical reasons (eg, cancer registry file data, with *International Classification of Diseases, Tenth Revision* codes only). In addition, some investigators may not have hypothesized the existence of differences in the etiology of seminoma and

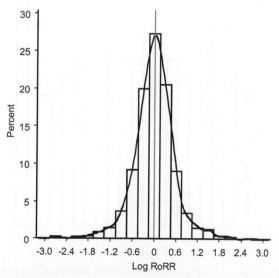

Fig. 3. Distribution of 1148 ratios of relative risk estimates. Log RoRR, logarithm of the ratios of relative risks estimates (RR$_{Seminoma}$ / RR$_{Nonseminoma}$).

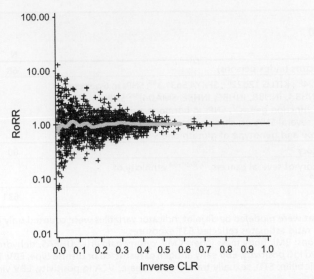

Fig. 4. Ratios of relative risk estimates by estimated precision of the ratio. Figure includes overall 1148 RoRR, that is, ratios of relative risks estimates ($RR_{Seminoma}$ / $RR_{Nonseminoma}$); bold gray line: parametric cubic spline smoother. CLR, confidence limit ratio.

nonseminoma and therefore did not differentiate between seminoma and nonseminoma in their analyses. Furthermore, a few investigators explicitly stated that they did not observe statistically significant differences between seminoma and nonseminoma and therefore did not report these histology-specific findings. However, hypothesis testing in epidemiology is generally problematic and becomes especially problematic if studies are underpowered, as many studies that we reviewed were.[95]

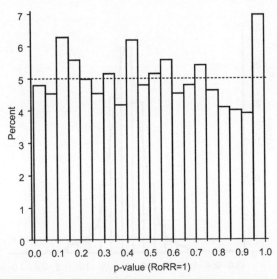

Fig. 5. P-value distribution of 1148 ratios of relative risk estimates. The horizontal line at 5% represents the p-value distribution if the null hypothesis of no histologic heterogeneity of RR estimates were true. RoRR, ratio of relative risk estimates ($RR_{Seminoma}$ / $RR_{Nonseminoma}$).

Comparison of histology-specific effect estimates across studies was complicated by the heterogeneity of testicular cancer subgroups. For example, 7 reports dealt with tumors in newborn and infants, and seminomatous and nonseminomatous tumors in adolescents and young adults. Another 3 studies dealt with all three WHO testicular cancer groups. However, the majority of studies (38 out of 73, or 52%) dealt only with seminomatous and nonseminomatous tumors of adolescents and young adults. A total of 7 studies explicitly excluded spermatocytic seminoma, whereas others did not. Some studies included mixed germ cell cancers within the group of nonseminomas, whereas others excluded them from analyses and some studies reported separate effect estimates for mixed germ cell cancers. If single histologic entities of nonseminoma germ cell cancers have different etiologies, the distribution of nonseminoma subtypes within the group of nonseminomas would influence RR estimation for nonseminomas as a whole group.

There are some limitations to the present study that deserve attention. First, many studies included small numbers of testicular cancer cases or events that resulted in imprecise histology-specific effect estimates. To address the question of histology-specific differences in RR estimates in the field of testicular cancer, study sizes have to be considerably increased in the future. Second, we did not conduct a formal assessment of the quality of the included studies and therefore could not include sensitivity analyses.

In conclusion, our results do not provide evidence in support of the hypothesis that seminoma and nonseminoma have different etiologies, or risk factors among adolescents and young men differ. To date, only descriptive epidemiologic features, such as incidence age patterns and incidence time trends of seminoma and nonseminoma, provide evidence suggesting different etiologies, especially among newborns, infants, and the elderly men.

REFERENCES

1. Woodward PJ, Mostofi FK, Talerman A, et al. Germ cell tumours. In: Eble JN, Sauter G, Epstein JI, et al, editors. Pathology and genetics of tumours of the urinary system and male genital organs. 1st edition. Lyon (France): IARC Press; 2004. p. 221–49.
2. McGlynn KA, Cook MB. Etiologic factors in testicular germ-cell tumors. Future Oncol 2009;5:1389–402.
3. Horwich A, Shipley J, Huddart R. Testicular germ-cell cancer. Lancet 2006;367: 754–65.
4. Oosterhuis JW, Looijenga LH. Testicular germ-cell tumours in a broader perspective. Nat Rev Cancer 2005;5:210–22.
5. Bray F, Richiardi L, Ekbom A, et al. Do testicular seminoma and nonseminoma share the same etiology? Evidence from an age-period-cohort analysis of incidence trends in eight European countries. Cancer Epidemiol Biomarkers Prev 2006;15:652–8.
6. Bray F, Ferlay J, Devesa SS, et al. Interpreting the international trends in testicular seminoma and nonseminoma incidence. Nat Clin Pract Urol 2006;3:532–43.
7. Liu S, Semenciw R, Waters C, et al. Clues to the aetiological heterogeneity of testicular seminomas and non-seminomas: time trends and age-period-cohort effects. Int J Epidemiol 2000;29:826–31.
8. Stang A, Jöckel KH. Etiologic conclusions from similar birth cohort effects. Cancer Epidemiol Biomarkers Prev 2006;15:1752–3.

9. Chia VM, Quraishi SM, Devesa SS, et al. International trends in the incidence of testicular cancer, 1973–2002. Cancer Epidemiol Biomarkers Prev 2010;19: 1151–9.
10. Aschim EL, Haugen TB, Tretli S, et al. Risk factors for testicular cancer–differences between pure non-seminoma and mixed seminoma/non-seminoma? Int J Androl 2006;29:458–67.
11. Xu Q, Pearce MS, Parker L. Incidence and survival for testicular germ cell tumor in young males: a report from the Northern Region Young Person's Malignant Disease Registry, United Kingdom. Urol Oncol 2007;25:32–7.
12. Stang A, Rusner C, Eisinger B, et al. Subtype-specific incidence of testicular cancer in Germany: a pooled analysis of nine population-based cancer registries. Int J Androl 2007;30:1–11.
13. Walsh TJ, Grady RW, Porter MP, et al. Incidence of testicular germ cell cancers in U.S. children: SEER program experience 1973 to 2000. Urology 2006;68: 402–5.
14. Stang A. Etiology of testicular germ cell tumors: lumping or splitting? A plea against lumping. Eur J Epidemiol 2009;24:65–7.
15. Grotmol T, Weiderpass E, Tretli S. Conditions in utero and cancer risk. Eur J Epidemiol 2006;21:561–70.
16. Akre O, Pettersson A, Richiardi L. Risk of contralateral testicular cancer among men with unilaterally undescended testis: a meta analysis. Int J Cancer 2009; 124:687–9.
17. Aschim EL, Grotmol T, Tretli S, et al. Is there an association between maternal weight and the risk of testicular cancer? An epidemiologic study of Norwegian data with emphasis on World War II. Int J Cancer 2005;116:327–30.
18. Kedem B, Kim EY, Voulgaraki A, et al. Two-dimensional semiparametric density ratio modeling of testicular germ cell data. Stat Med 2009;28:2147–59.
19. Chia VM, Li Y, Goldin LR, et al. Risk of cancer in first- and second-degree relatives of testicular germ cell tumor cases and controls. Int J Cancer 2009;124: 952–7.
20. Metcalfe S, Jones WG. Testicular cancer: B5, a new tumour marker. Urol Int 1987; 42:254–9.
21. Braun MM, Caporaso NE, Page WF, et al. Prevalence of a history of testicular cancer in a cohort of elderly twins. Acta Genet Med Gemellol (Roma) 1995;44: 189–92.
22. Prener A, Carstensen B. Month of birth and testicular cancer risk in Denmark. Am J Epidemiol 1990;131:15–9.
23. Stang A, Ahrens W, Baumgardt-Elms C, et al. Adolescent milk fat and galactose consumption and testicular germ cell cancer. Cancer Epidemiol Biomarkers Prev 2006;15:2189–95.
24. Subrahmaniam K. A primer in probability. 1st edition. New York: Dekker; 1979.
25. English PB, Goldberg DE, Wolff C, et al. Parental and birth characteristics in relation to testicular cancer risk among males born between 1960 and 1995 in California (United States). Cancer Causes Control 2003;14:815–25.
26. Richiardi L, Akre O, Bellocco R, et al. Perinatal determinants of germ-cell testicular cancer in relation to histological subtypes. Br J Cancer 2002;87:545–50.
27. Akre O, Ekbom A, Hsieh CC, et al. Testicular nonseminoma and seminoma in relation to perinatal characteristics. J Natl Cancer Inst 1996;88:883–9.
28. Akre O, Lipworth L, Tretli S, et al. Epstein-Barr virus and cytomegalovirus in relation to testicular-cancer risk: a nested case-control study. Int J Cancer 1999;82:1–5.

29. Holl K, Surcel HM, Koskela P, et al. Maternal Epstein-Barr virus and cytomegalo-virus infections and risk of testicular cancer in the offspring: a nested case-control study. APMIS 2008;116:816–22.
30. Prener A, Hsieh CC, Engholm G, et al. Birth order and risk of testicular cancer. Cancer Causes Control 1992;3:265–72.
31. Chia VM, Quraishi SM, Graubard BI, et al. Insulin-like growth factor 1, insulin-like growth factor-binding protein 3, and testicular germ-cell tumor risk. Am J Epidemiol 2008;167:1438–45.
32. Powles T, Bower M, Daugaard G, et al. Multicenter study of human immunodeficiency virus-related germ cell tumors. J Clin Oncol 2003;21:1922–7.
33. Coupland CA, Chilvers CE, Davey G, et al. Risk factors for testicular germ cell tumours by histological tumour type. United Kingdom Testicular Cancer Study Group. Br J Cancer 1999;80:1859–63.
34. Tolfvenstam T, Papadogiannakis N, Andersen A, et al. No association between human parvovirus B19 and testicular germ cell cancer. J Gen Virol 2002;83:2321–4.
35. Jacobsen R, Bostofte E, Engholm G, et al. Risk of testicular cancer in men with abnormal semen characteristics: cohort study. BMJ 2000;321:789–92.
36. Baker JA, Buck GM, Vena JE, et al. Fertility patterns prior to testicular cancer diagnosis. Cancer Causes Control 2005;16:295–9.
37. Hardell L, Carlberg M, Ohlson CG, et al. Use of cellular and cordless telephones and risk of testicular cancer. Int J Androl 2007;30:115–22.
38. Prener A, Engholm G, Jensen OM. Genital anomalies and risk for testicular cancer in Danish men. Epidemiology 1996;7:14–9.
39. Weir HK, Marrett LD, Kreiger N, et al. Pre-natal and peri-natal exposures and risk of testicular germ-cell cancer. Int J Cancer 2000;87:438–43.
40. Dusek L, Abrahamova J, Lakomy R, et al. Multivariate analysis of risk factors for testicular cancer: a hospital-based case-control study in the Czech Republic. Neoplasma 2008;55:356–68.
41. Nori F, Carbone P, Giordano F, et al. Endocrine-disrupting chemicals and testicular cancer: a case-control study. Arch Environ Occup Health 2006;61:87–95.
42. Patja K, Pukkala E, Sund R, et al. Cancer incidence of persons with Down syndrome in Finland: a population-based study. Int J Cancer 2006;118:1769–72.
43. McGlynn KA, Sakoda LC, Rubertone MV, et al. Body size, dairy consumption, puberty, and risk of testicular germ cell tumors. Am J Epidemiol 2007;165:355–63.
44. Moller H, Skakkebaek NE. Risk of testicular cancer in subfertile men: case-control study. BMJ 1999;318:559–62.
45. Doria-Rose VP, Biggs ML, Weiss NS. Subfertility and the risk of testicular germ cell tumors (United States). Cancer Causes Control 2005;16:651–6.
46. Hardell L, Bavel B, Lindstrom G, et al. In utero exposure to persistent organic pollutants in relation to testicular cancer risk. Int J Androl 2006;29:228–34.
47. Hardell L, van Bavel B, Lindstrom G, et al. Increased concentrations of polychlorinated biphenyls, hexachlorobenzene, and chlordanes in mothers of men with testicular cancer. Environ Health Perspect 2003;111:930–4.
48. Hardell L, Ohlson CG, Fredrikson M. Occupational exposure to polyvinyl chloride as a risk factor for testicular cancer evaluated in a case-control study. Int J Cancer 1997;73:828–30.
49. Garner MJ, Birkett NJ, Johnson KC, et al. Dietary risk factors for testicular carcinoma. Int J Cancer 2003;106:934–41.

50. Dieckmann KP, Hartmann JT, Classen J, et al. Tallness is associated with risk of testicular cancer: evidence for the nutrition hypothesis. Br J Cancer 2008;99: 1517–21.
51. Richiardi L, Askling J, Granath F, et al. Body size at birth and adulthood and the risk for germ-cell testicular cancer. Cancer Epidemiol Biomarkers Prev 2003;12: 669–73.
52. Cook MB, Zhang Y, Graubard BI, et al. Risk of testicular germ-cell tumours in relation to childhood physical activity. Br J Cancer 2008;98:174–8.
53. Littman AJ, Doody DR, Biggs ML, et al. Physical activity in adolescence and testicular germ cell cancer risk. Cancer Causes Control 2009;20:1281–90.
54. McGlynn KA, Zhang Y, Sakoda LC, et al. Maternal smoking and testicular germ cell tumors. Cancer Epidemiol Biomarkers Prev 2006;15:1820–4.
55. Daling JR, Doody DR, Sun X, et al. Association of marijuana use and the incidence of testicular germ cell tumors. Cancer 2009;115:1215–23.
56. Sigurdson AJ, Chang S, Annegers JF, et al. A case-control study of diet and testicular carcinoma. Nutr Cancer 1999;34:20–6.
57. Walcott FL, Hauptmann M, Duphorne CM, et al. A case-control study of dietary phytoestrogens and testicular cancer risk. Nutr Cancer 2002;44:44–51.
58. Bonner MR, McCann SE, Moysich KB. Dietary factors and the risk of testicular cancer. Nutr Cancer 2002;44:35–43.
59. Ekbom A, Richiardi L, Akre O, et al. Age at immigration and duration of stay in relation to risk for testicular cancer among Finnish immigrants in Sweden. J Natl Cancer Inst 2003;95:1238–40.
60. Beiki O, Granath F, Allebeck P, et al. Subtype-specific risk of testicular tumors among immigrants and their descendants in Sweden, 1960 to 2007. Cancer Epidemiol Biomarkers Prev 2010;19:1053–65.
61. Tarone RE, Hayes HM, Hoover RN, et al. Service in Vietnam and risk of testicular cancer. J Natl Cancer Inst 1991;83:1497–9.
62. Moller H. Work in agriculture, childhood residence, nitrate exposure, and testicular cancer risk: a case-control study in Denmark. Cancer Epidemiol Biomarkers Prev 1997;6:141–4.
63. Verreault R, Weiss NS, Hollenbach KA, et al. Use of electric blankets and risk of testicular cancer. Am J Epidemiol 1990;131:759–62.
64. Hayes RB, Brown LM, Pottern LM, et al. Occupation and risk for testicular cancer: a case-control study. Int J Epidemiol 1990;19:825–31.
65. Andersson E, Nilsson R, Toren K. Testicular cancer among Swedish pulp and paper workers. Am J Ind Med 2003;43:642–6.
66. Ohlson CG, Hardell L. Testicular cancer and occupational exposures with a focus on xenoestrogens in polyvinyl chloride plastics. Chemosphere 2000;40: 1277–82.
67. Rhomberg W, Schmoll HJ, Schneider B. High frequency of metalworkers among patients with seminomatous tumors of the testis: a case-control study. Am J Ind Med 1995;28:79–87.
68. Kristensen P, Andersen A, Irgens LM, et al. Testicular cancer and parental use of fertilizers in agriculture. Cancer Epidemiol Biomarkers Prev 1996;5:3–9.
69. Stenlund C, Floderus B. Occupational exposure to magnetic fields in relation to male breast cancer and testicular cancer: a Swedish case-control study. Cancer Causes Control 1997;8:184–91.
70. Pettersson A, Richiardi L, Cnattingius S, et al. Gestational hypertension, preeclampsia, and risk of testicular cancer. Cancer Res 2008;68:8832–6.

71. Wanderas EH, Grotmol T, Fossa SD, et al. Maternal health and pre- and perinatal characteristics in the etiology of testicular cancer: a prospective population- and register-based study on Norwegian males born between 1967 and 1995. Cancer Causes Control 1998;9:475–86.
72. Moller H, Skakkebaek NE. Testicular cancer and cryptorchidism in relation to prenatal factors: case-control studies in Denmark. Cancer Causes Control 1997; 8:904–12.
73. Westergaard T, Andersen PK, Pedersen JB, et al. Testicular cancer risk and maternal parity: a population-based cohort study. Br J Cancer 1998;77: 1180–5.
74. Richiardi I , Akre O, Lambe M, et al. Birth order, sibship size, and risk for germ-cell testicular cancer. Epidemiology 2004;15:323–9.
75. Moller H, Skakkebaek NE. Risks of testicular cancer and cryptorchidism in relation to socio-economic status and related factors: case-control studies in Denmark. Int J Cancer 1996;66:287–93.
76. Cook MB, Graubard BI, Rubertone MV, et al. Perinatal factors and the risk of testicular germ cell tumors. Int J Cancer 2008;122:2600–6.
77. Sabroe S, Olsen J. Perinatal correlates of specific histological types of testicular cancer in patients below 35 years of age: a case-cohort study based on midwives' records in Denmark. Int J Cancer 1998;78:140–3.
78. Tuomisto J, Holl K, Rantakokko P, et al. Maternal smoking during pregnancy and testicular cancer in the sons: a nested case-control study and a meta-analysis. Eur J Cancer 2009;45:1640–8.
79. Pettersson A, Akre O, Richiardi L, et al. Maternal smoking and the epidemic of testicular cancer–a nested case-control study. Int J Cancer 2007;120: 2044–6.
80. Coupland CA, Forman D, Chilvers CE, et al. Maternal risk factors for testicular cancer: a population-based case-control study (UK). Cancer Causes Control 2004;15:277–83.
81. Petridou E, Roukas KI, Dessypris N, et al. Baldness and other correlates of sex hormones in relation to testicular cancer. Int J Cancer 1997;71:982–5.
82. Holl K, Lundin E, Surcel HM, et al. Endogenous steroid hormone levels in early pregnancy and risk of testicular cancer in the offspring: a nested case-referent study. Int J Cancer 2009;124:2923–8.
83. Ramlau-Hansen CH, Olesen AV, Parner ET, et al. Perinatal markers of estrogen exposure and risk of testicular cancer: follow-up of 1,333,873 Danish males born between 1950 and 2002. Cancer Causes Control 2009;20:1587–92.
84. Cook MB, Graubard BI, Quraishi SM, et al. Genetic variants in the 8q24 locus and risk of testicular germ cell tumors. Hum Genet 2008;123:409–18.
85. Kanetsky PA, Mitra N, Vardhanabhuti S, et al. Common variation in KITLG and at 5q31.3 predisposes to testicular germ cell cancer. Nat Genet 2009; 41:811–5.
86. Purdue MP, Graubard BI, Chanock SJ, et al. Genetic variation in the inhibin pathway and risk of testicular germ cell tumors. Cancer Res 2008;68:3043–8.
87. Purdue MP, Sakoda LC, Graubard BI, et al. A case-control investigation of immune function gene polymorphisms and risk of testicular germ cell tumors. Cancer Epidemiol Biomarkers Prev 2007;16:77–83.
88. Figueroa JD, Sakoda LC, Graubard BI, et al. Genetic variation in hormone metabolizing genes and risk of testicular germ cell tumors. Cancer Causes Control 2008;19:917–29.

89. Rapley EA, Turnbull C, Al Olama AA, et al. A genome-wide association study of testicular germ cell tumor. Nat Genet 2009;41:807–10.

90. Vistisen K, Prieme H, Okkels H, et al. Genotype and phenotype of glutathione S-transferase mu in testicular cancer patients. Pharmacogenetics 1997;7: 21–5.

91. Dong C, Lonnstedt I, Hemminki K. Familial testicular cancer and second primary cancers in testicular cancer patients by histological type. Eur J Cancer 2001;37: 1878–85.

92. Bromen K, Stang A, Baumgardt-Elms C, et al. Testicular, other genital, and breast cancers in first-degree relatives of testicular cancer patients and controls. Cancer Epidemiol Biomarkers Prev 2004;13:1316–24.

93. Hemminki K, Chen B. Familial risks in testicular cancer as aetiological clues. Int J Androl 2006;29:205–10.

94. Kaijser M, Akre O, Cnattingius S, et al. Maternal lung cancer and testicular cancer risk in the offspring. Cancer Epidemiol Biomarkers Prev 2003;12:643–6.

95. Stang A, Poole C, Kuss O. The ongoing tyranny of statistical significance testing in biomedical research. Eur J Epidemiol 2010;25:225–30.

Imaging Studies for Germ Cell Tumors

S.A. Sohaib, MRCP, FRCR[a],*, G. Cook, FRCP, FRCR[b],
Dow-Mu Koh, MRCP, FRCR[a]

KEYWORDS

• Testicular cancer • CT • MRI • PET

In the management of patients with testicular germ cell tumors (TGCT), imaging plays a pivotal role. Although sonography of the testes is useful for the identification of a testicular mass, the definitive diagnosis of a testicular tumor is usually reliant on a biopsy or orchidectomy. Once the diagnosis of a testicular neoplasm is established, imaging is crucial for defining the presence and extent of metastatic disease, assessing disease response to treatment, evaluating the suitability of residual masses after chemotherapy for surgery, and detecting sites of relapse. Computed tomography (CT) remains the main radiologic technique for disease evaluation. However, other imaging techniques, such as chest radiography, MRI, positron emission tomography using 18-fluoro-2-deoxyglucose (FDG-PET), and ultrasound all have specific roles in the clinical management of these patients.

DIAGNOSIS

The diagnosis of GCT tumors is usually made on biopsy or at orchidectomy. TGCT most commonly presents as a painless palpable mass but occasionally may present with nonspecific symptoms, such as dull scrotal ache, pain, or acute fever. In patients with retroperitoneal metastases or disseminated disease, backache, malaise, lethargy, gynecomastia, and other systemic features may be the presenting symptoms.

Testicular ultrasound (which should be performed using a high-resolution 7.5-MHz probe) is used for the primary assessment of the testes to confirm the presence of a testicular mass (**Fig. 1**); to distinguish these from other scrotal abnormalities; and to screen for associated abnormalities, such as microlithiasis. Testicular ultrasound is also helpful for assessment in young male patients who present with metastatic disease, in whom an occult primary tumor of the testis is suspected. Ultrasound is

[a] Department of Diagnostic Radiology, Royal Marsden Hospital, Down Road, Sutton, Surrey SM2 5PT, England, UK
[b] Department of Nuclear Medicine, Royal Marsden Hospital, Down Road, Sutton, Surrey SM2 5PT, England, UK
* Corresponding author.

Hematol Oncol Clin N Am 25 (2011) 487–502
doi:10.1016/j.hoc.2011.03.014
0889-8588/11/$ – see front matter © 2011 Elsevier Inc. All rights reserved.

hemonc.theclinics.com

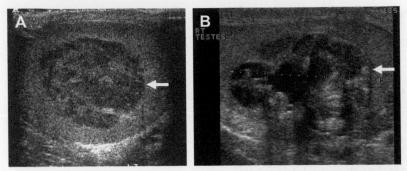

Fig. 1. TGCT tumors on ultrasound. Ultrasound images through the testes in two different patients showing mass lesion (*arrow*) in the testes. At pathology (*A*) seminoma and (*B*) non-seminomatous germ cell tumors were found.

also used to examine the contralateral testis of a patient confirmed to have testicular tumor, to identify the small number of patients who may present with bilateral synchronous tumors.

Sonographically, testicular tumors are usually well-defined and hypoechoic relative to the normal testicle, although some may display heterogeneous echo-texture, calcification, or cystic change.[1] Tumors may display increased vascularity on color and power Doppler with respect to surrounding normal testicular tissue but this is not specific and may not be demonstrable in small tumors. Ultrasound cannot reliably differentiate between tumor types, and for this purpose MRI may be useful.

MRI has been reported to be able to distinguish between seminoma and nonseminomatous GCT (NSGCT).[2] However, this may be of little practical value because appropriate management dictates orchidectomy to obtain detailed histopathology of the tumor, which is mandatory for primary treatment. Nevertheless, MRI of the scrotum may be useful if clinical and sonographic assessment cannot differentiate between an intratesticular or extratesticular mass.[3] A further role for MRI of the scrotum is the preoperative evaluation of the local extent of malignant testicular tumors in patients for whom testis-sparing surgery is planned, such as those with bilateral GCTs or tumor in a solitary testis.[4]

STAGING

Before initiating therapy, assessment of disease extent must be performed. Guidelines from the National Comprehensive Cancer Network and the European Germ Cell Cancer Consensus Group recommend that TNM staging be used (**Table 1**) and that patients with metastatic disease are further categorized using the International Germ Cell Cancer Collaborative Group classification, which stratifies patients into good, intermediate, and poor prognostic groups.[5–8] This latter classification is based on histology, location of primary tumor and metastases, and levels of serum markers (**Box 1**).[5] These guidelines also state that patients should have initial staging with a chest radiograph and CT of the abdomen and pelvis.[6,7] A CT of the chest is performed if the chest radiograph is abnormal or abdominopelvic CT shows metastatic disease.

PATTERN OF SPREAD

Knowledge of the spread of TGCT tumor is important to accurately stage these tumors.

Lymphatic drainage of the testes occurs along efferent lymphatic channels, which pass from the mediastinum of the testis through the internal inguinal ring accompanying the spermatic cord. They then join up to form major lymphatic channels that accompany the testicular vessels, and after crossing the ureter these lymphatics fan out to drain into the retroperitoneal lymph nodes. Left-sided tumors spread to the left paraaortic nodes and the preaortic nodes initially (**Figs. 2** and **3**). The upper paraaortic nodes, just below the renal vessels, are the most commonly involved first sites of spread in left-sided tumors. Right-sided tumors spread into the aortocaval nodes, the precaval nodes (see **Fig. 2**A), and the right paracaval and retrocaval nodes. Right-sided tumors spread preferentially to nodes below the right renal hilum, the first nodal site to be demonstrated frequently being an aortocaval node or a right paracaval node in the lower retroperitoneum.

Lymphatic spread may also occur to nodes lateral to the paracaval and paraaortic group, the so-called "echelon" node. Lymph node metastases lying on the anterior surface of the iliopsoas muscles are considered to represent echelon node deposits. These are an unusual site of disease, more frequently demonstrated at the time of relapse than at initial staging.

The consistency with which right-sided tumors spread to the right-sided retroperitoneal nodes and left-sided tumors to left-sided nodes is such that contralateral lymph node involvement in the absence of ipsilateral node involvement is very rare.[9] If a single enlarged node is demonstrated on the contralateral side and is the only possible evidence of metastatic disease, then histologic verification should be obtained before commencing systemic treatment. Crossover disease dissemination to contralateral nodes is unusual when ipsilateral nodes are less than 2 cm in diameter and is more frequently seen as lymphadenopathy becomes increasingly bulky, particularly with right-sided tumors. Direct spread to iliac or inguinal nodes alone is rare and usually associated with an identifiable predisposition, such as cryptorchidism or previous scrotal incision. However, pelvic nodes may become involved in the presence of bulky retroperitoneal lymphadenopathy because of retrograde lymph flow resulting from tumor obstruction. By a similar mechanism, nodes in the mesentery may also become involved, resulting in a "pseudolymphoma" appearance.

Lymph nodes above the renal hila are involved by direct spread from lower paraaortic nodes and extension of disease is then to the retrocrural lymph nodes. Supradiaphragmatic spread of testicular tumors occurs via the thoracic duct, which leads to involvement of the supraclavicular nodes and, occasionally, superior mediastinal and prevascular nodes. Direct spread through the diaphragm from the retroperitoneal space can lead to posterior mediastinal and subcarinal nodal involvement.

Hematogenous spread in testicular cancer is predominantly to the lungs. Multiple small metastases in a peripheral location are typical of NSGCT, but in seminoma pulmonary metastases tend to be larger lesions, when diagnosed, of at least 1 to 2 cm in diameter (**Fig. 4**). Other sites of metastases in patients with advanced aggressive tumors include the brain, bone, and liver. Brain metastases are more common in patients with trophoblastic teratomas (choriocarcinomas) than any other histologic type (**Fig. 5**). Other sites of hematogenous spread are rare and include the kidneys, adrenal glands, muscle, spleen, pericardium, pleura, and peritoneum. These unusual sites of disease are more frequently observed at the time of disease relapse in patients who have been previously treated.

CT

CT remains the imaging modality of choice for staging GCT. The effective use of CT relies on good technique and a detailed knowledge of the patterns of tumor spread,

Table 1
TNM staging classification of testicular tumors

	Primary Tumor
The extent of the primary tumor is classified after radical orchidectomy (pT)	
pTX	Primary tumor cannot be assessed (if no radical orchidectomy has been performed, TX is used)
pT0	No evidence of primary tumor (eg, histologic scar in testis)
pTis	Intratubular germ cell neoplasia
pT1	Tumor limited to testis and epididymis without vascular/lymphatic invasion; tumor may invade into the tunica albuginea but not tunica vaginalis
pT2	Tumor limited to testis and epididymus with vascular/lymphatic invasion, or tumor extending through tunica albuginea with involvement of tunica vaginalis
pT3	Tumor invades spermatic cord with or without vascular/lymphatic invasion
pT4	Tumor invades scrotum with or without vascular/lymphatic invasion
Regional Lymph Nodes	
Clinical Involvement	
NX	Regional nodes cannot be assessed
N0	No regional lymph node metastasis
N1	Metastasis with a lymph node mass ≤2 cm in greatest dimension or multiple lymph nodes none >2 cm in greatest dimension
N2	Metastasis with a lymph node mass >2 cm but <5 cm in greatest dimension, or multiple lymph nodes, any one mass >2 cm but ≤5 cm in greatest dimension
N3	Metastasis with a lymph node mass >5 cm in greatest dimension
Pathologic involvement	
pN0	No regional lymph node metastases
pN1	Metastasis with a lymph node mass ≤2 cm in greatest dimension and 5 or fewer positive nodes, none >2 cm in greatest dimension
pN2	Metastasis with a lymph node mass >2 cm but ≤5 cm in greatest dimensions; or more than five nodes positive, none >5 cm; or evidence of extranodal extension of tumor
pN3	Metastasis with a lymph node mass >5 cm in greatest dimension
Distant Metastases	
MX	Distant metastasis cannot be assessed
M0	No distant metastasis
M1	Distant metastasis
M1a	Nonregional lymph node or pulmonary metastasis
M1b	Distant metastasis other than to nonregional lymph nodes and lungs
Serum tumor markers (S)	
SX	Tumor marker studies not available or not performed
S0	Tumor marker levels within normal limits
S1	LDH <1.5 normal and HCG (mIu/ml) <5000 and AFP (g/ml) <1000
S2	LDH 1.5–10 normal or HCG (mIu/ml) 5000–50,000 or AFP (g/ml) 1000–10,000
S3	LDH >10 normal or HCG (mIu/ml) >50,000 or AFP (g/ml) >10,000
Stage Groupings	
• Stage I	pT1-4, N0, M0, SX

(continued on next page)

Table 1 *(continued)*	
	Primary Tumor
• Stage II	Any pT/Tx, N1-3, M0, SX
○ Stage IIA	Any pT/Tx, N1, M0, S0 Any pT/Tx, N1, M0, S1
○ Stage IIB	Any pT/Tx, N2, M0, S0 Any pT/Tx, N2, M0, S1
○ Stage IIC	Any pT/Tx, N3, M0, S0 Any pT/Tx, N3, M0, S1
• Stage III	Any pT/Tx, Any N, M1, SX
○ Stage IIIA	Any pT/Tx, Any N, M1a, S0 Any pT/Tx, Any N, M1a, S1
○ Stage IIIB	Any pT/Tx, N1-3, M0, S2 Any pT/Tx, Any N, M1a, S2
○ Stage IIIC	Any pT/Tx, N1-3, M0, S3 Any pT/Tx, Any N, M1a, S3 Any pT/Tx, Any N, M1b, Any S

Data from Sobin LH, Gospodarowicz MK, Wittekind CH, editors. TNM classification of malignant tumours. 7th edition. New York: Wiley-Liss; 2009.

the characteristic appearances of metastatic disease, and familiarity with potential diagnostic pitfalls.

Lymph node metastases vary in size from a single small node to huge intraabdominal retroperitoneal masses. Masses from seminoma are usually of soft tissue density but occasionally may contain areas of relatively low density because of central necrosis. However, large-volume masses of NSGCT are frequently heterogeneous in density, being composed of multiloculated complex cystic areas and soft tissue elements. Although the diagnosis of large-volume disease is readily made on CT, the diagnosis of small-volume metastatic disease may be extremely difficult.

Studies have been performed to assess the effect of different nodal size thresholds to ascribe the presence or absence of nodal disease.[10] Essentially, they confirm the general principle that reducing the lymph node diameter threshold used to determine malignancy, the likelihood of detecting positive nodes increases, but the specificity of the test decreases. It has been shown that using 10 to 15 mm as the upper limit of normal for nodal size measurement results in 44% of false-negative readings.[10] A further challenge of trying to define and standardize the upper limits of normal for nodal size measurement is that normal nodes in the superior retroperitoneum are smaller than those in the inferior retroperitoneum on CT.[11,12] Because the definition of normality varies between institutions, this translates to differences in clinical practice. In the authors' institution, a size threshold cut-off of 10 mm short-axis diameter is used to distinguish between normal and abnormal lymph nodes. Those measuring between 8 and 10 mm are regarded as suspicious. Nodal assessment based on size measurement must, however, be taken in context of the overall clinical assessment, such as serum marker levels, size, and laterality of the primary tumor. Thus, in a patient with a strong clinical suspicion for nodal disease, the presence of a borderline 8-mm retroperitoneal lymph node may warrant further investigation: tissue sampling; additional imaging, such as FDG-PET imaging (see later); or follow-up imaging.

Using a size criteria of 8 mm or larger in the maximum short-axis diameter to define a suspicious retroperitoneal node is associated with a high specificity but low

---

Box 1
International germ cell tumor consensus conference classification

- Nonseminoma
  - Good prognosis: all of the following
    - AFP <1000 ng/mL and HCG <5000 IU/L (1000 ng/mL) and LDH <1.5 upper limit of normal (N) and
    - Nonmediastinal primary
    - No nonpulmonary visceral metastases (NPVM)
  - Intermediate prognosis: all of the following
    - AFP 1000–10,000 ng/mL, or HCG 5000–50,000 IU/L, or LDH 1.5–10 N and
    - Nonmediastinal primary site and
    - No NPVM
  - Poor prognosis: any of the following
    - AFP >10,000 ng/mL or HCG >50,000 IU/L or LDH >10 N or
    - Mediastinal primary site <u>or</u>
    - NPVM
- Seminoma
  - Good prognosis
    - No NPVM
    - Any primary site
    - Normal AFP, any HCG, any LDH
  - Intermediate prognosis
    - NPVM present

Abbreviations: AFP, -fetoprotein; B-HCG, B-human gonadotrophin; CNS, central nervous system; LDH, lactate dehydrogenase.
Data from International germ cell consensus classification: a prognostic factor-based staging system for metastatic germ cell cancers. International germ cell cancer collaborative group. J Clin Oncol 1997;15:594–603.

---

sensitivity.[10] However, it is well established that between 25% and 30% of patients harbor occult microscopic metastases that cannot be detected by CT. False-negative examinations are inevitable, but the number of false-negative examinations can be minimized by reducing observer error and awareness of the limitations of imaging.

There are various well-known pitfalls in the diagnosis of retroperitoneal lymphadenopathy. These include mimickers of nodal disease, such as vascular anomalies (eg, gonadal veins, inferior vena cava (IVC) duplication, left-sided IVC, retroaortic and circumaortic renal vessels, and ascending lumbar communicating veins). These are usually apparent if intravenous contrast medium is given at CT and multiplanar reformats (MPR) are performed. Unopacified bowel loops may sometimes be mistaken for lymph nodes, particularly on the left side of the abdomen. Imaging with oral contrast, scanning the patient in a prone position, and performing MPR or MRI could be problem solving in such instances. Prominent crus of the diaphragm on CT may also be mistaken for nodal disease; again, review of the MPR should prevent this error.

CT is the most sensitive technique for the detection of pulmonary metastases and may also identify nodal spread to the supraclavicular fossa and mediastinum.

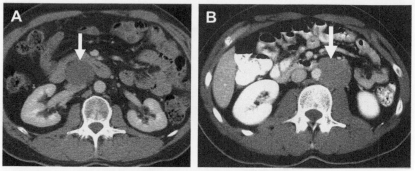

Fig. 2. Retroperitoneal adenopathy on CT. *(A)* Precaval node *(arrow)* in a patient with right-side GCT. *(B)* Left paraaortic adenopathy *(arrow)* in a man with a left testicular NSGCT. Right-sided testicular tumors usually metastasize to the aortocaval, retrocaval, or precaval region, whereas left-sided testicular tumors typically metastasize to the left paraaortic lymph nodes.

Mediastinal nodal disease usually occurs by direct contiguous spread of tumor via the thoracic duct into the posterior mediastinum through the diaphragmatic hiatus in seminomas. However, nodal tumor spread in NSGCT seems to be more variable. Nodal disease can involve the anterior mediastinum, aortopulmonary window, or hilar regions without evidence of spread to the posterior mediastinal or subcarinal lymph nodes. Similarly, tumor dissemination to the lymph nodes in the supraclavicular fossae and the neck is also more common in NSGCT. Pleural masses and effusions are a well-recognized feature of seminoma and are usually accompanied by other manifestations of metastatic spread. As in the assessment of retroperitoneal disease one needs to be aware of pitfalls in evaluating metastatic disease and understanding patterns of disease spread. For example, it is unusual to develop bilateral hilar

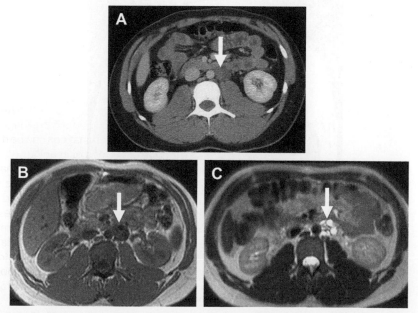

Fig. 3. Left-sided nodal disease. *(A)* CT and *(B)* T1-weighted and *(C)* T2-weighted MRIs in a man with a left testicular NSGCT show a 2.5-cm left paraaortic node *(arrows)*.

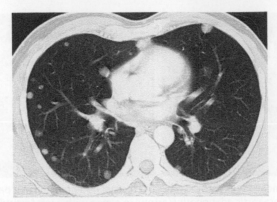

Fig. 4. Lung metastases. CT image showing multiple small pulmonary nodules in a patient with metastatic NSGCT.

adenopathy without any other evidence of disease elsewhere and one should consider such diagnosis as tuberculosis and sarcoidosis (**Fig. 6**).

CT of the brain is usually not undertaken as part of routine staging but is indicated in patients with high-risk factors (eg, very high serum -human chorionic gonadotropin or -fetoprotein) and in those with suspected metastatic disease on clinical grounds.[13] Brain metastases are usually hemorrhagic and are visible as lesions of high CT attenuation values on unenhanced scans. These metastases typically show enhancement after intravenous contrast medium administration (see **Fig 5**).

Metastases in other sites, such as the liver and bone, may be missed if these regions are not carefully scrutinized on the initial staging scan and at subsequent investigation.

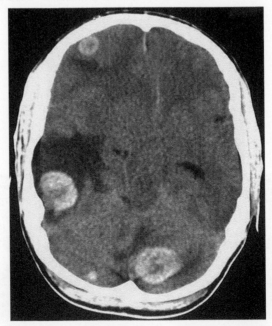

Fig. 5. Brain metastases. CT shows multiple brain metastases in a patient with malignant trophoblastic tumor.

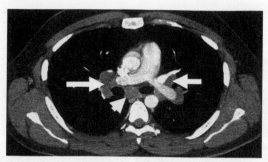

Fig. 6. Pitfalls in staging. A patient with TGCT and concomitant sarcoidosis. Apart from the bilateral hilar (*long arrows*) and mediastinal adenopathy (*short arrow*) there were no other sites of disease, making nodal involvement in the chest unlikely to be caused by metastatic GCT. Mediastinoscopy and biopsy showed the node was caused by sarcoidosis.

Unusual sites of disease in patients who relapse are not uncommon and it is important to be vigilant at scan review and scrutinize every abnormality. Where possible, previous CT studies in the same patient should always be available for comparison to ensure that subtle changes, particularly nodal enlargement, are detected early.

FDG-PET

The advantage of FDG-PET over CT is that it is a functional imaging technique that identifies metabolically active sites of disease and provides different information from anatomic imaging. Because of their higher metabolic rate, there is greater uptake of FDG tracer in malignant cells compared with normal tissue, which enables tumor to be detected, particularly at sites where CT is less sensitive (eg, the skeleton) or in some sub 1-cm lymph nodes that would not be considered positive by CT criteria. Aside from mature differentiated teratoma (which have a relatively low metabolic rate), most tumors (and their metastases) demonstrate avid FDG uptake. With respect to testicular tumors, seminomatous lesions have a significantly higher FDG uptake compared with NSGCT.[14]

Studies comparing FDG-PET with CT in the primary staging of GCT showed that FDG-PET is useful for detecting viable tumor in lesions that are visible on CT and may prevent false-positive diagnosis on CT in clinical stage II disease.[15] However, it does not consistently improve the staging in patients with clinical stage I disease. Although PET identifies some patients with disease not detected by CT (**Fig. 7**), the relapse rate in PET-negative patients is high, indicating that small volume and microscopic disease are missed.[15,16] Furthermore, FDG-PET is not able to confidently identify a mature teratoma and is generally considered insensitive for detecting intracerebral metastases in view of the poor contrast resulting from high normal uptake of FDG in the brain. A recent multicenter study concluded that using FDG-PET as a primary staging tool for NSGCT yielded only slightly better results than CT.[17] Both methods had a high specificity but false-negative findings were more frequent with CT. FDG-PET is mostly useful as a diagnostic tool in cases where the CT scan findings are equivocal.[17] FDG-PET is not recommended for the primary staging of TGCT.

Early studies suggested that there may be role of FDG-PET to identify patients likely to relapse after treatment of the primary tumor. A Danish pilot study in 46 patients with stage I NSGCT showed that FDG-PET could identify 70% of patients who subsequently relapsed with metastatic NSGCT.[18] Similar results were obtained in a German

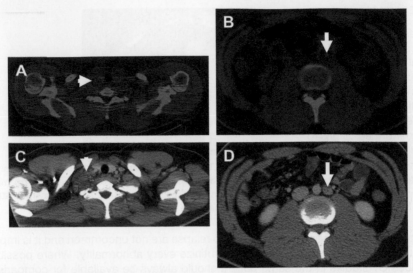

Fig. 7. FDG-PET in staging disease. (*A, B*) Fused color-coded FDG-PET-CT images and (*C, D*) contrast-enhanced CT in a patient with NSGCT (embryonal carcinoma) had a left paraaortic node (*long arrow*) detected on CT scan as the only site of metastatic disease. This node was also seen on FDG-PET but there was also evidence of small-volume right supraclavicular (*short arrow*) and upper mediastinal nodal (not illustrated here) involvement.

study in 50 patients.[19] The negative predictive value of the Danish study was 92%, which suggests that adjuvant treatment could potentially be avoided in most patients with stage NSGCT and a negative FDG-PET. This hypothesis (ie, to use of FDG-PET to predict relapse in patients with clinical stage I NSGCT) has been investigated by the Medical Research Council in the United Kingdom in the TE22 study.[20] The study, conducted in 111 patients, showed that although FDG-PET identified a proportion of patients with disease not detectable by CT, the relapse rate among FDG-PET–negative patients remained high (33 of the 87 on surveillance relapsed). The study results suggest that FDG-PET scanning is not a reliable method of identifying stage I patients at risk of relapse to replace other treatment options in this setting.[20]

MRI

MRI, despite recent technical developments with faster acquisitions, is still not routinely used for disease staging. This is in part because of its longer examination times, higher cost, and lesser availability compared with CT. However, MRI is useful for the detection and characterization of central nervous system disease, and musculoskeletal and hepatic metastases. MRI is particularly useful for assessing involvement of the IVC by tumor.[21] MRI may also be valuable as a problem-solving technique in the presence of equivocal CT findings.

For the detection of retroperitoneal lymph nodes MRI relies on the same size criteria as in CT to identify malignant nodes. Therefore, MRI has the same important limitation (ie, inability to identify disease in normal-sized nodes or distinguish reactive from malignant enlarged nodes). Nevertheless, as there is increasing awareness of the potential detrimental effects of ionizing radiation from CT examinations, there may be an argument to perform more MRI studies for the serial follow-up of these patients to minimize radiation exposure. A prospective study of 52 patients with TGCT showed that MRI (see **Fig. 3**) is comparable with CT for detection of nodal disease.[22]

CHEST RADIOGRAPHS

Chest radiographs are used in the staging and follow-up of testicular cancer patients because lung metastases greater than 1 cm can be detected and monitored, mediastinal masses can be evaluated, and pleurally based tumors and effusions can also be recognized. They provide a valuable cost-effective, low-radiation method of follow-up compared with chest CT. The greater sensitivity of CT often leads to false-positive findings.[23,24] In a large retrospective study of 182 patients with seminoma a 10% false-positive rate at initial staging with chest CT was found.[24] A chest CT should be performed to characterize any abnormality in chest radiographs or if the staging abdominal CT is abnormal.[25]

Ultrasound

On ultrasound, the retroperitoneum is difficult to visualize because of overlying bowel gas and intraabdominal fat and small-volume nodal disease is likely to be missed. Ultrasound is not routinely used for staging but only used in specific clinical situations as a problem-solving technique, such as in the investigation of focal liver lesions demonstrated on staging CT when it has not been possible to reach a definitive diagnosis. Ultrasound is also useful to guide the biopsy of retroperitoneal masses, liver lesions, or masses at other sites.

ASSESSMENT OF TUMOR RESPONSE AND RESIDUAL AND RECURRENT DISEASE

CT remains the primary imaging modality in the follow-up of patients with GCTs. However, there is a growing awareness of radiation exposure from diagnostic imaging investigation, especially in young patients.[26] The potential benefit of repeated scanning must be weighed against the financial and health costs of more frequent scans. For example, an abdominal CT gives a radiation dose equivalent to 1000 chest radiographs (10 mSv vs 0.01 mSv).[26] The lifetime risk of developing a second malignancy in a 20-year-old man after a CT of the abdomen and pelvis has been estimated as being between 1:500 and 1:1000.[27]

Modern CT scanners are becoming dose efficient using technologic advances, such as variable dose modulation and new image reconstruction algorithms.[28,29] Despite this it is important to keep the dose as low as reasonably achievable (ALARA principle). Possible approaches to reducing radiation exposure in patients with GCTs include keeping imaging with CT or PET to a minimum, only imaging the body region required, using chest radiograph where it suffices over chest CT, using lower-dose CT techniques, or using imaging with nonionizing radiation. A recent study showed that MRI and CT were equivalent in terms of detection of retroperitoneal disease.[22] Currently, the Medical Research Council in the United Kingdom is conducting a trial in stage I seminoma patients (TRISST Trial) to compare MRI with CT as follow-up methods.[22] Other investigators have studied low-dose CT techniques in patients with stage 1 testicular cancer managed by surveillance. They showed that the low-dose protocol provided diagnostically acceptable images for at least 99% of patients and achieved mean dose reduction of 55% compared with the standard dose protocol.[30]

In assessing tumor response to treatment, reduction in the size of metastases is the main change on CT indicating response to therapy even though malignant cells may persist within the residuum (Fig. 8). Interval CT scanning during and after completion of therapy is important to assess response. In addition to size, CT can show morphologic changes (eg, after chemotherapy, cystic and fatty change are associated with mature differentiated teratoma).[31–33] However, these morphologic changes are not specific

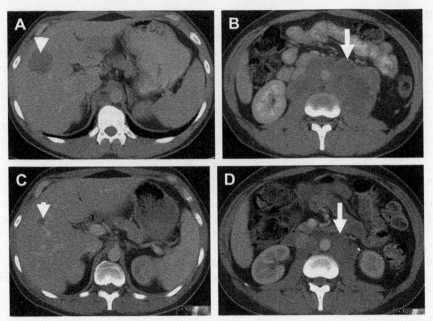

Fig. 8. Response to chemotherapy. (*A, B*) Prechemotherapy and (*C, D*) postchemotherapy axial CT images in a patient with stage IV NSGCT showing the response in the large retroperitoneal nodal (*long arrows*) and liver (*short arrows*) metastasis.

enough to determine management. In those patients with large-volume residual masses, CT and MRI have been shown to be useful in planning an operative approach.[34]

Seminoma is extremely sensitive to chemotherapy and radiotherapy, such that a residual mass posttreatment usually only consists of fibrosis and necrosis. FDG-PET has a role for the assessment of residual masses in patients with seminoma after chemotherapy. In a recent large prospective study (SEMPET trial), where FDG-PET was used to assess residual tumors in patients with seminoma treated with chemotherapy, FDG-PET imaging was found to be more accurate than other imaging modalities. In this study, FDG-PET was performed in all patients with residual masses greater than 1 cm within 4 to 12 weeks of completing chemotherapy. The results were compared with histology of tumor viability and CT evidence of disease progression. FDG-PET correctly identified all cases of residual tumor in lesions greater than 3 cm and in 95% of cases in lesions less than 3 cm. This gave an overall specificity and sensitivity for 100% and 80%, respectively, for FDG-PET, compared with 74% and 70% for CT. Because there were no false-positive results, it was suggested that a positive FDG-PET scan, even in small lesions, was highly specific for viable tumor.[35] However, the experience published from Indiana University reported slightly different findings.[36] In a retrospective review of 24 FDG-PET scans, it was found that cases with negative scans correlated with no viable disease and all patients with residual disease had positive FDG-PET studies. However, there were four positive cases on FDG-PET imaging that led to surgical resections of the residual masses, but these revealed only fibrosis, necrosis, or inflammation (false-positive) at histology. Based on their findings, the authors recommended that a negative FDG-PET scan is likely to indicate a low likelihood of persistent seminoma after chemotherapy (**Fig. 9**), whereas a positive PET scan does not translate to a high probability of persistent seminoma in the residual nodal masses.[36]

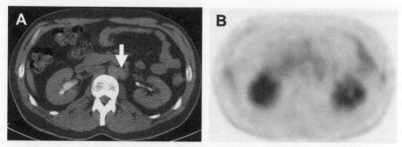

Fig. 9. Residual mass following chemotherapy treatment for seminoma. (*A*) Noncontrast CT shows the residual 1.5-cm retroperitoneal mass (*arrow*). (*B*) Corresponding FDG-PET image shows no activity in the residual mass. Subsequent follow-up has shown no evidence of recurrent disease.

In NSGCT, assessment of residual masses using FDG-PET can potentially differentiate between viable disease and fibrosis.[14,37–39] The sensitivity and specificity of FDG-PET in the largest series (70 scans in 55 men) was 88% and 95%, respectively, with high negative predictive value of 90% and positive predictive value of 96%. The positive predictive value achieved using FDG-PET is clearly superior compared with CT in this circumstance (56%).[37] However, its use may be limited in this clinical setting because differentiated teratoma has variable low or no uptake and cannot be easily

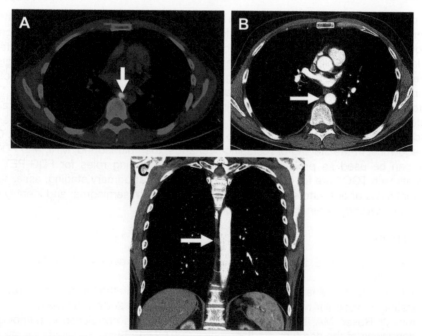

Fig. 10. Recurrent disease on FDG-PET. A man previously treated for metastatic NSGCT had a slowly rising tumor marker level but no apparent disease on contrast-enhanced CT. (*A*) FDG-PET-CT images were performed and the fused color-coded FDG-PET-CT images show increased uptake in a node in the posterior mediastinum (*arrow*). This small node can in retrospect be seen on the (*B*) contrast-enhanced CT images (*arrow*) and is more easily discernable on the (*C*) coronal reformatted image (*arrow*).

distinguished from fibrosis or necrosis. Patients with residual differentiated teratoma require surgery because there is a risk of developing malignant change. Therefore, the crucial decision of whether a residual lesion after chemotherapy requires surgery is not aided when FDG-PET study shows low or no uptake. Residual viable disease as indicated by FDG avid lesion indicates the need for further therapy.

Detection of recurrent disease is reliant on careful follow-up using a combination of clinical assessment, serum markers, chest radiographs, and abdominal CT. Follow-up protocols vary depending on the type of tumor, stage, treatments administered, and individual institutions. They are based on the known patterns of disease relapse in TGCT.[40,41] FDG-PET has been investigated for the detection of recurrent disease and may have a possible role in patients with raised tumor markers but no visible active disease on other imaging, such as CT (**Fig. 10**). A retrospective study of 47 scans in 55 patients performed for the assessment of residual masses (18 with raised tumor markers) and 23 studies for the investigation of raised tumor markers in the presence of normal CT scans was performed.[37] FDG-PET identified a site of disease in all but one case and five false-negative FDG-PET results were found. Out of the false-negatives, three cases had no abnormality on any imaging modality. During follow-up of these patients, it was found that FDG-PET scans were the first imaging modality to identify the site of recurrence. Hence, it was suggested that in the presence of raised tumor marker levels and negative imaging (including negative FDG-PET), the most appropriate follow-up imaging may be to repeat FDG-PET imaging.

SUMMARY

The diagnosis of TGCT is made by tissue biopsy or at orchidectomy even though ultrasound is the primary imaging modality for the evaluation of testicular mass lesions. Scrotal MRI can be used to differentiate between an intratesticular versus an extratesticular mass where clinical and sonographic assessment is inadequate. For staging patients with TGCT, CT remains the imaging modality of choice. Modern multidetector CT provides detailed anatomic information of disease spread. Knowledge of the pattern of spread and potential pitfalls in imaging are important to accurately stage these patients. CT is also the primary imaging modality to assess response and residual disease after treatment, and to identify recurrent disease. If findings at CT are equivocal in the staging or restaging scenarios, then ultrasound, MRI, and FDG-PET can be used as problem-solving tools. The emerging roles for FDG-PET in patients with TGCT are for evaluating equivocal nodes at primary staging; assessing residual mass after treatment, particularly in patients with seminoma; and identifying sites of recurrence when findings are occult on CT.

REFERENCES

1. Carkaci S, Ozkan E, Lane D, et al. Scrotal sonography revisited. J Clin Ultrasound 2010;38:21.
2. Tsili AC, Tsampoulas C, Giannakopoulos X, et al. MRI in the histologic characterization of testicular neoplasms. AJR Am J Roentgenol 2007;189:W331.
3. Kim W, Rosen MA, Langer JE, et al. US MR imaging correlation in pathologic conditions of the scrotum. Radiographics 2007;27:1239.
4. Tsili AC, Argyropoulou MI, Giannakis D, et al. MRI in the characterization and local staging of testicular neoplasms. AJR Am J Roentgenol 2010;194:682.
5. International germ cell consensus classification: a prognostic factor-based staging system for metastatic germ cell cancers. International Germ cell cancer collaborative group. J Clin Oncol 1997;15:594–603.

6. Krege S, Beyer J, Souchon R, et al. European consensus conference on diagnosis and treatment of germ cell cancer: a report of the second meeting of the European Germ Cell Cancer Consensus group (EGCCCG): part I. Eur Urol 2008;53:478.

7. Krege S, Beyer J, Souchon R, et al. European consensus conference on diagnosis and treatment of germ cell cancer: a report of the second meeting of the European Germ Cell Cancer Consensus Group (EGCCCG): part II. Eur Urol 2008;53:497.

8. Sobin LH, Gospodarowicz MK, Wittekind CH, editors. TNM classification of malignant tumours. 7th edition. New York: Wiley-Liss; 2009.

9. Dixon AK, Ellis M, Sikora K. Computed tomography of testicular tumours: distribution of abdominal lymphadenopathy. Clin Radiol 1986;37:519.

10. Hilton S, Herr HW, Teitcher JB, et al. CT detection of retroperitoneal lymph node metastases in patients with clinical stage I testicular nonseminomatous germ cell cancer: assessment of size and distribution criteria. AJR Am J Roentgenol 1997;169:521.

11. Dorfman RE, Alpern MB, Gross BH, et al. Upper abdominal lymph nodes: criteria for normal size determined with CT. Radiology 1991;180:319.

12. Magnusson A. Size of normal retroperitoneal lymph nodes. Acta Radiol Diagn (Stockh) 1983;24:315.

13. Fossa SD, Bokemeyer C, Gerl A, et al. Treatment outcome of patients with brain metastases from malignant germ cell tumors. Cancer 1999;85:988.

14. Cremerius U, Effert PJ, Adam G, et al. FDG PET for detection and therapy control of metastatic germ cell tumor. J Nucl Med 1998;39:815.

15. Albers P, Bender H, Yilmaz H, et al. Positron emission tomography in the clinical staging of patients with stage I and II testicular germ cell tumors. Urology 1999; 53:808.

16. Spermon JR, Geus-Oei LF, Kiemeney LA, et al. The role of (18)fluoro-2-deoxyglucose positron emission tomography in initial staging and re-staging after chemotherapy for testicular germ cell tumours. BJU Int 2002;89:549.

17. de Wit M, Brenner W, Hartmann M, et al. [18F]-FDG-PET in clinical stage I/II nonseminomatous germ cell tumours: results of the German Multicentre Trial. Ann Oncol 2008;19:1619.

18. Lassen U, Daugaard G, Eigtved A, et al. Whole-body FDG-PET in patients with stage I non-seminomatous germ cell tumours. Eur J Nucl Med Mol Imaging 2003;30:396.

19. Cremerius U, Wildberger JE, Borchers H, et al. Does positron emission tomography using 18-fluoro-2-deoxyglucose improve clinical staging of testicular cancer? Results of a study in 50 patients. Urology 1999;54:900.

20. Huddart RA, O'Doherty MJ, Padhani A, et al. 18fluorodeoxyglucose positron emission tomography in the prediction of relapse in patients with high-risk, clinical stage I nonseminomatous germ cell tumors: preliminary report of MRC Trial TE22–the NCRI testis tumour clinical study group. J Clin Oncol 2007;25:3090.

21. Ng CS, Husband JE, Padhani AR, et al. Evaluation by magnetic resonance imaging of the inferior vena cava in patients with non-seminomatous germ cell tumours of the testis metastatic to the retroperitoneum. Br J Urol 1997;79:942.

22. Sohaib SA, Koh DM, Barbachano Y, et al. Prospective assessment of MRI for imaging retroperitoneal metastases from testicular germ cell tumours. Clin Radiol 2009;64:362.

23. Fernandez EB, Colon E, McLeod DG, et al. Efficacy of radiographic chest imaging in patients with testicular cancer. Urology 1994;44:243.

24. Horan G, Rafique A, Robson J, et al. CT of the chest can hinder the management of seminoma of the testis; it detects irrelevant abnormalities. Br J Cancer 2007;96: 882.

25. See WA, Hoxie L. Chest staging in testis cancer patients: imaging modality selection based upon risk assessment as determined by abdominal computerized tomography scan results. J Urol 1993;150:874.
26. Brenner DJ, Hall EJ. Computed tomography: an increasing source of radiation exposure. N Engl J Med 2007;357:2277.
27. Smith-Bindman R, Lipson J, Marcus R, et al. Radiation dose associated with common computed tomography examinations and the associated lifetime attributable risk of cancer. Arch Intern Med 2009;169:2078.
28. McCollough CH, Bruesewitz MR, Kofler JM Jr. CT dose reduction and dose management tools: overview of available options. Radiographics 2006;26:503.
29. Sagara Y, Hara AK, Pavlicek W, et al. Abdominal CT: comparison of low-dose CT with adaptive statistical iterative reconstruction and routine-dose CT with filtered back projection in 53 patients. AJR Am J Roentgenol 2010;195:713.
30. O'Malley ME, Chung P, Haider M, et al. Comparison of low dose with standard dose abdominal/pelvic multidetector CT in patients with stage 1 testicular cancer under surveillance. Eur Radiol 2010;20:1624.
31. Connor S, Guest P. Conversion of multiple solid testicular teratoma metastases to fatty and cystic liver masses following chemotherapy: CT evidence of "maturation." Br J Radiol 1999;72:1114.
32. Lentini JF, Love MB, Ritchie WG, et al. Computed tomography in retroconversion of hepatic metastases from immature ovarian teratoma. J Comput Assist Tomogr 1986;10:1060.
33. Moskovic E, Jobling T, Fisher C, et al. Retroconversion of immature teratoma of the ovary: CT appearances. Clin Radiol 1991;43:402.
34. Sugawara Y, Zasadny KR, Grossman HB, et al. Germ cell tumor: differentiation of viable tumor, mature teratoma, and necrotic tissue with FDG PET and kinetic modeling. Radiology 1999;211:249.
35. De Santis M, Becherer A, Bokemeyer C, et al. 2-18fluoro-deoxy-D-glucose positron emission tomography is a reliable predictor for viable tumor in postchemotherapy seminoma: an update of the prospective multicentric SEMPET trial. J Clin Oncol 2004;22:1034.
36. Lewis DA, Tann M, Kesler K, et al. Positron emission tomography scans in postchemotherapy seminoma patients with residual masses: a retrospective review from Indiana University Hospital. J Clin Oncol 2006;24:e54.
37. Hain SF, O'Doherty MJ, Timothy AR, et al. Fluorodeoxyglucose positron emission tomography in the evaluation of germ cell tumours at relapse. Br J Cancer 2000; 83:863.
38. Oechsle K, Hartmann M, Brenner W, et al. [18F]Fluorodeoxyglucose positron emission tomography in nonseminomatous germ cell tumors after chemotherapy: the German Multicenter Positron Emission Tomography Study Group. J Clin Oncol 2008;26:5930.
39. Stephens AW, Gonin R, Hutchins GD, et al. Positron emission tomography evaluation of residual radiographic abnormalities in postchemotherapy germ cell tumor patients. J Clin Oncol 1996;14:1637.
40. Flechon A, Culine S, Theodore C, et al. Pattern of relapse after first line treatment of advanced stage germ-cell tumors. Eur Urol 2005;48:957.
41. Kondagunta GV, Sheinfeld J, Motzer RJ. Recommendations of follow-up after treatment of germ cell tumors. Semin Oncol 2003;30:382.

Management of Stage I Testicular Seminoma

Gary Mok, MD, FRCPC[a], Padraig Warde, MB, FRCPC[b],*

KEYWORDS

- Seminoma • Surveillance • Radiation • Chemotherapy
- Stage I

Testicular cancer is a rare tumor accounting for only 1% to 2% of all cancers in men.[1] An American Caucasian man has an estimated 0.2% cumulative lifetime risk for developing testicular cancer.[2] Despite the relative rarity of this tumor, it is still the most common solid tumor in young men aged 20 to 35 years and the incidence has increased by 61% from 1973 to 2003, with the majority of the rise caused by seminomas rather than nonseminomas.[3] In 2010, there was an estimated 8480 new diagnoses and 350 deaths from testicular cancer in the United States.[4] Approximately 60% of testicular cancers will have seminoma histology and 80% of these men, or approximately 4300 men, will have disease confined to the testicle (stage I).[5] Thus, stage I seminoma is the most common presentation of testicular cancer.

Adjuvant treatment options for stage I seminoma include surveillance, radiation, and chemotherapy. Historically, adjuvant radiation had been the treatment of choice with excellent cure rates and overall survival rates. Chemotherapy has recently emerged as an alternative option, although longer follow-up is required to ensure that long-term relapse rates and toxicities are acceptable in comparison to radiation. Despite excellent results for both adjuvant chemotherapy and radiotherapy (RT), many concerns have been raised in regards to the potential long-term toxicities, such as secondary cancers, gonadal toxicity, and cardiac toxicity.

To minimize the burden of treatment, there has been a shift away from adjuvant treatments for stage I testicular seminomas toward surveillance protocols for seminoma survivors. This article reviews the evidence for all adjuvant treatment options for stage I testicular seminomas with a particular focus on surveillance.

The authors have nothing to disclose.

[a] Radiation Medicine Program, Princess Margaret Hospital, 610 University Avenue, Toronto, ON M5G 2M9, Canada

[b] Department of Radiation Oncology, University of Toronto, FitzGerald Building, 150 College Street, Room 106, Toronto, ON M5S 3S2, Canada

* Corresponding author.

E-mail address: padraig.warde@rmp.uhn.on.ca

Hematol Oncol Clin N Am 25 (2011) 503–516
doi:10.1016/j.hoc.2011.03.008

hemonc.theclinics.com

INITIAL EVALUATION AND MANAGEMENT

The initial management of a testicular mass or suspected testicular seminoma includes a full history and physical examination. A testicular ultrasound is helpful in differentiating between a solid mass and a potential hydrocele. After confirmation of a solid testicular mass, an inguinal orchidectomy should be performed rather than testicular biopsy. Histology of the testicular mass will guide further adjuvant treatments. Routine laboratory testing includes a complete blood count (CBC); creatinine; and tumor markers, including βHCG, AFP, and LDH. A computed tomography (CT) scan of the abdomen and pelvis and a chest radiograph should be obtained to complete staging. If the CT abdomen and pelvis demonstrates metastatic lymph nodes, a CT scan of the thorax should be included to better evaluate for lung metastases.

SURVEILLANCE

There is now mature data demonstrating that patients with stage I seminoma enrolled in surveillance protocols have a relapse rate of 15% to 20% (**Table 1**).[6–14] The largest series of patients placed on a surveillance protocol is from Canada with 421 patients with a median follow-up of 8.2 years and a 5-year relapse-free rate of 85.5%.[7] Similarly, the Danish Testicular Cancer Study Group (DATECA) reported on 394 patients with a median follow-up of 60 months and a relapse rate of 17%.[8] Interestingly, 2 independent Japanese studies report lower relapse rates of 10% to 11%, which may represent differences in tumor biology compared with North American and European data.[13,14] The most common site of relapse was the para-aortic lymph nodes in 82% and 89% of all relapses in the Danish and Canadian series, respectively.[7,8] Relapses are typically detected at 12 to 18 months in most series; however, late relapses more than 4 years from orchidectomy have been reported.[15] Ultimately, patients managed with surveillance can expect excellent cause-specific survival rates approaching 100%, which is attributable to highly effective salvage radiation or chemotherapy. A review of the Princess Margaret Hospital (PMH) database demonstrated a 6-fold decrease in treatment episodes per patient in patients managed with surveillance (0.16) compared with patients managed with adjuvant RT (1.05).[16]

Table 1
Outcomes for patients with stage I seminoma enrolled on surveillance programs

Author	Year	Median Follow-up (mo)	Number of Patients	Relapse (Number of Patients)	Relapse (%)	Cause-Specific Survival (%)
Horwich et al[10]	1992	62	103	17	16.5	100.0
Ramakrishnan et al[11]	1992	44	72	13	18.0	100.0
Von der Maase et al[12]	1993	48	261	49	18.8	98.9
Oliver et al[6]	2001	98	110	21	19.0	100.0
Germa-Lluch et al[9]	2002	33	233	38	16.0	100.0
Daugaard et al[8]	2003	60	394	69	17.5	100.0
Warde et al[7]	2005	98	421	64	15.2	99.7
Yoshida et al[14]	2009	124	64	7	11.0	98.4
Kamba et al[13]	2010	45	186	19	10.0	100.0

Predictors of Relapse

The identification of tumor and patient characteristics for predicting tumor relapse has evolved over the past decade. The PMH has reported tumor size and patient age as key predictors for relapse, whereas small vessel invasion approached statistical significance.[17] The Royal Marsden Hospital reported vascular or lymphatic invasion as the only significant risk factor.[10] To better identify these risk factors, 638 patients were pooled and analyzed from the databases of the Royal Marsden Hospital, DATECA, PMH, and the Royal London Hospital. On multivariate analysis, only tumor size greater than 4 cm and rete testis invasion were significant predictors for relapse following orchidectomy. A 5-year relapse rate of 12.2% was observed if neither risk factor was present compared with 15.9% and 31.5% if one or both risk factors were present.[18] A validation of this risk-stratification model was performed using 687 patients with stage I seminoma managed with surveillance from the Copenhagen National Hospital, PMH, and British Columbia Cancer Agency. This study found that tumor size remained the only predictor for relapse on univariate analysis, whereas rete testis invasion was no longer statistically significant.[19]

Risk-Adapted Models

Using the prognostic model based on the risk factors (tumor size >4 cm and rete testis invasion) identified earlier, the Spanish Germ Cell Cancer Cooperative Study Group has reported a risk-adapted management approach for stage I seminoma.[20] Patients with no risk factors were considered low-risk and were managed on a surveillance protocol. Patients with a single risk factor had an intermediate risk of relapse, whereas patients with both risk factors were considered to be at high-risk for relapse. Both intermediate and high-risk groups were treated with 2 cycles of adjuvant carboplatin. This study confirmed the findings of the multi-institutional pooled analysis that low-risk patients had a small risk of relapse.[18]

This current risk-adapted approach is problematic because it does not sufficiently identify patients at risk of relapse. Patients in the high-risk group have a predicted 30% relapse rate, which still results in 70% of patients receiving unnecessary treatment. Furthermore, a recent pooled analysis was unable to validate this prognostic model and one of the prognostic factors, rete testis invasion, is no longer a predictor of relapse.[19] The current standard practice at the PMH is to offer surveillance protocol as the management option of choice for all patients with stage I seminoma. Treatment with either radiation or chemotherapy is reserved in the event of a relapse.

Surveillance Schedule

An optimal surveillance schedule has yet to be universally adopted. However, evidence-based recommendations have been published regarding the frequency of follow-up based on the risk of relapse per year. These guidelines suggest increased surveillance with CT scans for the first few years following orchidectomy when the risk of relapse is the highest at 5% per year.[21] Screening becomes less frequent as the risk of relapse decreases until the 10th year when routine screening is discontinued. These recommendations have been adopted by the European Germ Cell Cancer Consensus Group (EGCCCG).[22,23] The National Comprehensive Cancer Network (NCCN) guidelines are similar with 3 to 4 abdominopelvic CT scans annually for the first 3 years, then every 6 months for the next 4 years and then annually until 10 years of follow-up have been completed.[24] The recommendations adopted by the EGCCCG for the follow-up and investigations for patients managed with surveillance, radiation and carboplatin are included in **Tables 2** and **3**.[21]

Table 2
Recommended frequency of follow-up in stage I seminoma

Annual Hazard Rate (%)	Frequency	Surveillance	Extended Field RT	Para-Aortic RT	Carboplatin x1
>5.0	3x/y	First to second y	NA	NA	NA
1.0–5.0	2x/y	Third to fourth y	First to third y	First to third y	First to third y
0.3–1.0	1x/y	5th–10th y	Fourth to sixth y	Fourth to sixth y	Limited data
<0.3	Cease	After 10 y	After 6 y	After 6 y	

Abbreviation: NA, not applicable.

CT Screening Radiation Exposure

Despite efforts to diminish potential risks from adjuvant treatments by placing patients on surveillance protocols, concerns remain in regards to the potential toxicities associated with radiation exposure for patients undergoing routine and frequent CT scans. Over the course of 10 years of follow-up, patients on the EGCCCG program would receive 15 CT scans, whereas patients on the NCCN guidelines would receive 21 scans. An average abdominopelvic CT scan exposes patients to approximately 10 to 20 mSV.[25,26] Over the course of follow-up, patients may receive up to 420 mSV of radiation on a surveillance protocol.

The stochastic effects of radiation, the induction of cancer or a germ line mutation, increase in probability as dose increase. These effects are not considered to have a minimum threshold radiation dose and therefore the risk of carcinogenesis still exists even in individuals who are exposed to low doses of radiation. Data from Japanese atomic bomb survivors have been used to model radiation dose to organs from radiation exposure. This model estimates that 0.6% to 2.0% of all cancers in the United States are attributable to radiation exposure from CT imaging.[27,28] Although some may view this as an overestimation, this data remains the best available estimate of the carcinogenic risk of radiation exposure from CT scans. Based on retrospective data, the risk of radiation-induced carcinogenesis is thought be higher in younger patients, which is of particular concern in the seminoma patient population who are typically in their third or fourth decade of life at diagnosis.[29,30]

Current research efforts to reduce radiation exposure in seminoma survivors are underway. In the United Kingdom, the Medical Research Council (MRC) is conducting the TE24 clinical study to evaluate magnetic resonance imaging (MRI) screening as an alternative to conventional CT scans for detection of relapse. The PMH has established an investigational low-dose CT scan protocol, which decreases radiation exposure for each CT scan by approximately 50%.[31] Reduction of radiation exposure comes at the expense of degraded image quality, but in the majority of cases the quality is sufficient to detect relapse. In the future, low-dose CT scans or MRI scans may be incorporated into future surveillance protocols. Elimination of routine imaging

Table 3
Recommended investigations during follow-up for stage I seminoma

Investigation	Surveillance	Extended-Field RT	Para-Aortic RT	Carboplatin x1
CT abdomen	Yes	No	No	Yes
CT pelvis	Yes	No	Yes	Yes
Chest radiograph	Yes	Yes	Yes	Yes

of the pelvic lymph at low risk of relapse may lead to a form of targeted imaging where solely the para-aortic lymph nodes are monitored on a regular basis, although this approach remains to be validated. MR lymphography is becoming increasingly used in a variety of different cancer sites to increase the specificity and sensitivity of lymph node metastasis.[32–34] There may be a role for MR lymphography in the surveillance setting for future patients with seminomas.

ADJUVANT RADIOTHERAPY

Historically, adjuvant retroperitoneal radiotherapy had been the standard treatment for stage I seminoma following an inguinal orchidectomy. Most institutional series report 10-year overall survival rates of ranging from 92% to 99%. Data from large, single institutional or multi-institutional experiences report relapse rates ranging from 3.5% to 5.0% (Table 4).[7,13,35–39] Relapses are almost always found outside the treatment field and are most commonly found in the mediastinum, lungs, and the left supraclavicular fossa. A minority of patients may relapse in the inguinal lymph nodes and typically have predisposing risk factors, such as prior inguinal or scrotal surgery. In-field relapses are highly unusual and if suspected should be biopsied to rule out a nonseminomatous etiology. In the event of a supradiaphragmatic relapse, chemotherapy is the treatment of choice and cure rates approach 100%.

Volume of Radiation

Traditional radiation volumes following inguinal orchidectomy for stage I testicular seminoma included the para-aortic and pelvic lymph nodes. In most studies, the superior limit of the radiation field was at the T10-11 vertebral body.[37,40] Care should be taken to avoid placing cardiac tissue in the radiation field. The low incidence of pelvic lymph node involvement led to a randomized controlled trial by the Medical Research Council Testicular Study Group comparing para-aortic and pelvic irradiation to para-aortic irradiation alone in 478 subjects with stage I seminoma.[37] There was a 4% relapse rate in subjects treated with para-aortic radiation compared with 3.4% in subjects treated with extended field radiation. All relapses in the para-aortic and pelvic radiotherapy arm were in supradiaphragmatic sites, whereas 1.6% of subjects in the para-aortic radiation arm relapsed in the pelvis. The time to first normal post-radiotherapy sperm count was significantly longer in the extended field group; however, this difference declined over time and at 3 years from the start of radiotherapy.[37]

This trial demonstrated that para-aortic radiation provides excellent results; however, a small, but non-negligible risk of pelvic failure remains. Data from the

Table 4
Outcomes for adjuvant retroperitoneal radiotherapy in stage I seminoma

Author	Years of Study	Number of Patients	Relapse (%)	Cause-Specific Survival (%)
Santoni et al[38]	(1970–1999)	487	4.3	99.4
Bayens et al[35]	(1975–1985)	132	4.5	99.0
Hültenschmidt et al[39]	(1978–1992)	188	1.0	100.0
Coleman et al[36]	(1980–1995)	144	4.2	100.0
Warde et al[7]	(1981–2002)	283	5.0	100.0
Kamba et al[13]	(1985–2006)	182	4.9	99.5
Fossa et al[37]	(1989–1993)	242	3.7	100.0

Christie Hospital in Manchester, where there was no routine evaluation of the pelvic lymph nodes after para-aortic radiation, demonstrated that the median size of the pelvic lymph nodes at time of detection of relapse was 5 cm (range 2.5–9.0 cm).[41] To maximize the probability of cure, early detection of relapse is essential and if only the para-aortic lymph nodes are irradiated, then routine evaluation of the pelvis by CT imaging is still necessary.

Dose of Radiation

Traditional adjuvant radiation doses have ranged from 25 to 35 Gy for stage testicular seminoma in the past. The Medical Research Council conducted a noninferiority randomized clinical trial (TE18) in 625 patients comparing 30 Gy in 15 fractions to 20 Gy in 10 fractions. The majority of patients received para-aortic irradiation only (88.1% in the 30-Gy group and 88.7% in the 20-Gy group). Five-year relapse rates were similar in both groups at 3.0% for the 30-Gy arm and 3.6% in the 20-Gy arm.[42]

Upon closure of this trial, an additional 469 patients, for a total of 1094 patients, were added from a second trial comparing adjuvant chemotherapy to adjuvant radiotherapy (TE19/30,982). Within the adjuvant radiotherapy arm, the dose was selected by a second randomization to either 30 Gy or 20 Gy. The results of the combined TE18 and T19 trials were presented at the American Society of Clinical Oncology (ASCO) 2008 annual meeting. The 5-year relapse rates were 4.9% and 3.0%, for the 30 Gy and 20 Gy groups, respectively.[43] If adjuvant radiotherapy is to be used, a dose of 20 Gy in 10 fractions or a biologically equivalent dose is effective for reducing the risk of relapse.

Radiation Toxicity

In the acute setting, lethargy, nausea, vomiting, and diarrhea can be experienced by patients undergoing retroperitoneal radiotherapy. Nausea and vomiting can be managed effectively with a wide range of antiemetics, whereas diarrhea can be controlled with medications to suppress bowel motility.

Essentially all patients with stage I seminoma are expected to be long-term survivors and thus, there is mounting evidence that the burden of long-term toxicities may outweigh the potential benefits of adjuvant radiotherapy. Multiple institutions have demonstrated an increased risk of cardiac disease or cardiac-associated mortality in seminoma survivors treated with adjuvant radiation.[44,45] The MD Anderson experience reported mortality rates for 453 men treated with infradiaphragmatic radiotherapy with at least 15 years of follow-up. The cardiac-specific standardized mortality risk ratio 15 years after treatment was 1.80 (95% confidence interval [CI] 1.01–2.98).[44] The Royal Marsden Hospital published similar findings demonstrating an increased cardiovascular mortality risk ratio of 2.4 (95% CI 1.04–5.45) in 992 men treated with infradiaphragmatic radiotherapy compared with men who were placed on a surveillance protocol.[45] A pooled analysis from Norway of 386 patients with seminoma with a median follow-up of 18 years demonstrated hazard ratios of 2.1 and 2.3 for coronary artery disease and atherosclerotic disease, respectively.[46] Although the pathogenesis of cardiovascular disease in seminoma survivors treated with radiation is unknown, it is suspected that low-grade inflammation and elevated levels of high-sensitivity C-reactive protein detected in these survivors may drive the atherosclerotic process.[47]

The testicular germinal epithelium is highly sensitive to ionizing radiation. Scatter radiation within the pelvis may impair spermatogenesis and impact fertility. Reducing the radiotherapy target volume to the para-aortic chains can reduce the mean dose of radiation to the contralateral testicle to 0.09 Gy compared with 0.32 Gy for extended field radiation. Despite this reduction of dose, sperm counts are still reduced 1 year following treatment.[48] Data from the MRC randomized trial comparing radiation treatment volumes demonstrated a shorter time to normal sperm counts for the para-aortic–only arm compared with the extended-field arm (13 months vs 20 months). However, at 3 years the sperm counts were not significantly different.[37] Testicular shielding has been shown to decrease radiation dose to the contralateral testis regardless if the patient is treated with extended field or para-aortic radiation.[49] Total protection of the contralateral testis from radiation exposure cannot be guaranteed and sperm banking should be offered to all men undergoing radiotherapy who wish to preserve fertility.

Several studies have documented an increased second malignancy risk in seminoma survivors treated with adjuvant radiation. The largest study conducted by the National Cancer Institute collected data from 10,534 patients with irradiated seminoma (all stages) from 14 population-based registries.[50] Using a matched cohort analysis from corresponding general population registries, the overall relative risk of a second nontesticular malignancy was 2.0 (95% CI 1.8–2.2). For a 35-year-old patient with seminoma, the cumulative 40-year risk of a second malignancy was 36%, compared with 23% in the general population. These results were confirmed by a Dutch study involving 1354 long-term survivors treated with infradiaphragmatic radiotherapy. The risk of a second malignancy in these patients was 2.6-fold higher than the normal population.[51] Using a dose-modeling study, the risk of a second malignancy is thought to be reduced when treating with para-aortic irradiation compared with extended-field irradiation.[52] However, a risk of second malignancy still exists compared with individuals who are not irradiated.

In summary, adjuvant radiotherapy is highly effective in reducing relapse for stage I testicular seminoma, but survival is not improved compared with other strategies. Pre-irradiation sperm banking should be offered to patients wishing to preserve fertility. A radiation dose of 20 Gy to the retroperitoneal lymph nodes is sufficient and a radiation field encompassing the para-aortic lymph nodes is equivalent to extended field radiation. If the pelvic lymph nodes are omitted from the treatment field, a risk of pelvic relapse still exists and interval CT scans of the pelvis are still required. In addition to monitoring for relapse, follow-up should include assessment for possible complications of radiation treatment including cardiac disease, fertility issues, and second malignancies.

ADJUVANT CHEMOTHERAPY

There have been multiple publications demonstrating the efficacy of carboplatin in the adjuvant setting as an alternative to adjuvant radiotherapy. All have used either 1 or 2 cycles of carboplatin. If chemotherapy is to be used, the area under the curve (AUC) of 7 formula is the preferred dosing regimen compared with the older formula dosing to body-surface area (450 mg/m^2). This change in clinical practice has occurred for 2 primary reasons: (1) the AUC of 7 more reliably delivers the intended carboplatin dose compared with body surface area formulas; and consequently (2) all of the contemporary studies now use AUC of 7 dosing for carboplatin.[53] The first carboplatin phase I trial treated 78 patients with stage I seminoma with adjuvant carboplatin. Fifty-three patients received 2 cycles of carboplatin and 25 received 1 cycle. During a median 44-month follow-up time, there was 1 relapse for the entire group.[54] The remaining studies are summarized in **Table 5** and demonstrate relapse rates ranging from 1.8% to 8.6%.[6,20,54–59]

The MRC has published the results of a randomized controlled trial comparing a single cycle of carboplatin to adjuvant radiotherapy in 1477 men with stage I seminoma. This trial randomized patients to radiotherapy or adjuvant chemotherapy in

Table 5
Results of adjuvant carboplatin studies for stage I seminoma

Author	Year	Carboplatin Treatment	Median FU (mo)	Number of Patients	Relapse (%)	Sites of Relapse	5-Year Disease-Free Survival (%)
Oliver et al[54]	1994	1 cycle	29	25	0.0	—	100.0
		2 cycles	51	53	1.9	N/A	100.0
Krege et al[57]	1997	2 cycles	28	43	0.0	—	100.0
Dieckmann et al[56]	2000	1 cycle	48	93	8.6	Para-aortic region	91.1
		2 cycles	45	32	0.0	—	100.0
Oliver et al[6]	2001	1 cycle	52	146	0.7	N/A	100.0
		2 cycles	128	57	1.8	N/A	96.5
Aparicio et al[58]	2003	2 cycles	52	60	3.3	Retroperitoneum	96.6
Oliver et al[55]	2005	1 cycle	48	560	5.2	Retroperitoneal lymph nodes, para-aortic nodes	94.8
Aparicio et al[20]	2005	2 cycles	34	214	3.3	Retroperitoneum, spermatic cord	100.0
Argirovic[59]	2005	2 cycles	48	163	1.8	Retroperitoneum	100.0

Abbreviation: N/A, not available.

a 5:3 ratio; therefore, 904 patients received radiotherapy and 573 received carboplatin. Patients randomized to radiotherapy were further randomized to either 30 Gy or 20 Gy. There was no randomization for the field of irradiation, although 85% (668 patients) received para-aortic irradiation, whereas 15% (118 patients) received para-aortic and pelvic irradiation. The chemotherapy consisted of a single-cycle of carboplatin using an AUC of 7.[55] An update of the data with a median of 6.5 years of follow-up was presented at the 2008 annual ASCO meeting and demonstrated 5-year relapse rates in the radiotherapy and carboplatin arms of 4.0% and 5.3%, respectively. The retroperitoneum was the most common site of relapse accounting for 67% of all relapses. An unexpected benefit of carboplatin was observed with the 5-year rate of contralateral primary germ cell tumors reduced from 1.96% in the radiotherapy arm to 0.54% In carboplatin arm.[60]

Chemotherapy Toxicity

The long-term toxicities of carboplatin exposure are largely unknown. Platinum-based chemotherapy is associated with an increased risk of cardiovascular disease and second malignancy in testicular cancer survivors.[61] Data from Norway with a median 19-year follow-up, demonstrate an increased risk for coronary artery disease and atherosclerotic disease with respective hazard ratios of 5.7 and 4.7 in 364 subjects with seminoma treated with bleomycin, etoposide, and cisplatin chemotherapy compared with age-matched male population controls.[46] Furthermore, there is evidence that platinum can still be detected in the urine and serum in treated subjects at levels up to 1000-fold higher than nonexposed controls.[62–64] It remains to be seen if similar effects will be seen in patients treated with carboplatin.

A prospective study of 199 patients treated with adjuvant carboplatin reported no long-term toxicities in regards to cardiovascular disease or second malignancy compared with the UK general population over a median follow-up of 9 years.[65] In comparison to the radiotherapy data, more than 10,000 patients with irradiated seminoma, many of whom had more than 20 years of follow-up, were collected from multiple population-based tumor registries to estimate the risks of radiation-induced cancer.[50] The cardiovascular toxicity data from both MD Anderson and Royal Marsden Hospital, demonstrated that the risk of cardiovascular disease was mainly elevated at more than 10 years following radiation.[44,45] It appears that the number of patients and length of follow-up from a single study would be insufficient to conclusively elucidate the true long-term toxicities of carboplatin. This scenario may be analogous to the mid 1990s when it was prematurely concluded after short follow-up that there was no excess risk of second malignancy following radiotherapy for seminoma. Clearly, longer follow-up will be required to better define the long-term toxicities of current adjuvant carboplatin studies.

In summary, 1 to 2 cycles of adjuvant carboplatin postorchidectomy is comparable to adjuvant radiotherapy in terms of relapse free survival. Although the long-term toxicities of carboplatin have not been well characterized, it cannot be assumed that no reports of long-term toxicities equates to a safer therapeutic option. The predominant site of relapse in patients treated with adjuvant chemotherapy is in the retroperitoneum, thus routine surveillance with CT scans of the abdomen and pelvis are still required following treatment.

RETROPERITONEAL LYMPH NODE DISSECTION

Retroperitoneal lymph node dissection (RPLND) may be an appropriate alternative in rare instances where patients are unable to comply with surveillance and unable to

Table 6
Biologically effective doses for tumor control and late normal tissue toxicity

Fractionation Regimen	BED Tumor Control	BED Late Normal Tissue Effects
20 Gy in 10 fractions (2.0 Gy/fraction)	24.0	40.0
25 Gy in 20 fractions (1.25 Gy/fraction)	28.1	40.6
25 Gy in 15 fractions (1.67 Gy/fraction)	29.2	45.8

Abbreviation: BED, biologically effective dose.

receive radiotherapy or chemotherapy. Patients with a genetic instability disorder, inflammatory bowel disease, or prior retroperitoneal radiotherapy are generally not candidates for radiotherapy. RPLND may also be appropriate in patients with concurrent or previous malignancy for whom histologic examination of lymph nodes is essential to plan treatment. Dissection of the retroperitoneal lymph nodes is a technically difficult surgical procedure and can be associated with significant morbidity.

MANAGEMENT OF RELAPSE

Most patients who relapse during postorchiectomy surveillance can be treated successfully with radiotherapy alone. In both the Danish and PMH series, approximately 10% of patients treated with salvage radiotherapy experienced a second relapse.[7,12] Patients with centrally located, small volume relapses are suitable for salvage radiotherapy. Although the success of salvage radiotherapy requires early detection with routine CT scans to maximize the probability of successful salvage treatments. Large, bulky relapses or lateralized relapses are best treated with chemotherapy and are typically treated with 3 cycles of bleomycin, etoposide and cisplatin (BEP) at the PMH. Men with stage I seminoma who relapse after radiation therapy or after single-agent carboplatin are treated with either 3 or 4 cycles of BEP chemotherapy, depending on whether they have good-risk or intermediate-risk disease at the time of relapse.

Stage I seminoma that relapses in the retroperitoneum during postorchiectomy surveillance is treated with extended field radiation fields encompassing the para-aortic and pelvic lymph nodes as previously described in the "Adjuvant radiation" section. The dose of radiation at the PMH is 25 Gy in 20 fractions to para-aortic and pelvic lymph nodes, whereas gross recurrent disease is concomitantly boosted to an additional 10 Gy for a total of 35 Gy. This treatment regimen is one of many, although it is preferred at PMH because it is associated with less acute radiation-induced nausea and may allow for better tumor control compared with other fractionation schedules (**Table 6**).

An anatomic variation, such as horseshoe kidneys or disease that overlies a large portion of kidney or liver, may cause significant toxicity to normal organs if treated with radiotherapy. In these scenarios, chemotherapy is usually preferred over radiotherapy.

SUMMARY

Over the past 30 years, testicular seminoma has become a model for a curable malignancy with long-term survival of nearly 100% regardless of management strategy chosen following orchidectomy. In fact, approximately 80% to 85% of all patients with stage I seminoma are cured with an inguinal orchidectomy alone. Surveillance is increasingly becoming the management option of choice as the awareness of the associated long-term risks of adjuvant treatments increases. The Canadian Germ Cell Cancer Consensus Group, Société International d'Urologie, and the European Society of Medical Oncology have all published guidelines with surveillance as the primary management option in men diagnosed with stage I testicular seminoma.[66–68]

Despite excellent survival rates, there remains much work to improve the care for seminoma survivors. Current research efforts are focused on maintaining excellent cure rates while minimizing the long-term toxicities of treatments or surveillance. Clinical risk factors are not sufficient predictors for relapse and current research initiatives are concentrating on identifying molecular markers. If successful, future risk-adapted management approaches may incorporate both clinical and molecular markers to more accurately identify patients at risk of relapse. Optimal surveillance follow-up strategies to minimize radiation exposure during screening have yet to be determined. These strategies may include decreasing the number of CT scans over the course of follow-up or identifying alternatives to conventional CT scans, such as low-dose CTs or MRI scans.

REFERENCES

1. Manecksha R, Fitzpatrick J. Epidemiology of testicular cancer. BJU Int 2009; 104(9):1329–33.
2. Sokoloff M, Joyce G, Wise M. Testis cancer. J Urol 2007;177(6):2030–41.
3. Shah M, Devessa S, Zhu K, et al. Trends in testicular germ cell tumours by ethnic group in the United States. Int J Androl 2007;30(4):206–13.
4. Jemal A, Siegel R, Xu J, et al. Cancer statistics, 2010. CA Cancer J Clin 2010; 60(5):277–300.
5. Warde P, Sturgeon J, Gospodarowicz M. Testicular cancer. In: Gunderson L, Tepper J, editors. Clinical radiation oncology. Philadelphia: Churchill Livingstone; 2000. p. 844–62.
6. Oliver R, Boubilkova L, Ong J. Fifteen-year follow-up of Anglian Germ Cell Cancer group adjuvant studies of carboplatin as an alternative to radiation or surveillance for stage I seminoma. Proc Am Sc Clin Oncol 2001;20:780.
7. Warde P, Chung P, Sturgeon J, et al. Should surveillance be considered the standard of care in stage I seminoma? J Clin Oncol (Meeting abstracts) 2005;23(16): 4520.
8. Daugaard G, Petersen P, Rorth M. Surveillance in stage I testicular cancer. APMIS 2003;111(1):76–85.
9. Germa-Lluch J, Garcia del Muro X, Maroto P, et al. Clinical pattern and therapeutic results achieved in 1490 patients with germ-cell tumors of the testis: the experience of the Spanish Germ-Cell Cancer Group (GG). Eur Urol 2002;42(6): 553–62.
10. Horwich A, Alsanjari N, A'Hern R, et al. Surveillance following orchidectomy for stage I testicular seminoma. Br J Cancer 1992;65(5):775–8.
11. Ramakrishnan S, Champion A, Dorreen M, et al. Stage I seminoma of the testis: Is post-orchiectomy surveillance a safe alternative to routine postoperative radiotherapy? Clin Oncol (R Coll Radiol) 1992;4(5):284–6.
12. von der Maase H, Specht L, Jacobsen G, et al. Surveillance following orchidectomy for stage I seminoma of the testis. Eur J Cancer 1993;29A(14):1931–4.

13. Kamba T, Kamoto T, Okubo K, et al. Outcome of different post-orchiectomy management for stage I seminoma: Japanese multi-institutional study including 425 patients. Int J Urol 2010;17:980–8.
14. Yoshida T, Kakimoto K, Takezawa K, et al. Surveillance following orchiectomy for stage I testicular seminoma: long-term outcome. Int J Urol 2009;16:756–9.
15. Chung P, Parker C, Panzarella T, et al. Surveillance in stage I testicular seminoma - risk of late relapse. Can J Urol 2002;9(5):1637–40.
16. Leung E, Warde P, Panzarella T, et al. Total treatment burden in stage 1 seminoma patients. J Clin Oncol 2010;28(Suppl 15):A4534.
17. Warde P, Gospodarowicz M, Banarjee D, et al. Prognostic factors for relapse in stage I testicular seminoma treated with surveillance. J Urol 1997;157(5):1705–10.
18. Warde P, Specht L, Horwich A, et al. Prognostic factors for relapse in stage I seminoma managed by surveillance: a pooled analysis. J Clin Oncol 2002; 20(22):4448–52.
19. Chung P, Daugaard G, Tyldesley S, et al. Prognostic factors for relapse in stage I seminoma managed with surveillance: a validation study. J Clin Oncol 2010; 28(Suppl 15):A4535.
20. Aparicio J, Germa J, Del Muro X, et al. Risk-adapted management for patients with clinical stage I seminoma: the second Spanish Germ Cell Cancer Cooperative Group study. J Clin Oncol 2005;23(34):8717–23.
21. Martin J, Panzarella T, Zwahlen D, et al. Evidence-based guidelines for following stage I seminoma. Cancer Res 2007;109(11):2248–56.
22. Krege S, Beyer J, Souchon R, et al. European consensus conference on diagnosis and treatment of germ cell cancer: a report of the second meeting of the European Germ Cell Cancer Consensus Group (EGCCCG): part I. Eur Urol 2008;53(3):478–96.
23. Krege S, Beyer J, Souchon R, et al. European consensus conference on diagnosis and treatment of germ cell cancer: a report of the second meeting of the European Germ Cell Cancer Consensus Group (EGCCCG): part II. Eur Urol 2008;53(3):496–513.
24. The NCCN Clinical Practice Guidelins in Oncology (NCCN GuidelinesTM) Testicular Cancer (Version 1.2010). 2010 National Comprehensive Cancer Network, Inc. Available at: www.NCCN.org. Accessed March 14, 2011.
25. Schrimpton P, Hillier M, Lewis M, et al. National survey of doses from CT in the UK: 2003. Br J Radiol 2006;79:968–80.
26. Mettler F, Huda W, Yoshizumi T, et al. Effective doses in radiology and diagnostic nuclear medicine: a catalog. Radiology 2008;248:254–63.
27. Brenner D, Hall EJ. Computed tomography - an increasing sourve of radiation exposure. N Engl J Med 2007;357(22):2277–84.
28. Berrington de Gonzalez A, Darby S. Risk of cancer from diagnostic X-rays: estimates for the UK and 14 other countries. Lancet 2004;363:345–51.
29. Tarin T, Sonn G, Shinghal R. Estimating the risk of cancer associated with imaging related radiation during surveillance for stage I testicular cancer using computerized tomography. J Urol 2009;181:627–33.
30. Health risks from exposure to low levels of ionizing radiation: BEIR VII, phase 2. Washington, DC: National Academies; 2006.
31. O'Malley M, Chung P, Haider M, et al. Comparison of low dose with standard dose abdominal/pelvic multidetector CT in patients with stage I testicular cancer under surveillance. Eur Radiol 2010;20:1624–30.
32. Narayanan P, Iyngkaran T, Sohaib A, et al. Pearls and pitfalls of MR lymphography in gynecologic malignancy. Radiographics 2009;29(4):1057–69.

33. Desemo W, Debats O, Rozema T, et al. Comparison of nodal risk formula and MR lymphography for predicting lymph node involvement in prostate cancer. Int J Radiat Oncol Biol Phys 2010. [Epub ahead of print].
34. Heesakkers R, Jager G, Hovels A, et al. Prostate cancer: detection of lymph node metastases outside the routine surgical area with ferumoxtran-10-enhanced MR imaging. Radiology 2009;251(2):408–14.
35. Bayens Y, Helle P, Van Putten W, et al. Orchidectomy followed by radiotherapy in 176 stage I and II testicular seminoma patients: benefits of a 10-year follow-up study. Radiother Oncol 1992;25(2):97–102.
36. Coleman J, Coleman R, Turner A, et al. The management and clinical course of testicular seminoma: 15 years' experience at a single institution. Clin Oncol 1998;10(4):237–41.
37. Fossa S, Horwich A, Russell J, et al. Optimal planning target volume for stage I testicular seminoma: a Medical Research Council randomized trial. Medical Research Council Testicular Tumor Working Group. J Clin Oncol 1999;17(4):1146–54.
38. Santoni R, Barbera F, Bertoni F, et al. Stage I seminoma of the testis: a bi-institutional retrospective analysis of patients treated with radiation therapy only. BJU Int 2003;92(1):47–52.
39. Hultenschmidt B, Budach V, Genters K, et al. Results of radiotherapy for 230 patients with stage I-II seminomas. Strahlenther Onkol 1996;172(4):186–92.
40. Classen J, Schmidberger J, Meisner C, et al. Para-aortic irradiation for stage I testicular seminoma: results of a prospective study in 675 patients. A trial of the German cancer study group (GTCSG). Br J Cancer 2004;90(12):2305–11.
41. Logue J, Harris M, Livsey J, et al. Short course para-aortic radiation for stage I seminoma of the testis. Int J Radiat Oncol Biol Phys 2003;57(5):1304–9.
42. Jones W, Fossa S, Mead G, et al. Randomized trial of 30 versus 20 Gy in the adjuvant treatment of stage I testicular seminoma: a report on Medical Research Council Trial TE18, European Organization for the Research and Treatment of Cancer Trial 20942 (ISRCTN18525328). J Clin Oncol 2005;23(6):1200–8.
43. Mead G, Fossa S, Oliver R, et al. Relapse patterns in 2, 466 stage 1 seminoma patients entered into Medical Research Council randomised trials. J Clin Oncol 2008;26:A5020.
44. Zagars G, Ballo M, Lee A, et al. Mortality after cure of testicular seminoma. J Clin Oncol 2004;22(4):640–7.
45. Huddart R, Norman A, Shahidi M, et al. Cardiovascular disease as a long-term complication of treatment for testicular cancer. J Clin Oncol 2003;21(8):1513–23.
46. Haugnes H, Wethal T, Aass ND, et al. Cardiovascular risk factors and morbidity in long-term survivors of testicular cancer: a 20-year follow-up study. J Clin Oncol 2010;29:4649–57.
47. Wethal T, Kjekshus J, Roislien J, et al. Treatment-related differences in cardiovascular risk factors in long-term survivors of testicular cancer. J Cancer Surviv 2007; 1(1):8–16.
48. Jacobsen K, Olsen D, Fossa K, et al. External beam abdominal radiotherapy in patients with seminoma stage I: field type, testicular dose, and spermatogenesis. Int J Radiat Oncol Biol Phys 1997;38(1):95–102.
49. Bieri S, Rouzaud M, Miralbell R. Seminoma of the testis: is scrotal shielding necessary when radiotherapy is limited to the para-aortic nodes? Radiother Oncol 1999;50:349–53.
50. Travis L, Fossa S, Schonfeld S, et al. Second cancers among 40576 testicular cancer patients: focus on long-term survivors. J Natl Cancer Inst 2005;97(18): 1354–65.

51. van den Belt-Dusebout A, de Wit R, Gietema J, et al. Treatment-specific risks of second malignancies and cardiovascular disease in 5-year survivors of testicular cancer. J Clin Oncol 2007;25(28):4370–8.

52. Zwahlen D, Martin J, Millar J, et al. Effect of radiotherapy volume and dose on secondary cancer risk in stage I testicular seminoma. Int J Radiat Oncol Biol Phys 2008;70(3):853–8.

53. Sculier J, Paesmans M, Thiriaux J, et al. A comparison of methods of calculation for estimating carboplatin AUC with a retrospective pharmacokinetic-pharmacodynamic analysis in patients with advanced non-small cell lung cancer. Eur J Cancer 1999; 35(9):1314–9.

54. Oliver R, Edmonds PO, Ong JY, et al. Pilot studies of 2 and 1 course carboplatin as adjuvant for stage I seminoma: should it be tested in a randomized trial against radiotherapy? Int J Radiat Oncol Biol Phys 1994;29(1):3–8.

55. Oliver R, Mason M, Mead G, et al. Radiotherapy versus single-dose carboplatin in adjuvant treatment of stage I seminoma: a randomised trial. Lancet 2005; 366(9482):293–300.

56. Dieckmann K, Bruggeboes B, Pichlmeier U, et al. Adjuvant treatment of clinical stage I seminoma: is a single course of carboplatin sufficient? Urology 2000; 55(1):102–6.

57. Krege S, Kalund G, Otto T, et al. Phase II study: adjuvant single-agent carboplatin therapy for clinical stage I seminoma. Eur Urol 1997;31(4):405–7.

58. Aparicio J, Garcia del Muro X, Maroto P, et al. Multicenter study evaluating a dual policy of postorchidectomy surveillance and selective adjuvant single-agent carboplatin for patients with clinical stage I seminoma. Ann Oncol 2003;14(6): 867–72.

59. Agirovic D. Germ cell testicular tumors in clinical stage A and normal values of serum tumor markers post-orchiectomy: the experience in the management of 300 consecutive patients. J BUON 2005;10(2):195–200.

60. Oliver R, Mead G, Fogarty P, et al. Radiotherapy versus carboplatin for stage I seminoma: updated analysis of the MRC/EORTC randomized trial. J Clin Oncol 2008;26:A1.

61. Pliarchpoulou K, Pectasides D. Late complications of chemotherapy in testicular cancer. Cancer Treat Rev 2010;36:262–7.

62. Gietema J, Meinardi M, Messerschmidt J, et al. Circulating plasma platinum more than 10 years after cisplatinum treatment for testicular cancer. Lancet 2000; 355(9209):1075–6.

63. Brouwers E, Huitema A, Beijnen J, et al. Long-term platinum retention after treatment with cisplatin and oxaliplatin. BMC Clin Pharmacol 2008;8:7.

64. Gerl A, Schierl R. Urinary excretion of platinum in chemotherapy-treated long-term survivors of testicular cancer. Acta Oncol 2000;39(4):519–22.

65. Powles T, Robinson D, Shamash J, et al. The long-term risks of adjuvant carboplatin treatment for stage I seminoma of the testis. Ann Oncol 2008;19:443–7.

66. Schmoll H, Jordan K, Huddart R, et al. Testicular seminoma: ESMO clinical recommendations for diagnosis, treatment and follow-up. Ann Oncol 2009; 20(Suppl 4):iv83–8.

67. Warde P, Huddart R, Bolton D, et al. Consensus guidelines for the management of localised seminoma, stage I/II. Shanghai (China): International Consultation on Urologic Diseases; 2009. International Consultation on Urologic Diseases.

68. Wood L, Kollmannsberger C, Jewett M, et al. Canadian consensus guidelines for the management of testicular germ cell cancer. Can Urol Assoc J 2010;4(2): e19–38.

Stage I Nonseminomatous Germ Cell Tumor of the Testis: More Questions than Answers?

Thomas Powles, MRCP, MD

KEYWORDS

- Nonseminomatous germ cell cancer • Surveillance
- Adjuvant therapy

An increasing proportion of patients with germ cell tumors are presenting with stage I disease.[1] This trend may be partly because of increased awareness among young men. Stage I seminoma occurs more frequently than nonseminoma; however, the unifying factor for both conditions is the excellent outcome after orchiectomy irrespective of subsequent treatments. For example, in a recent study with 740 patients with stage I nonseminomatous germ cell tumors (NSGCTs) showed no NSGCT-related deaths.[2] This finding underlines the challenging nature of prospective randomized studies in this rare disease, because current standard treatment results in disease-specific survival of nearly 100%.

The treatment options after orchiectomy include adjuvant chemotherapy, retroperitoneal lymph node dissection (RPLND), and surveillance. These options have all become accepted standards of care, based predominantly on numerous single-arm descriptive studies (**Tables 1–3**). The lack of randomized data favoring one treatment has resulted in standard treatment pathways differing among institutions and countries, with Europe leaning toward surveillance and adjuvant chemotherapy and North America recommending surveillance or RPLND.[3–8]

Most patients with stage I NSGCTs will not experience relapse after orchiectomy. Therefore, adjuvant treatment in most individuals is without benefit and potentially harmful,[8–10] making a stratified approach to treatment based on the identification of risk factors associated with relapse an attractive prospect.[2,4,7] The two factors that are most consistently associated with relapse include lymphovascular invasion and

St Bartholomew's Hospital, Barts and The London NHS Trust, Charterhouse Square, London EC1A7BE, UK
E-mail address: Thomas.Powles@bartsandthelondon.nhs.uk

Hematol Oncol Clin N Am 25 (2011) 517–527
doi:10.1016/j.hoc.2011.03.013
0889-8588/11/$ – see front matter © 2011 Published by Elsevier Inc.

hemonc.theclinics.com

Table 1
Summary of studies investigating RPLND in stage I NSGCTs

Study (y)	Number of Patients	Stage II at Pathology	Relapse Rate for Pathology Stage I[a]	Relapse Rate for Pathology Stage II[a]	Overall Survival
Donohue et al,[31] 1993	379	112 (30%)	12%	34%	99%
Hermans et al,[14] 2000	292	66 (32%)	10%	23%	NA
Albers et al,[11] 2003	182	62 (28%)	18%	25%	NA
Nicolai et al,[15] 2004	322	60 (19%)	NA	NA	99%
Stephenson et al,[18] 2005	309	91 (30%)	7%	34%	99%

[a] This includes only those patients who did not go on to receive post-RPLND adjuvant chemotherapy.

of embryonal carcinoma at histology.[4,8,11–20] However, even with this knowledge, a group with a greater than 50% risk of relapse is difficult to identify.

Finally, this article addresses survivorship issues associated with stage I NSGCT. Given that cure rates approach 100%, decisions about treatment must take short- and long-term toxicity into account. Surgery and chemotherapy both have established short-and long-term risks, which range from bowel obstruction and loss of antegrade ejaculation after RPLND to the development of cardiovascular disease and second cancers after chemotherapy.[7,21–26] These factors militate in favor of surveillance. However, even the surveillance group is exposed to risk, particularly from the radiation exposure associated with repeated cross-sectional imaging, which can occur up to 12 times over a 5-year period.[2,8,27]

CLINICAL STAGE I DISEASE

Clinical stage I disease is defined as no evidence of disease on CT of the chest, abdomen, and pelvis and normal serum tumor markers (α-fetoprotein [AFP], human chorionic gonadotropin [HCG], and lactate dehydrogenase [LDH]). Patients with persistently elevated makers after orchiectomy are considered to have metastatic disease, and chemotherapy is recommended.[4,28] The results for RPLND in patients with elevated serum tumor markers have been disappointing because relapses outside of the surgical field have been frequent.[4,29]

Table 2
Surveillance for patients with stage I NSGCT

Study (y)	Number of Patients	Years of Follow-Up	Relapse Rate	Overall Survival[a]
Read et al,[9] 1992	373	5	100 (27%)	98%
Colls et al,[10] 1999	248	4.5	70 (28%)	98%
Francis et al,[71] 2000	183	5	52 (28%)	99%
Daugaard et al,[72] 2003	349	5	86 (29%)	100%
Ernst et al,[73] 2005	194	4.5	57 (29%)	100%
Oliver et al,[5] 2004	234	3.0	71 (30%)	98%
Sturgeon et al,[8] 2011	371	6.3	104 (28%)	99%

[a] At the time of publication.

Table 3						
Summary of studies investigating adjuvant chemotherapy in high-risk stage I NSGCT						
Study (y)	Number	Chemotherapy Regimen	Number of Cycles	Years of Follow-Up	Relapses	Testis Cancer Deaths
Cullen et al,[7] 1996	116	BEP	2	4	2 (2%)	2%
Oliver et al,[5] 2004	28	BEP	2	3	1 (4%)	4%
Chevreau et al,[74] 2004	40	BEP	2	10	0 (0%)	0%
Pont et al,[75] 1996	42	BEP	2	6	2 (5%)	3%
Tanstad et al,[2] 2009	157	BEP	1	5	5 (3%)	0%
Oliver et al,[5] 2004	47	BEP	1	3	3 (7%)	0%
Klepp et al,[76] 2003	57	PVB	2	3	1 (2%)	0%
Dearnley et al,[56] 2005	115	BOP	2	6	2 (2%)	1%

Abbreviations: B, bleomycin; E, etoposide; O, vincristine; P, cisplatin; V, vinblastine.

The retroperitoneal lymph nodes are the commonest site (>70%) of metastatic spread in NSGCTs. Lymph nodes larger than 1 cm are considered abnormal. However, borderline lymph nodes 8 to 10 mm in the primary landing zones may be worthy of more frequent investigation or intervention.[24,30] These primary landing zones include the paracaval, precaval, interaortocaval and preaortic nodes for right-sided tumors, and the para-aortic, preaortic, and interaortocaval nodes for left-sided tumors.[31]

Understaging of the retroperitoneum with CT occurs in 25% to 30% of patients, even with modern scanners. 18-Fluoroudeoxyglucose–positron emission tomography (FDG-PET)/CT has not helped further characterize these nodes and cannot be recommended in the routine staging for this disease.[32] RPLND gives more accurate data than CT scanning regarding retroperitoneal involvement. However, RPLND is associated with morbidity and is not considered necessary to complete staging.

PROGNOSTIC FACTORS FOR STAGE I NSGCT

During the 1980s, an investigation of more than 250 patients with stage I NSGCT showed several histologic factors that predisposed to relapse, including tumor invasion of testicular veins, lymphatic invasion by the tumor, absence of yolk sac elements, and the presence of embryonal cell carcinoma within the cancer. The absence of any of these factors resulted in a 100% 3-year relapse-free survival, whereas the presence of three or four factors was associated with a 58% relapse rate over the same period.[33] These data were successfully externally validated in a larger cohort.[9]

Subsequent investigators simplified the prognostic index through combining the presence of venous and lymphatic invasion as only one prognostic factor. This factor, along with the proportion of the tumor that consisted of embryonal carcinoma, became the most important factors over the next 2 decades.[8,12–18] However, positive predictive values for relapse in high-risk groups remain less than 70%.[11]

A more recent retrospective analysis of 23 publications between 1979 and 2001 investigated prognostic factors in more than 2500 patients with stage I NSCGT.[20] Lymphovascular invasion remained the most significant prognostic factor (odds ratio [OR], 5.2; 95% CI, 4.0–6.8). Other factors, such as the presence of embryonal carcinoma in the primary tumor (OR, 2.9; 95% CI, 2.0–4.4) and a high pathologic stage of the tumor (OR, 2.6; 95% CI, 1.8–3.8), were also of significance.

Other makers such as MIB-1, p53, bcl-2, cathepsin D, and E-cadherin have been investigated in this setting with mixed results, although they have not been established in routine use.[8,13,20,34–37]

RPLND FOR STAGE I NSGCT

Except for choriocarcinoma, NSGCTs follow a predictable pattern of metastasis. The landing zones within the retroperitoneum are the most commonly affected sites. RPLND not only accurately differentiates between stage I and II disease but also significantly reduces the probability of systemic relapse. Relapse within the retroperitoneal field after RPLND occurs in fewer than 1% of patients at centers of excellence, and overall survival is roughly 99% at 5 years.[4,11,14,15,38] This approach appears safe and successful, with relatively few long-term side effects (retrograde ejaculation being the notable exception). RPLND also has the potential advantage of removal of chemotherapy-resistant teratoma, which is present in 30% of patients with stage II disease. Surgical removal of teratoma is required because it can undergo malignant transformation or become inoperable.[39,40] The absence of teratoma in the primary tumor does not equate with absence in the retroperitoneal lymph nodes, making who is most likely to benefit from surgery difficult to predict.[41,42] A major downside to RPLND is that relapse can occur outside the retroperitoneum in approximately 5% to 10% of patients with pathologic stage I disease.[43]

RPLND for clinical stage I disease is safe with relatively few long-term side effects. Series published from Indiana University and Cleveland Clinic reported no perioperative deaths or permanent disability. Major complications were reported in only 2% to 3% of patients.[25,44] The most significant long-term side effect with RPLND is the loss of antegrade ejaculation, which occurs in fewer than 5% of patients whose surgery is performed by a highly experienced surgeon. Other complications, which occur in approximately 1% of patients, include small bowel obstruction, wound infections, or lymphocele. It has been speculated that these excellent results are partly from the experience of the centers and the high volume of surgery, because most series have been reported by high-volume centers.[45,46] These results seem to not be reproducible in the community setting.[43]

Randomized prospective data from the German group compares one cycle of bleomycin, etoposide, platinum (BEP) with RPLND for treating clinical stage I disease.[43] Both cancer centers and community-based hospitals participated, and 61 centers accrued a total of 382 subjects. The results showed that after a median follow-up of more than 4 years, none of the patients had died of germ cell tumors. However, 15 patients had experienced recurrence (2 in the chemotherapy arm vs 13 in the RPLND arm; P<.005). The 13 recurrences in the RPLND arm were observed within 17 months of therapy, with 5 (3%) of these relapses occurring in the RPLND field.

A modified ipsilateral nerve-sparing RPLND was allowed in this study, which may account for the relatively high relapse rate within the retroperitoneum (3%). It is also of note that such a low relapse rate was achieved with a single cycle of BEP chemotherapy, which is not generally considered chemotherapy standard of care.[3,47] Overall, this study confirmed that chemotherapy results in a lower relapse rate than RPLND and supported the position that RPLND is best performed in specialist centers rather than in community hospitals.[48]

SURVEILLANCE FOR STAGE I NSGCT

Surveillance after orchiectomy is an attractive option, particularly in the absence of high-risk features, when the chances of relapse are less than 20% (see **Table 2**).[2,5,8,49,50]

It is also an option in the high-risk setting because only approximately 50% of these patients relapse.[8,16,50] Overall survival for surveillance is indistinguishable from the results seen with adjuvant treatments (98%–100%), resulting in some institutions pursuing a surveillance program for all patients with stage I NSGCT. When relapses occur, they do so in predicable anatomic locations and mostly within 2 years of orchiectomy (median time to relapse, 7 months). Late relapses in patients with stage I NSGCT undergoing surveillance are uncommon, occurring in 0% to 3% of men.[9,17,51–54] Serum tumor markers are frequently elevated in patients with metastatic NSGCT, facilitating the detection of relapse and reducing the dependence on imaging studies. Together these factors make surveillance an attractive option for potentially all patients.

Cross-sectional imaging with CT identifies 48% to 53% of relapses, whereas raised serum tumor makers are responsible for indentifying 29% to 39% of relapses in these patients.[2,49] Therefore, guidelines regarding the follow-up of these patients tend to focus on frequent cross-sectional imaging over the first 2 years.[3] Subsequent imaging between years 2 and 5 varies depending on the treatment center. Serum tumor makers are measured regularly during this period. Guidance for follow-up varies a great deal depending on the individual institution and required clarification. Some recommend cross-sectional imaging every 3 to 6 months for up to 5 years, whereas others reduce the frequency of imaging and stop this follow-up much sooner.[2,5,8,49] A prospective study compared two and five CT scans over the first 2 years of follow-up after orchiectomy.[49] The results showed that a less-frequent imaging protocol did not predispose to an increased risk of relapse with more advanced disease. In view of the risk associated with radiation exposure, it seems wise to follow the guidance of this study to perform fewer scans.

The main concern with surveillance is the comparatively high risk of relapse, especially in high-risk patients. Waiting until relapse also results in a significant proportion of patients requiring RPLND after chemotherapy, because many patients do not experience a radiologic complete remission with chemotherapy for metastatic disease.[5,45,55] Teratoma (40%) and viable tumor (10%) are frequently seen at surgery in this setting.[41]

Overall surveillance seems safe and very attractive, provided that patients comply with follow-up and cross-sectional imaging protocols. The lack of randomized data in this area should not discourage clinicians from pursuing this approach, especially in patients with low-risk disease. Recent data suggest that a less-frequent cross-sectional imaging may not have a detrimental effect on relapse.

ADJUVANT CHEMOTHERAPY FOR STAGE I NSGCT

The success of cisplatin-based combination chemotherapy in metastatic germ cell tumors prompted the testis cancer community to investigate these drugs in the adjuvant setting in high-risk stage I NSGCT (see **Table 3**).[6] **Table 3** shows that several different regimens have been used in selected patients (usually in a high-risk subgroup). Inconsistency exists on the number of cycles of chemotherapy administered and regimens used. Three studies require particular attention, the first of which describes two cycles of adjuvant BEP chemotherapy, which is still considered the gold standard regimen.[7] In this Medical Research Council study, 116 high-risk patients (>50% chance of relapse) with stage I NSGCT were given two 21-day cycles of cisplatin, 20 mg/m^2/d for 5 days; bleomycin, 30 mg weekly (3 doses); and etoposide, 120 mg/m^2/d for 3 days (modified BEP). After 4 years of follow-up, only two patients had experienced relapse. Although the short-term toxicity was low, the longer-term toxicity remains uncertain and concerning.[5,22,23,56–58] Two cycles of standard BEP became the standard adjuvant chemotherapy regimen based on these results.

Other investigators have reduced the number of cycles of BEP to one.[2,43] This practice has the theoretical benefit of reduced toxicity; however, there is no direct comparison in terms of efficacy between one and two cycles, and it would seem unlikely that two versus one cycle will have a major impact on long-term toxicity. The largest study to report on one cycle of BEP includes a high-risk group (presence of lymphovascular invasion).[2] Results are comparable with two cycles of BEP.[7] Once again, follow-up was short, and long-term follow-up data are lacking. With relapse-free survival rates at approximately 95% for both regimens, a randomized study in this setting seems unrealistic because the number of patients required to prove noninferiority would be huge.

The final study investigates two cycles of cisplatin and bleomycin with vincristine instead of etoposide (BOP).[56] Etoposide is seen as a potentially unattractive agent in the adjuvant setting because it is associated with alopecia, myelosuppression, and, like cisplatin, the development of leukemia.[59,60] Indirect comparisons suggested the results for BOP were comparable with two cycles of BEP in terms of efficacy; however, high levels of neuropathy were seen with BOP, and the investigators concluded that BOP has no advantages over BEP. Concerns have been expressed that adjuvant therapy may delay time to relapse, extending the follow-up period; however, this does not seem to be the case.[61,62]

Overall, these phase II studies show that cisplatin-based chemotherapy reduces the risk of relapse in a high-risk population from approximately 50% to less than 10% (<5% in most series). This finding is attractive, but without accurate long-term follow-up data addressing the risk of late toxicity, chemotherapy cannot be recommended as standard of care for unselected patients, particularly in light of the documented increased risk of cardiovascular disease, fertility issues, neurologic toxicity, metabolic syndromes, and second cancers associated with longer courses of chemotherapy for testis cancer.[22,23,58,63-69]

A STRATIFIED APPROACH TO THE MANAGEMENT OF STAGE I NSGCT

Although adjuvant strategies in stage I NSGCT reduce the risk of relapse, no randomized data show improved outcomes compared with surveillance. Both adjuvant approaches are associated with risk; therefore, caution must be used before these treatments are administered to an unselected population. After all, because only a minority of the population will experience relapse, treating the whole population will result in most patients receiving treatment unnecessarily. Although the prognostic factors are far from perfect, they are able to identify patients with a poor outcome.[8]

A prospective study using a stratified design investigated adjuvant chemotherapy (BEP × 1) in a high-risk population (the presence of lymphovascular invasion).[2] Patients who were not deemed high-risk were allowed to choose between surveillance and adjuvant BEP. Surveillance in the low-risk group (n = 338) resulted in a 11.5% relapse at 6 years, whereas one cycle of BEP was associated with a 3.5% risk of relapse in the high-risk group. None of the patients died of testis cancer. This approach has merit because the overall risk of relapse is less than 10%. Nevertheless, this 10% risk is still significant, and standardized follow-up regimens with CT scans (and the risks associated with them) are required. Therefore, the overall benefit of this approach in a compliant patient remains debatable.

Urologists at the Cleveland Clinic recommend RPLND rather than adjuvant chemotherapy in patients with high-risk stage I NSGCT.[48] They advocate surveillance for patients with low-risk features, and RPLND for those with evidence of lymphovascular invasion or embryonal carcinoma, or with retroperitoneal adenopathy of 5 mm or greater in the primary landing zone.[46]

Because of the debate between adjuvant therapy and surveillance, decision analysis models have been investigated in this setting.[70] The models incorporate cancer outcomes, treatment-related morbidity, and patient preference. The models provide quality-adjusted survival for each treatment option. Overall, the difference in quality-adjusted survival scores for the three treatment groups was low. Moreover, patients were surprisingly tolerant of treatment-related morbidity. Patients preferred surveillance if the risk of relapse was less than approximately one-third. Active treatment was preferred in the remaining patients with a higher risk. The average scores for RPLND and chemotherapy varied significantly, depending on the model used. Overall, these data emphasize the attractive nature of surveillance for a low-risk population. They also underline the ongoing difficulty in choosing between chemotherapy and RPLND as adjuvant therapy.

SUMMARY

All three treatment options for stage I NSGCT have similar survival outcomes (see **Tables 1–3**) and all have a potential role in the management of this disease. Surveillance seems particularly attractive in the low-risk setting. At the other extreme, two cycles of BEP chemotherapy is considered by many to be overtreatment, especially because patients with good-risk metastatic disease according to the International Germ Cell Cancer Collaborative Group require only three cycles of BEP.

Patients should be informed of the treatment options and ultimately be instrumental in the decision-making process. Compliance during follow-up is essential, especially for patients undergoing surveillance. Recent data suggest that less-frequent imaging during follow-up is safe, further reducing risk for these patients.[49]

REFERENCES

1. Powles TB, Bhardwa J, Shamash J, et al. The changing presentation of germ cell tumours of the testis between 1983 and 2002. BJU Int 2005;95(9):1197–200.
2. Tandstad T, Dahl O, Cohn-Cedermark G, et al. Risk-adapted treatment in clinical stage I nonseminomatous germ cell testicular cancer: the SWENOTECA management program. J Clin Oncol 2009;27(13):2122–8.
3. Krege S, Beyer J, Souchon R, et al. European consensus conference on diagnosis and treatment of germ cell cancer: a report of the second meeting of the European Germ Cell Cancer Consensus group (EGCCCG): part I. Eur Urol 2008;53(3):478–96.
4. Stephenson AJ, Bosl GJ, Motzer RJ, et al. Retroperitoneal lymph node dissection for nonseminomatous germ cell testicular cancer: impact of patient selection factors on outcome. J Clin Oncol 2005;23(12):2781–8.
5. Oliver RT, Ong J, Shamash J, et al. Long-term follow-up of Anglian Germ Cell Cancer Group surveillance versus patients with Stage 1 nonseminoma treated with adjuvant chemotherapy. Urology 2004;63(3):556–61.
6. Cullen M, James N. Adjuvant therapy for stage I testicular cancer. Cancer Treat Rev 1996;22(4):253–64.
7. Cullen MH, Stenning SP, Parkinson MC, et al. Short-course adjuvant chemotherapy in high-risk stage I nonseminomatous germ cell tumors of the testis: a Medical Research Council report. J Clin Oncol 1996;14(4):1106–13.
8. Sturgeon JF, Moore MJ, Kakiashvili DM, et al. Non-risk-adapted surveillance in clinical stage I nonseminomatous germ cell tumors: the Princess Margaret Hospital's experience. Eur Urol 2011;59(4):556–62.

9. Read G, Stenning SP, Cullen MH, et al. Medical Research Council prospective study of surveillance for stage I testicular teratoma. Medical Research Council Testicular Tumors Working Party. J Clin Oncol 1992;10(11):1762–8.

10. Colls BM, Harvey VJ, Skelton L, et al. Late results of surveillance of clinical stage I nonseminoma germ cell testicular tumours: 17 years' experience in a national study in New Zealand. BJU Int 1999;83(1):76–82.

11. Albers P, Siener R, Kliesch S, et al. Risk factors for relapse in clinical stage I non-seminomatous testicular germ cell tumors: results of the German Testicular Cancer Study Group Trial. J Clin Oncol 2003;21(8):1505–12.

12. Alexandre J, Fizazi K, Mahe C, et al. Stage I non-seminomatous germ-cell tumours of the testis: identification of a subgroup of patients with a very low risk of relapse. Eur J Cancer 2001;37(5):576–82.

13. Heidenreich A, Sesterhenn IA, Mostofi FK, et al. Prognostic risk factors that identify patients with clinical stage I nonseminomatous germ cell tumors at low risk and high risk for metastasis. Cancer 1998;83(5):1002–11.

14. Hermans BP, Sweeney CJ, Foster RS, et al. Risk of systemic metastases in clinical stage I nonseminoma germ cell testis tumor managed by retroperitoneal lymph node dissection. J Urol 2000;163(6):1721–4.

15. Nicolai N, Miceli R, Artusi R, et al. A simple model for predicting nodal metastasis in patients with clinical stage I nonseminomatous germ cell testicular tumors undergoing retroperitoneal lymph node dissection only. J Urol 2004;171(1):172–6.

16. Roeleveld TA, Horenblas S, Meinhardt W, et al. Surveillance can be the standard of care for stage I nonseminomatous testicular tumors and even high risk patients. J Urol 2001;166(6):2166–70.

17. Sogani PC, Perrotti M, Herr HW, et al. Clinical stage I testis cancer: long-term outcome of patients on surveillance. J Urol 1998;159(3):855–8.

18. Stephenson AJ, Bosl GJ, Bajorin DF, et al. Retroperitoneal lymph node dissection in patients with low stage testicular cancer with embryonal carcinoma predominance and/or lymphovascular invasion. J Urol 2005;174(2):557–60 [discussion: 60].

19. Sweeney CJ, Hermans BP, Heilman DK, et al. Results and outcome of retroperitoneal lymph node dissection for clinical stage I embryonal carcinoma–predominant testis cancer. J Clin Oncol 2000;18(20):358–62.

20. Vergouwe Y, Steyerberg EW, Eijkemans MJ, et al. Predictors of occult metastasis in clinical stage I nonseminoma: a systematic review. J Clin Oncol 2003;21(22):4092–9.

21. Heidenreich A, Albers P, Hartmann M, et al. Complications of primary nerve sparing retroperitoneal lymph node dissection for clinical stage I nonseminomatous germ cell tumors of the testis: experience of the German Testicular Cancer Study Group. J Urol 2003;169(5):1710–4.

22. Fossa SD, Gilbert E, Dores GM, et al. Noncancer causes of death in survivors of testicular cancer. J Natl Cancer Inst 2007;99(7):533–44.

23. Travis LB, Fossa SD, Schonfeld SJ, et al. Second cancers among 40,576 testicular cancer patients: focus on long-term survivors. J Natl Cancer Inst 2005;97(18):1354–65.

24. Stephenson AJ, Sheinfeld J. Management of patients with low-stage nonseminomatous germ cell testicular cancer. Curr Treat Options Oncol 2005;6(5):367–77.

25. Subramanian VS, Nguyen CT, Stephenson AJ, et al. Complications of open primary and post-chemotherapy retroperitoneal lymph node dissection for testicular cancer. Urol Oncol 2010;28(5):504–9.

26. Baniel J, Sella A. Complications of retroperitoneal lymph node dissection in testicular cancer: primary and post-chemotherapy. Semin Surg Oncol 1999;17(4):263–7.

27. Brenner DJ, Hall EJ. Computed tomography–an increasing source of radiation exposure. N Engl J Med 2007;357(22):2277–84.

28. Gilligan TD, Seidenfeld J, Basch EM, et al. American Society of Clinical Oncology Clinical Practice Guideline on uses of serum tumor markers in adult males with germ cell tumors. J Clin Oncol 2010;28(20):3388–404.

29. Davis BE, Herr HW, Fair WR, et al. The management of patients with nonseminomatous germ cell tumors of the testis with serologic disease only after orchiectomy. J Urol 1994;152(1):111–3 [discussion: 114].

30. Leibovitch L, Foster RS, Kopecky KK, et al. Improved accuracy of computerized tomography based clinical staging in low stage nonseminomatous germ cell cancer using size criteria of retroperitoneal lymph nodes. J Urol 1995;154(5):1759–63.

31. Donohue JP, Zachary JM, Maynard BR. Distribution of nodal metastases in nonseminomatous testis cancer. J Urol 1982;128(2):315–20.

32. Oechsle K, Hartmann M, Brenner W, et al. [18F]Fluorodeoxyglucose positron emission tomography in nonseminomatous germ cell tumors after chemotherapy: the German multicenter positron emission tomography study group. J Clin Oncol 2008;26(36):5930–5.

33. Fernandez EB, Colon E, McLeod DG, et al. Efficacy of radiographic chest imaging in patients with testicular cancer. Urology 1994;44(2):243–8 [discussion: 248–9].

34. Spermon JR, Roeleveld TA, van der Poel HG, et al. Comparison of surveillance and retroperitoneal lymph node dissection in stage I nonseminomatous germ cell tumors. Urology 2002;59(6):923–9.

35. Albers P, Miller GA, Orazi A, et al. Immunohistochemical assessment of tumor proliferation and volume of embryonal carcinoma identify patients with clinical stage A nonseminomatous testicular germ cell tumor at low risk for occult metastasis. Cancer 1995;75(3):844–50.

36. Leibovitch I, Foster RS, Kopecky KK, et al. Identification of clinical stage A nonseminomatous testis cancer patients at extremely low risk for metastatic disease: a combined approach using quantitative immunohistochemical, histopathologic, and radiologic assessment. J Clin Oncol 1998;16(1):261–8.

37. Pectasides D, Papaxoinis G, Nikolaou M, et al. Analysis of 7 immunohistochemical markers in male germ cell tumors demonstrates the prognostic significance of p53 and MIB-1. Anticancer Res 2009;29(2):737–44.

38. Donohue JP, Thornhill JA, Foster RS, et al. Retroperitoneal lymphadenectomy for clinical stage A testis cancer (1965 to 1989): modifications of technique and impact on ejaculation. J Urol 1993;149(2):237–43.

39. Motzer RJ, Amsterdam A, Prieto V, et al. Teratoma with malignant transformation: diverse malignant histologies arising in men with germ cell tumors. J Urol 1998;159(1):133–8.

40. Logothetis CJ, Samuels ML, Trindade A, et al. The growing teratoma syndrome. Cancer 1982;50(8):1629–35.

41. Sheinfeld J. Nonseminomatous germ cell tumors of the testis: current concepts and controversies. Urology 1994;44(1):2–14.

42. Vergouwe Y, Steyerberg EW, Foster RS, et al. Validation of a prediction model and its predictors for the histology of residual masses in nonseminomatous testicular cancer. J Urol 2001;165(1):84–8 [discussion: 88].

43. Albers P, Siener R, Krege S, et al. Randomized phase III trial comparing retroperitoneal lymph node dissection with one course of bleomycin and etoposide plus

cisplatin chemotherapy in the adjuvant treatment of clinical stage I nonseminomatous testicular germ cell tumors: AUO trial AH 01/94 by the German Testicular Cancer Study Group. J Clin Oncol 2008;26(18):2966–72.

44. Baniel J, Foster RS, Rowland RG, et al. Complications of primary retroperitoneal lymph node dissection. J Urol 1994;152(2 Pt 1):424–7.

45. de Wit R, Fizazi K. Controversies in the management of clinical stage I testis cancer. J Clin Oncol 2006;24(35):5482–92.

46. Choueiri TK, Stephenson AJ, Gilligan T, et al. Management of clinical stage I nonseminomatous germ cell testicular cancer [abstract]. Urol Clin North Am 2007; 34(2):137–48.

47. Schmoll HJ, Jordan K, Huddart R, et al. Testicular non-seminoma: ESMO Clinical Practice Guidelines for diagnosis, treatment and follow-up. Ann Oncol 2010; 21(Suppl 5):v147–54.

48. Stephenson AJ, Klein EA. Surgical management of low-stage nonseminomatous germ cell testicular cancer. BJU Int 2009;104(9 Pt B):1362–8.

49. Rustin GJ, Mead GM, Stenning SP, et al. Randomized trial of two or five computed tomography scans in the surveillance of patients with stage I nonseminomatous germ cell tumors of the testis: Medical Research Council Trial TE08, ISRCTN56475197–the National Cancer Research Institute Testis Cancer Clinical Studies Group. J Clin Oncol 2007;25(11):1310–5.

50. Kollmannsberger C, Moore C, Chi KN, et al. Non-risk-adapted surveillance for patients with stage I nonseminomatous testicular germ-cell tumors: diminishing treatment-related morbidity while maintaining efficacy. Ann Oncol 2010;21(6): 1296–301.

51. Shahidi M, Norman AR, Dearnaley DP, et al. Late recurrence in 1263 men with testicular germ cell tumors. Multivariate analysis of risk factors and implications for management. Cancer 2002;95(3):520–30.

52. Gels ME, Hoekstra HJ, Sleijfer DT, et al. Detection of recurrence in patients with clinical stage I nonseminomatous testicular germ cell tumors and consequences for further follow-up: a single-center 10-year experience. J Clin Oncol 1995;13(5): 1188–94.

53. Oldenburg J, Fossa SD. Late relapse of nonseminomatous germ cell tumours. BJU Int 2009;104(9 Pt B):1413–7.

54. Oldenburg J, Martin JM, Fossa SD. Late relapses of germ cell malignancies: incidence, management, and prognosis. J Clin Oncol 2006;24(35):5503–11.

55. Stephenson AJ, Bosl GJ, Motzer RJ, et al. Nonrandomized comparison of primary chemotherapy and retroperitoneal lymph node dissection for clinical stage IIA and IIB nonseminomatous germ cell testicular cancer. J Clin Oncol 2007; 25(35):5597–602.

56. Dearnaley DP, Fossa SD, Kaye SB, et al. Adjuvant bleomycin, vincristine and cisplatin (BOP) for high-risk stage I non-seminomatous germ cell tumours: a prospective trial (MRC TE17). Br J Cancer 2005;92(12):2107–13.

57. Kondagunta GV, Sheinfeld J, Mazumdar M, et al. Relapse-free and overall survival in patients with pathologic stage II nonseminomatous germ cell cancer treated with etoposide and cisplatin adjuvant chemotherapy. J Clin Oncol 2004;22(3):464–7.

58. Fossa SD, Oldenburg J, Dahl AA. Short- and long-term morbidity after treatment for testicular cancer. BJU Int 2009;104(9 Pt B):1418–22.

59. Travis LB, Andersson M, Gospodarowicz M, et al. Treatment-associated leukemia following testicular cancer. J Natl Cancer Inst 2000;92(14):1165–71.

60. Travis LB, Holowaty EJ, Ergfeldt KB, et al. Risk of leukemia after platinum-based chemotherapy for ovarian cancer. N Engl J Med 1999;340:351–7.
61. Westermann DH, Schefer H, Thalmann GN, et al. Long-term followup results of 1 cycle of adjuvant bleomycin, etoposide and cisplatin chemotherapy for high risk clinical stage I nonseminomatous germ cell tumors of the testis. J Urol 2008;179(1):163–6.
62. Gilbert DC, Norman AR, Nicholl J, et al. Treating stage I nonseminomatous germ cell tumours with a single cycle of chemotherapy. BJU Int 2006;98(1):67–9.
63. Kollmannsberger C, Kuzcyk M, Mayer F, et al. Late toxicity following curative treatment of testicular cancer. Semin Surg Oncol 1999;17(4):275–81.
64. van den Belt-Dusebout AW, de Wit R, Gietema JA, et al. Treatment-specific risks of second malignancies and cardiovascular disease in 5-year survivors of testicular cancer. J Clin Oncol 2007;25(28):4370–8.
65. van den Belt-Dusebout AW, Nuver J, de Wit R, et al. Long-term risk of cardiovascular disease in 5-year survivors of testicular cancer. J Clin Oncol 2006;24(3):467–75.
66. Huddart RA, Norman A, Moynihan C, et al. Fertility, gonadal and sexual function in survivors of testicular cancer. Br J Cancer 2005;93(2):200–7.
67. Glendenning JL, Barbachano Y, Norman AR, et al. Long-term neurologic and peripheral vascular toxicity after chemotherapy treatment of testicular cancer. Cancer 2010;116(10):2322–31.
68. Huddart RA, Norman A, Shahidi M, et al. Cardiovascular disease as a long-term complication of treatment for testicular cancer. J Clin Oncol 2003;21(8):1513–23.
69. Wethal T, Kjekshus J, Roislien J, et al. Treatment-related differences in cardiovascular risk factors in long-term survivors of testicular cancer. J Cancer Surviv 2007;1(1):8–16.
70. Nguyen CT, Fu AZ, Gilligan TD, et al. Defining the optimal treatment for clinical stage I nonseminomatous germ cell testicular cancer using decision analysis. J Clin Oncol 2010;28(1):119–25.
71. Francis R, Bower M, Brunstrom G, et al. Surveillance for stage I testicular germ cell tumours: management of stage I testis cancer. Eur J Cancer 2000;36:1925–32.
72. Daugaard G, Petersen PM, Rorth M. Surveillance in stage I testicular cancer. APMIS 2003;111:76–83.
73. Ernst DS, Brasher P, Venner PM, et al. Compliance and outcome of patients with stage 1 non-seminomatous germ cell tumors (NSGCT) managed with surveillance programs in seven Canadian centres. Can J Urol 2005;12:2575–80.
74. Chevreau C, Mazerolles C, Soulie M, et al. Long-term efficacy of two cycles of BEP regimen in high-risk stage I nonseminomatous testicular germ cell tumors with embryonal carcinoma and/or vascular invasion. Eur Urol 2004;46:209–14.
75. Pont J, Albrecht W, Postner G, et al. Adjuvantchemotherapy for high-risk clinical stage I nonseminomatoustesticular germ cell cancer: long-term results of a prospective trial. J Clin Oncol 1996;14:441–8.
76. Klepp O, Dahl O, Cavallin-Stahl E, et al. Risk-adapted, brief adjuvant chemotherapy in clinical stage 1 (CS1) nonseminomatous germ cell testicular cancer (NSGCT). Proc Am Soc Clin Oncol 2003;22:399 [abstract: 1604].

Stage II Seminomas and Nonseminomas

Peter W.M. Chung, MBChB, FRCPC[a,b,*], Philippe Bedard, MD, FRCPC[c,d]

KEYWORDS

- Seminoma • Nonseminoma • Stage II • Chemotherapy
- Radiation therapy

In 2008, there were more than 52,000 new patients and 9000 deaths from testicular cancer worldwide.[1] The incidence continues to increase in most populations across the world but this seems to be confined mostly to the populations of European ancestry.[2] The incidence of seminoma is slightly higher than that of nonseminoma, and overall about 15% to 20% of patients present with evidence of infradiaphragmatic retroperitoneal lymphadenopathy.

Evaluation of the patient should include scrotal examination and ultrasonography to image the testis; determination of the serum tumor markers (α-fetoprotein [AFP], human chorionic gonadotropin [hCG], and lactate dehydrogenase [LDH]); and computed tomography (CT) scan of the thorax, abdomen, and pelvis. The role of other imaging modalities, such as magnetic resonance imaging and positron emission tomography (PET), for routine initial assessment is yet to be established. Tumor markers should be measured before radical inguinal orchiectomy. Occasionally, testis-sparing surgery may be performed in suitable patients. Patients with abnormal preoperative serum tumor markers should have these repeated postoperatively to aid in stage categorization. An elevated serum AFP level is considered to be associated with nonseminoma regardless of the primary pathology unless an alternative non–germ cell explanation is likely, and such patients should be managed as having a nonseminoma.

The TNM classification system should be used for staging and to determine the appropriate management. Generally, patients with retroperitoneal lymph node involvement and normal or low-level abnormality of the tumor markers are considered to have stage II disease.[3] Options for management after orchiectomy include radiation

The authors have nothing to disclose.

[a] Radiation Medicine Program, Princess Margaret Hospital, 610 University Avenue, Toronto, ON, M5G 2M9 Canada

[b] Department of Radiation Oncology, University of Toronto, Toronto, ON, Canada

[c] Department of Medical Oncology/Haematology, Princess Margaret Hospital, 610 University Avenue, Toronto, ON, M5G 2M9 Canada

[d] Department of Medicine, University of Toronto, Toronto, ON, Canada

* Corresponding author. Radiation Medicine Program, Princess Margaret Hospital, 610 University Avenue, Toronto, ON, M5G 2M9 Canada

E-mail address: peter.chung@rmp.uhn.on.ca

Hematol Oncol Clin N Am 25 (2011) 529–541
doi:10.1016/j.hoc.2011.03.009
0889-8588/11/$ – see front matter © 2011 Elsevier Inc. All rights reserved.

therapy (RT) or combination chemotherapy in patients with seminoma and combination chemotherapy in those with nonseminoma, with retroperitoneal lymph node dissection (RPLND) reserved for select patients as either primary or postchemotherapy management. Overall outcomes for men who are diagnosed with stage II disease are excellent, with survival expected to exceed 95%, and patient involvement in management decision making is important, particularly because the associated short- and long-term toxicities of treatment add to the overall burden that these patients must bear.[4,5] These and other survivorship issues are beyond the scope of this article and will be discussed elsewhere, but they continue to fuel some of the controversy with respect to the optimal management of the individual patient.

STAGE II SEMINOMA

After orchiectomy, about 15% of patients have enlarged retroperitoneal lymph nodes. Of these patients, 70% have small bulk disease, with lymph nodes that are 5 cm or smaller (clinical stage IIA/B). Pathologic stage II disease is generally not seen in patients with seminoma because retroperitoneal lymphadenectomy has seldom been used as the primary management. Due to the small number of patients with stage II disease, there is a lack of randomized controlled trials, and thus, treatment decisions have been guided by reports from single institutions in which patients have been managed with a uniform policy. The 2 main treatment options for stage II seminoma are RT to the retroperitoneal (para-aortic and iliac) lymph node chain or combination cisplatin-based chemotherapy. Prophylactic mediastinal radiation (PMI) was previously practiced in some institutions, although the benefit of this approach was somewhat controversial. PMI has been abandoned with the advent of effective chemotherapy and evidence that PMI was associated with unacceptable long-term toxicity.[6]

The bulk of retroperitoneal lymphadenopathy is the single most important prognostic factor in patients with stage II disease. Lymph node size was the only factor that predicted recurrence in 95 patients with stage II seminoma treated with RT at the Princess Margaret Hospital between 1981 and 1999.[7] The 5-year relapse-free rate in patients with nodal disease of 5 cm or less (stage IIA/B) was 91% (7 of 79 patients), compared with 44% (9 of 16 patients) in patients with bulkier disease (stage IIC). Relapses mostly occurred outside the radiation field. In this series, 6 patients died of the disease. In 31 patients who received primary chemotherapy for stage II disease, 23 had stage IIC disease. Relapses were reported in 2 patients, 1 of whom was salvaged by second-line chemotherapy. These results are consistent with other series, in which the relapse rates ranged from 6% to 13.5%, that were reported in patients with small bulk stage II disease, thus supporting the use of primary RT in this setting.[8–10] Given the increase in failure after RT for bulky retroperitoneal disease (stage IIC) and that not all patients with recurrent disease were salvaged, primary chemotherapy is recommended for this subset.

As relapses almost always occur outside the radiation field, there seems to be an increased risk of distant micrometastasis in patients with stage IIC disease; the overall tumor burden should also be considered when choosing the management options, for example, a patient with multiple involved nodes extending craniocaudally along the para-aortic chain with a maximum diameter of 3.5 cm would be classified as having stage IIB disease. The risk of micrometastasis in such a patient may be higher than that in a patient with a solitary node of 3.5 cm, and thus, chemotherapy may be preferred over RT if the overall tumor burden is greater.[7] Other factors to consider are situations in which excess morbidity induced by radiation might be anticipated, such as the need to encompass a large volume of the kidney or liver to adequately treat a laterally positioned nodal mass. A similar problem might be caused in cases of abnormal anatomy, such as a horseshoe or pelvic kidney. In such situations, chemotherapy may again be preferred.

RT technique for stage II seminoma is similar to that used for stage I disease. Whereas para-aortic RT alone (excluding the pelvic nodes from the treatment volume) has been established as a treatment option for stage I disease, it has not been confirmed for stage II disease. Traditionally, a so-called dogleg-shaped RT field extending from the T10/T11 intervertebral space down to the ipsilateral obturator foramen has been used for stage II seminoma. More recently, attempts have been made to reduce this volume, recognizing that the lower internal and external iliac nodes are usually not a part of the lymphatic drainage of the testis (in the absence of prior scrotal/inguinal surgery) and thus do not need to be included in the treated volume.[8] Thus, the radiation volume should include the gross tumor as well as the para-aortic and ipsilateral common iliac lymph nodes, which allows the inferior border of the field to usually end at the acetabulum (**Fig. 1**). Although there is some variation, typically a dose of 25 Gy in 20 daily fractions plus a boost of 10 Gy to gross lymphadenopathy can be delivered either concurrently in 20 fractions or sequentially in 5 to 8 fractions.[7]

The combination of carboplatin and RT has been proposed to reduce the risk of relapse associated with RT alone in patients with stage IIA/B seminoma.[11] An updated report of this experience described 62 patients treated with 1 to 2 courses of carboplatin 4 to 6 weeks before RT.[12] Since 1997, 29 patients have been treated with 1 course of carboplatin before RT to the para-aortic nodes alone, and no relapses have been observed. Further study of this treatment option is warranted before it can

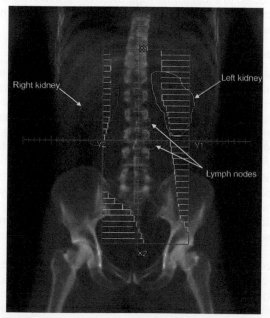

Fig. 1. Radiation field to encompass both macroscopic and microscopic nodal disease within the para-aortic and ipsilateral iliac chain for a patient with a left-sided stage II seminoma.

be accepted as standard practice, but it is attractive in that the rate of relapse outside the RT field may be lowered and the RT volume may be reduced. This option may allow patients to be cured while avoiding combination chemotherapy and potentially reducing the risk of late radiation–associated toxicity.

When chemotherapy is recommended as a primary treatment (or for relapse), 3 cycles of bleomycin, etoposide, and cisplatin (BEP) or 4 courses of EP (etoposide and cisplatin) are considered as standard options, which is based largely on trials of chemotherapy for good-prognosis germ cell tumors according to the International Germ Cell Consensus Classification (IGCCC) criteria.[13–16] Although there was a trend toward more favorable outcomes for BEP in these trials, most patients had nonseminoma histology, and it is not clear if this can be directly applied to patients with stage II seminoma. A prospective trial of cisplatin-based chemotherapy as an alternative to RT reported on 72 men with stage IIA/B seminoma with resultant 5-year relapse-free survival of 95%.[17] All the relapses occurred in those with stage IIB disease. Although these results are excellent, it is debatable if the incremental toxicity of combination chemotherapy is worthwhile for most patients compared with RT alone. When combination chemotherapy is chosen as the management in older men or those with poor pulmonary function, it may be preferable to omit bleomycin.

The role of carboplatin alone in IGCCC good-prognosis seminoma has been investigated in 2 randomized trials; a pooled analysis of these trials showed inferior outcomes for carboplatin and suggested that cisplatin-based combination chemotherapy remains the standard.[18] In addition, carboplatin alone cannot be recommended as the treatment option for stage IIA/B seminoma based on a phase II trial that reported an overall failure rate of 18% at a median follow-up of 28 months.[19]

Although many of these approaches have the aim of improving outcomes while also attempting to minimize toxicity, none have been completely successful in demonstrating an improvement. As overall disease-specific survival of patients with stage II seminoma is expected to exceed 95% regardless of the initial mode of management, only very small increases in disease control will likely be possible in the future and may well be at the expense of an increase in toxicity.

Residual Mass After RT or Chemotherapy

A residual mass seen on imaging after treatment is completed is not uncommon especially in those patients who initially present with a large nodal mass. Such masses most often contain fibrosis or necrotic material with only a few containing active tumor. Occasionally, nonseminoma elements may cause a persistent mass after therapy even in patients who have pure seminoma only in the primary tumor. RPLND in seminoma is technically challenging and associated with a higher acute morbidity after previous therapy.[20]

Options for patients with residual masses in the posttreatment setting may include observation, surgical excision, or RT (after previous chemotherapy). PET has been advocated by some to aid in decision making but is somewhat controversial. Surgical resection of a residual mass should not rely solely on a positive scan as the presence of false positives may result in unnecessary treatment with its attendant morbidity.[21–23]

As an illustration of the difficulty of surgical resection in residual masses after chemotherapy, in a published series of 55 patients, only 32 (58%) had a formal RPLND and 23 (42%) had multiple intraoperative biopsies performed, because the residual mass was deemed unresectable.[24] Of 27 patients who had a residual mass larger than 3 cm, 8 (30%) had residual viable tumor, of whom 2 had teratoma. No patients with tumors smaller than 3 cm had viable tumor. The investigators recommended resection or biopsy of masses of 3 cm or larger. Contrary to this, other investigators suggest continued observation as long as the retroperitoneal mass continues to decrease in size after treatment.[25]

RT has been used for residual masses after chemotherapy in men with seminoma, but the Medical Research Council Testicular Tumor Working Party published a retrospective pooled analysis evaluating the role of RT.[26] Of 123 patients with a residual abdominal mass, 56% received consolidative RT, with no significant difference in outcome regardless of the use of RT. Given the surgical data showing a low likelihood of the presence of viable tumor in this setting, the conclusion that routine RT was not indicated is not surprising.

The use of 3 cm as a cutoff point when considering observation of a residual mass would seem to be reasonable. For those with a more bulky residual mass, immediate surgery and observation (and treatment of increasing size) are the options. The use of PET scan together with size criteria may also aid decision making in this situation.

STAGE II NONSEMINOMA

Clinical stage II nonseminoma (CS-II) refers to patients who have enlarged lymph nodes by size criteria at the time of radiographic staging, whereas pathologic stage II nonseminoma (PS-II) refers to patients with pathologic confirmation of nodal involvement after an RPLND. Although stage II only accounts for 19% of all nonseminoma diagnoses,[27] the optimal management of this stage grouping is widely debated,[28–35] which is, in large part, because of the excellent expected 5-year survival of patients diagnosed with stage II nonseminoma of more than 96%.[27]

There are 3 general treatment strategies available for patients with stage II nonseminoma: primary retroperitoneal lymph node dissection (pRPLND) alone, pRPLND followed by adjuvant chemotherapy, and primary chemotherapy followed by, in the event of residual masses, retroperitoneal lymph node dissection (pcRPLND) (**Fig. 2**). Patients with stage IIA disease (largest lymph node ≤2 cm) and negative tumor makers are a unique group, in whom close surveillance after orchiectomy may be entertained because a significant proportion of these patients have benign adenopathy. Clinical decision making for all patients with stage II nonseminoma must balance an understanding of disease biology against the expected efficacy of the available treatment strategies and their attendant long-term toxicities.

In the landmark randomized controlled trial of observation versus adjuvant chemotherapy after orchiectomy and pRPLND for patients with involved retroperitoneal lymph nodes, the rate of relapse in the observation arm was 49% compared with 2% in the adjuvant chemotherapy arm.[36] However, there was no difference in survival between the 2 arms, because the observed patients were successfully salvaged with chemotherapy. There was a trend toward a greater risk of relapse with more extensive nodal involvement: 40% with microscopic nodal involvement, 53% with macroscopic nodal involvement of less than 2 cm, and 60% with nodal involvement of more than 2 cm. It should be noted, however, that one-third of the patients had elevated tumor markers after orchiectomy. In the modern era, patients with elevated markers would generally be treated with primary chemotherapy than with pRPLND because of the elevated risk of systemic progression associated with persistent tumor marker elevation after orchiectomy.[37]

Patients with enlarged small-volume lymph nodes (1–2 cm) at the time of radiographic staging (CS-IIA) and normal tumor markers after orchiectomy present a unique management dilemma. The differential diagnosis for nodal enlargement includes

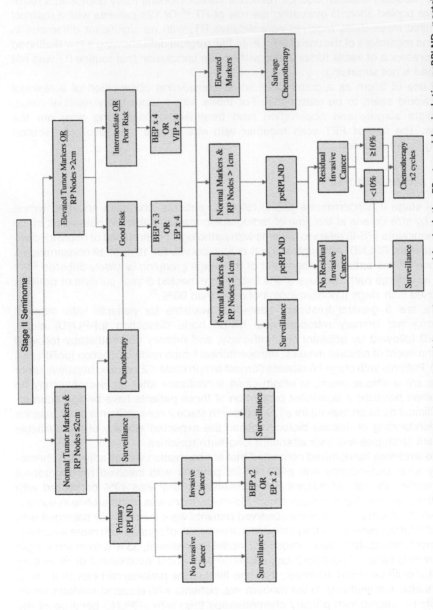

Fig. 2. Algorithm for management of Stage II nonseminoma. BEP, bleomycin-etoposide-cisplatin; EP, etoposide-cisplatin; pcRPLND, postchemotherapy RPLND; RP, retroperitoneal; VIP, etoposide-ifosphamide-cisplatin.

viable germ cell cancer (PS-II), teratoma, or benign lymph node enlargement. Although there is pathologic confirmation of tumor stage, pRPLND is associated with a risk of overtreatment, because 10% to 40% of patients will be found to have uninvolved lymph nodes at the time of surgery (PS-I).[38–40] As a result, close surveillance with repeat imaging and tumor marker assessment every 6 weeks until normalization of the nodes is an option for patients with CS-IIA disease and normal serum tumor markers after orchiectomy.[28,29,35]

For patients with PS-stage IIA disease and normal pre-RPLND tumor markers, the risk of relapse is approximately 10% to 15%. Management options include surveillance with full-course chemotherapy at relapse or adjuvant chemotherapy with 2 cycles of BEP or EP.[41,42] Most institutions recommend surveillance to reduce the risk of unnecessary chemotherapy for patients who are cured with pRPLND alone.

By comparison, the risk of relapse for patients with PS-IIB and PS-IIC after RPLND is substantially higher at 35% to 50% and 60% to 85%, respectively.[43–46] As a result, patients with PS-IIB and PS-IIC are usually treated with 2 cycles of adjuvant chemotherapy after RPLND, which reduces the risk of relapse to less than 5%.[36,42,47] Relapses after adjuvant chemotherapy for PS-II disease occur almost exclusively outside the retroperitoneum.

With improvements in cross-sectional imaging, patients with large involved retroperitoneal lymph nodes are now more easily identified before RPLND (CS-IIB and CS-IIC). There are no randomized clinical trials that compare pRPLND followed by adjuvant chemotherapy with primary chemotherapy for stage II disease. Comparative series suggests no difference in disease-specific survival for either approach.[31,39] Recognition of risk factors associated with systemic progression after RPLND, such as lymph node size greater than 2 cm, multiple enlarged lymph nodes, and elevated AFP or hCG level, has led to an increasing use of primary chemotherapy for patients with CS-IIB and CS-IIC disease over time.[31] Primary chemotherapy for patients with stage II disease is associated with a complete response rate of 60% to 78%.[39,48–50] A consensus definition of complete response does not exist, but most guidelines suggest that pcRPLND is recommended for retroperitoneal masses larger than 1 cm.[28,29,35] Necrotic debris or fibrosis is found in approximately 40% to 45% of patients with pcRPLND, immature teratoma in 40% to 45%, and viable germ cell tumor in 10% to 15%.[51] PET after chemotherapy is not helpful in differentiating necrosis or fibrosis from other histologies.[52] Although histologically benign, immature teratoma may grow and produce local complications. It is also associated with late viable germ cell relapses and may transform to carcinomatous or sarcomatous malignancies. When viable germ cell tumor is encountered at pcRPLND, additional chemotherapy is generally recommended to reduce the risk of systemic relapse.[28,29,35]

An area of ongoing controversy is the management of patients with complete response after primary chemotherapy. Many authors suggest observation,[28,35,50,53,54] because the risk of isolated retroperitoneal progression is less than 5% with long-term follow-up. In addition, pcRPLND is associated with a 6% to 8% risk of retrograde ejaculation, and the risk of pulmonary postoperative complications is increased with prior bleomycin exposure. Patients who had relapse during surveillance can subsequently be salvaged.[53,54] Others recommend pcRPLND for all patients with stage II disease, arguing that radiologic response is not a reliable predictor of fibrosis or necrosis, and the incidence of teratoma identified at pcRPLND is similar for patients with residual masses larger than 1 cm versus those with residual masses of 1 cm or smaller by CT after primary chemotherapy.[31,34,55] Regardless, cause-specific survival with either approach is excellent, and as such, patient preference should be taken into account during the decision-making process with discussion of the toxicities of surgery and radiation exposure associated with continued CT imaging.

Duration of Primary Chemotherapy

Most patients who are treated with primary chemotherapy for stage II nonseminoma are classified as good prognosis by the IGCCC criteria: AFP less than 1000 ng/mL, hCG less than 5000 IU/L, LDH less than 1.5 upper limit of normal, and no nonpulmonary visceral metastases.[13] A landmark study of the Southeastern Cancer Study Group (SECSG) established 4 cycles of BEP as the standard for patients with disseminated germ cell tumors.[45] The BEP regimen based on the SECSG or Indiana protocol (cisplatin 20 mg/m^2; etoposide 100 mg/m^2 on days 1–5; and bleomycin 30 IU on days 1, 8, and 15 for every 3 weeks) has remained the gold standard for treatment to this day. A subsequent study by the same research group demonstrated that 3 cycles of BEP were equally effective and less toxic compared with 4 cycles of BEP for patients with a favorable risk profile, defined according to their prognostic staging system that classified all patients with stage II disease as favorable risk.[56] A joint study by the European Organisation of Research and Treatment of Cancer (EORTC) and the Medical Research Council (MRC) further established the equivalence of 3 cycles of BEP to 3 cycles of BEP followed by 1 cycle of EP for patients with good-prognosis disease defined by the IGCCC criteria.[57] This study involved a 2 × 2 factorial design, with a second randomization of BEP to either the 5-day Indiana regimen or a 3-day regimen (cisplatin 50 mg/m^2 on days 1–2 and etoposide 165 mg/m^2 on days 1–5) for 681 of the 812 patients included in this trial. Three cycles of BEP administered by the 5- or 3-day schedule had equivalent progression-free survival, although the condensed BEP regimen was associated with greater nausea and ototoxicity.

Role of Bleomycin

Bleomycin-induced pneumonitis is a rare potentially fatal toxicity of bleomycin therapy, the risk of which increases with higher cumulative bleomycin exposure.[58] Three cycles of BEP delivers a total bleomycin dose of 270 IU. Various trials have examined whether bleomycin can be omitted in regimens for advanced germ cell tumors. A study from the Eastern Cooperative Oncology Group randomized 178 patients with favorable-risk advanced germ cell tumors to 3 cycles of BEP versus 3 cycles of EP.[16] The failure-free survival and overall survival were inferior in the EP arm. The EORTC randomized 419 patients with good-prognosis disease by the IGCCC criteria to 4 cycles of BEP versus 4 cycles of EP. The EP arm experienced a lower rate of complete response (87% vs 95%, $P = .0075$), although there were no differences in time to progression or overall survival. Of note, the dose of etoposide (360 mg/m^2) administered with each cycle of therapy was lower than what is now considered standard for both BEP and EP (etoposide 500 mg/m^2).

A large retrospective series of patients with IGCCC good-risk disease treated with 4 cycles of EP showed excellent outcomes.[32] The Genito-Urinary Group of the French Federation of Cancer Centers randomized 270 patients with good-risk disease defined by the Institut Gustav Roussy prognostic model to 3 cycles of BEP using the Indiana regimen versus 4 cycles of EP (cumulative etoposide dose of 500 mg/m^2).[49] In the French trial, both regimens achieved a similar rate of favorable response, defined as normal serum tumor markers and no residual radiographic disease after chemotherapy or pathologic complete response observed at pcRPLND. There was also no difference in 4-year event-free survival

(91% vs 86%, $P = .14$) and 4-year overall survival (5 vs 12 deaths, $P = .096$) for the primary comparison. However, in the subset of IGCCC good-risk patients, there was a trend toward improved 4-year event-free survival for 3 cycles of BEP (93% vs 86%, $P = .052$).

Cumulative exposure to bleomycin also seems to be important. The Australian and New Zealand Germ Cell Trials Group recently reported long-term follow-up from a trial that randomized 166 patients with good-risk disease according to Memorial Sloan Kettering Cancer Center criteria to 3 cycles of $B_{90}E_{500}P$ (cumulative bleomycin dose of 270 IU) versus 4 cycles of $B_{30}E_{360}P$ (cumulative bleomycin dose of 120 IU).[59] After a median follow-up of 8.5 years, the group assigned to a higher cumulative dose of bleomycin experienced improved overall survival (8-year survival 92% vs 83%, $P = .037$). The 4 cycles of $B_{30}E_{360}P$ also received a lower cumulative dose and dose intensity of etoposide, which may confound the interpretation of the importance of bleomycin dosing in this study. Based on these findings, 3 cycles of BEP should be the preferred regimen, with 4 cycles of EP reserved for patients with contraindications to bleomycin.[28,29,35,60]

Role of Carboplatin

Although less nephrotoxic and neurotoxic than cisplatin, carboplatin should not routinely be substituted for cisplatin in patients with good-risk disease. A MRC/EORTC trial randomized 598 patients with good-risk nonseminoma to 4 cycles of BEP (with 30 IU of bleomycin and 360 mg/m^2 of etoposide per cycle) or the identical regimen with carboplatin substituted for cisplatin (CEB).[61] Patients allocated to CEB were less likely to achieve complete response (87% vs 94%, $P = .009$), which translated into inferior 1-year failure-free survival (77% vs 91%, $P = .001$) and 3-year overall survival (90% vs 97%, $P = .003$). A randomized trial of 4 cycles of CEB versus 3 cycles of BEP (with 120 IU of bleomycin and 500 mg/m^2 of etoposide per cycle) showed a similar rate of complete response but an increased risk of relapse with CEB.[62] Likewise, more relapses were observed after 4 cycles of carboplatin and etoposide (CE) compared with 4 cycles of EP.[14]

SUMMARY

In patients with stage II seminoma, RT is the treatment of choice for those with stage IIA and low-volume stage IIB disease, with combination chemotherapy (either 3 cycles of BEP or 4 cycles of EP) being preferred for more advanced disease. In those with stage II nonseminoma, RPLND (with or without chemotherapy) is a treatment option for small-volume stage IIA disease, with combination chemotherapy consisting of 3 cycles of BEP being preferred for more advanced disease. Cancer cure in this population of patients is excellent, thus further efforts are required to characterize and reduce the risk of long-term sequelae of treatment. Long-term follow-up is essential to deal with the issues of screening for and management of late effects. Thus, research into cancer survivorship together with reduction of treatment burden in patients with testicular cancer is warranted to provide the sought after cure without compromise in this disease.

REFERENCES

1. Ferlay J, Shin HR, Bray F, et al. Estimates of worldwide burden of cancer in 2008: GLOBOCAN 2008. Int J Cancer 2010;127:2893–917.
2. Purdue MP, Devesa SS, Sigurdson AJ, et al. International patterns and trends in testis cancer incidence. Int J Cancer 2005;115(5):822–7.

3. Sobin LH, Gospodarowicz MK, Wittekind C, editors. TNM classification of malignant tumors. 7th edition. Oxford (UK): Wiley-Blackwell; 2009. p. 310.
4. Gospodarowicz M. Testicular cancer patients: considerations in long-term follow-up. Hematol Oncol Clin North Am 2008;22(2):245–55, vi.
5. Travis L, Beard C, Allan J, et al. Testicular cancer survivorship: research strategies and recommendations. J Natl Cancer Inst 2010;102(15):1114–30.
6. Zagars GK, Ballo MT, Lee AK, et al. Mortality after cure of testicular seminoma. J Clin Oncol 2004;22(4):640–7.
7. Chung PW, Gospodarowicz MK, Panzarella T, et al. Stage II testicular seminoma: patterns of recurrence and outcome of treatment. Eur Urol 2004;45(6):754–9 [discussion: 759–60].
8. Classen J, Schmidberger H, Meisner C, et al. Radiotherapy for stages IIA/B testicular seminoma: final report of a prospective multicenter clinical trial. J Clin Oncol 2003;21(6):1101–6.
9. Vallis KA, Howard GC, Duncan W, et al. Radiotherapy for stages I and II testicular seminoma: results and morbidity in 238 patients. Br J Radiol 1995;68(808):400–5.
10. Zagars GK, Pollack A. Radiotherapy for stage II testicular seminoma. Int J Radiat Oncol Biol Phys 2001;51(3):643–9.
11. Patterson H, Norman AR, Mitra SS, et al. Combination carboplatin and radiotherapy in the management of stage II testicular seminoma: comparison with radiotherapy treatment alone. Radiother Oncol 2001;59(1):5–11.
12. Gilbert DC, Vanas NJ, Beesley S, et al. Treating IIA/B seminoma with combination carboplatin and radiotherapy. J Clin Oncol 2009;27(12):2101–2 [author reply: 2102–3].
13. International Germ Cell Consensus Classification: a prognostic factor-based staging system for metastatic germ cell cancers. International Germ Cell Cancer Collaborative Group. J Clin Oncol 1997;15(2):594–603.
14. Bajorin D, Sarosdy M, Pfister D, et al. Randomized trial of etoposide and cisplatin versus etoposide and carboplatin in patients with good-risk germ cell tumors: a multiinstitutional study. J Clin Oncol 1993;11(4):598–606.
15. Bosl GJ, Geller NL, Bajorin D, et al. A randomized trial of etoposide + cisplatin versus vinblastine + bleomycin + cisplatin + cyclophosphamide + dactinomycin in patients with good-prognosis germ cell tumors. J Clin Oncol 1988;6(8):1231–8.
16. Loehrer PJ Sr, Johnson D, Elson P, et al. Importance of bleomycin in favorable-prognosis disseminated germ cell tumors: an Eastern Cooperative Oncology Group trial. J Clin Oncol 1995;13(2):470–6.
17. Garcia-del-Muro X, Maroto P, Guma J, et al. Chemotherapy as an alternative to radiotherapy in the treatment of stage IIA and IIB testicular seminoma: a Spanish Germ Cell Cancer Group Study. J Clin Oncol 2008;26(33):5416–21.
18. Bokemeyer C, Kollmannsberger C, Stenning S, et al. Metastatic seminoma treated with either single agent carboplatin or cisplatin-based combination chemotherapy: a pooled analysis of two randomised trials. Br J Cancer 2004;91(4):683–7.
19. Krege S, Boergermann C, Baschek R, et al. Single agent carboplatin for CS IIA/B testicular seminoma. A phase II study of the German Testicular Cancer Study Group (GTCSG). Ann Oncol 2006;17(2):276–80.
20. Mosharafa AA, Foster RS, Leibovich BC, et al. Is post-chemotherapy resection of seminomatous elements associated with higher acute morbidity? J Urol 2003; 169(6):2126–8.
21. Becherer A, De Santis M, Karanikas G, et al. FDG PET is superior to CT in the prediction of viable tumour in post-chemotherapy seminoma residuals. Eur J Radiol 2005;54(2):284–8.

22. Ganjoo KN, Chan RJ, Sharma M, et al. Positron emission tomography scans in the evaluation of postchemotherapy residual masses in patients with seminoma. J Clin Oncol 1999;17(11):3457–60.
23. Hinz S, Schrader M, Kempkensteffen C, et al. The role of positron emission tomography in the evaluation of residual masses after chemotherapy for advanced stage seminoma. J Urol 2008;179(3):936–40 [discussion: 940].
24. Herr HW, Sheinfeld J, Puc HS, et al. Surgery for a post-chemotherapy residual mass in seminoma. J Urol 1997;157(3):860–2.
25. Culine S, Droz JP. Optimal management of residual mass after chemotherapy in advanced seminoma: there is time for everything. J Clin Oncol 1996;14(10):2884–5.
26. Duchesne GM, Stenning SP, Aass N, et al. Radiotherapy after chemotherapy for metastatic seminoma—a diminishing role. MRC Testicular Tumour Working Party. Eur J Cancer 1997;33(6):829–35.
27. Biggs M, Schwartz S. Cancer of the testis. In: Young JL, Ries LA, Keel GE, et al, editors. Cancer survival among adults: US SEER Program, 1988–2001. Bethesda (MD): National Cancer Institute; 2007. p. 165–70.
28. Schmoll H, Jordan K, Huddart R, et al. Testicular non-seminoma: ESMO clinical practice guidelines for diagnosis, treatment and follow-up. Ann Oncol 2010; 21(Suppl 5):v147.
29. Wood L, Kollmannsberger C, Jewett M, et al. Canadian consensus guidelines for the management of testicular germ cell cancer. Can Urol Assoc J 2010;4(2):e19.
30. Motzer RJ, Agarwal N, Beard C, et al. Testicular cancer. J Natl Compr Canc Netw 2009;7(6):672–93.
31. Stephenson A, Bosl G, Motzer R, et al. Nonrandomized comparison of primary chemotherapy and retroperitoneal lymph node dissection for clinical stage IIA and IIB nonseminomatous germ cell testicular cancer. J Clin Oncol 2007; 25(35):5597.
32. Kondagunta GV, Bacik J, Bajorin D, et al. Etoposide and cisplatin chemotherapy for metastatic good-risk germ cell tumors. J Clin Oncol 2005;23(36):9290–4.
33. Einhorn L, Foster R. Bleomycin, etoposide, and cisplatin for three cycles compared with etoposide and cisplatin for four cycles in good-risk germ cell tumors: is there a preferred regimen? J Clin Oncol 2006;24(16):2597.
34. Oldenburg J, Alfsen GC, Lien HH, et al. Postchemotherapy retroperitoneal surgery remains necessary in patients with nonseminomatous testicular cancer and minimal residual tumor masses. J Clin Oncol 2003;21(17):3310–7.
35. Krege S, Beyer J, Souchon R, et al. European consensus conference on diagnosis and treatment of germ cell cancer: a report of the second meeting of the European Germ Cell Cancer Consensus group (EGCCCG): part I. Eur Urol 2008;53(3):478–96.
36. Williams S, Stablein D, Einhorn L, et al. Immediate adjuvant chemotherapy versus observation with treatment at relapse in pathological stage II testicular cancer. N Engl J Med 1987;317(23):1433–8.
37. Rabbani F, Sheinfeld J, Farivar-Mohseni H, et al. Low-volume nodal metastases detected at retroperitoneal lymphadenectomy for testicular cancer: pattern and prognostic factors for relapse. J Clin Oncol 2001;19(7):2020.
38. Stephenson A, Bosl G, Bajorin D, et al. Retroperitoneal lymph node dissection in patients with low stage testicular cancer with embryonal carcinoma predominance and/or lymphovascular invasion. J Urol 2005;174(2):557–60.
39. Weissbach L, Bussar-Maatz R, Flechtner H, et al. RPLND or primary chemotherapy in clinical stage IIA/B nonseminomatous germ cell tumors? Eur Urol 2000;37(5):582–94.

40. Sheinfeld J, Motzer R, Rabbani F, et al. Incidence and clinical outcome of patients with teratoma in the retroperitoneum following primary retroperitoneal lymph node dissection for clinical stages I and IIA nonseminomatous germ cell tumors. J Urol 2003;170(4):1159–62.

41. Behnia M, Foster R, Einhorn LH, et al. Adjuvant bleomycin, etoposide and cisplatin in pathological stage II non-seminomatous testicular cancer. The Indiana University experience. Eur J Cancer 2000;36(4):472–5.

42. Kondagunta GV, Sheinfeld J, Mazumdar M, et al. Relapse-free and overall survival in patients with pathologic stage II nonseminomatous germ cell cancer treated with etoposide and cisplatin adjuvant chemotherapy. J Clin Oncol 2004;22(3):464–7.

43. Donohue J, Thornhill J, Foster R, et al. The role of retroperitoneal lymphadenectomy in clinical stage B testis cancer: the Indiana University experience (1965 to 1989). J Urol 1995;153(1):85–9.

44. Donohue J, Thornhill J, Foster R, et al. Clinical stage B non-seminomatous germ cell testis cancer: the Indiana University experience (1965–1989) using routine primary retroperitoneal lymph node dissection. Eur J Cancer 1995;31(10):1599–604.

45. Williams S, Birch R, Einhorn L, et al. Treatment of disseminated germ-cell tumors with cisplatin, bleomycin, and either vinblastine or etoposide. N Engl J Med 1987;316(23):1435–40.

46. Pizzocaro G, Piva L, Salvioni R, et al. Adjuvant chemotherapy in resected stage-II nonseminomatous germ cell tumors of testis. In which cases is it necessary? Eur Urol 1984;10(3):151–8.

47. Weissbach L, Hartlapp J. Adjuvant chemotherapy of metastatic stage II nonseminomatous testis tumor. J Urol 1991;146(5):1295.

48. Logothetis C, Swanson D, Dexeus F, et al. Primary chemotherapy for clinical stage II nonseminomatous germ cell tumors of the testis: a follow-up of 50 patients. J Clin Oncol 1987;5(6):906.

49. Culine S, Kerbrat P, Kramar A, et al. Refining the optimal chemotherapy regimen for good-risk metastatic nonseminomatous germ-cell tumors: a randomized trial of the Genito-Urinary Group of the French Federation of Cancer Centers (GETUG T93BP). Ann Oncol 2007;18(5):917–24.

50. Kuczyk M, Machtens S, Stief C, et al. Management of the post-chemotherapy residual mass in patients with advanced stage non-seminomatous germ cell tumors (NSGCT). Int J Cancer 1999;83(6):852–5.

51. Toner G, Panicek D, Heelan R, et al. Adjunctive surgery after chemotherapy for nonseminomatous germ cell tumors: recommendations for patient selection. J Clin Oncol 1990;8(10):1683.

52. Oechsle K, Hartmann M, Brenner W, et al. [18F] Fluorodeoxyglucose positron emission tomography in nonseminomatous germ cell tumors after chemotherapy: the German multicenter positron emission tomography study group. J Clin Oncol 2008;26(36):5930–5.

53. Ehrlich Y, Brames MJ, Beck SDW, et al. Long-term follow-up of cisplatin combination chemotherapy in patients with disseminated nonseminomatous germ cell tumors: is a postchemotherapy retroperitoneal lymph node dissection needed after complete remission? J Clin Oncol 2010;28(4):531–6.

54. Kollmannsberger C, Daneshmand S, So A, et al. Management of disseminated nonseminomatous germ cell tumors with risk-based chemotherapy followed by response-guided postchemotherapy surgery. J Clin Oncol 2010;28(4):537–42.

55. Bosl G, Motzer R. Weighing risks and benefits of postchemotherapy retroperitoneal lymph node dissection: not so easy. J Clin Oncol 2010;28(4):519.

56. Einhorn L, Williams S, Loehrer P, et al. Evaluation of optimal duration of chemo-therapy in favorable-prognosis disseminated germ cell tumors: a Southeastern Cancer Study Group protocol. J Clin Oncol 1989;7(3):387.
57. De Wit R, Roberts J, Wilkinson P, et al. Equivalence of three or four cycles of bleo-mycin, etoposide, and cisplatin chemotherapy and of a 3- or 5-day schedule in good-prognosis germ cell cancer: a randomized study of the European Organi-zation for Research and Treatment of Cancer Genitourinary Tract Cancer Coop-erative Group and the Medical Research Council. J Clin Oncol 2001;19(6):1629.
58. Sleijfer S. Bleomycin-induced pneumonitis. Chest 2001;120(2):617.
59. Grimison PS, Stockler MR, Thomson DB, et al. Comparison of two standard chemotherapy regimens for good-prognosis germ cell tumors: updated analysis of a randomized trial. J Natl Cancer Inst 2010;102(16):1253–62.
60. Nichols C, Kollmannsberger C. Alternatives to standard BEP × 3 in good-prognosis germ cell tumors—you bet your life. J Natl Cancer Inst 2010;102(16):1214–5.
61. Horwich A, Sleijfer D, Fossa S, et al. Randomized trial of bleomycin, etoposide, and cisplatin compared with bleomycin, etoposide, and carboplatin in good-prognosis metastatic nonseminomatous germ cell cancer: a Multiinstitutional Medical Research Council/European Organization for Research and Treatment of Cancer Trial. J Clin Oncol 1997;15(5):1844.
62. Bokemeyer C, Kohrmann O, Tischler J, et al. A randomized trial of cisplatin, eto-poside and bleomycin (PEB) versus carboplatin, etoposide and bleomycin (CEB) for patients with 'good-risk' metastatic non-seminomatous germ cell tumors. Ann Oncol 1996;7(10):1015–21.

First-Line Chemotherapy of Disseminated Germ Cell Tumors

Craig Nichols, MD[a],*, Christian Kollmannsberger, MD[b]

KEYWORDS

• Chemotherapy • Germ cell • Cisplatin • Testicular cancer

The development of effective chemotherapy has been the defining event in the history of testicular cancer treatment. The discovery of cisplatin-based chemotherapy created a massive inflection that sharply defined the relatively grim precisplatin era from the astonishing postcisplatin era. The ripple effects of this discovery continue today with the rewriting of management of early-stage germ cell tumors to surveillance-based programs. This article reviews the discovery, development, and delivery of cisplatin-based chemotherapy; expected outcomes of chemotherapy treatment; remaining controversies in primary chemotherapy treatment of disseminated disease; and practical management tips for delivery of bleomycin, etoposide, and cisplatin (BEP) and after chemotherapy treatment.

ERA OF DISCOVERY (1960s–1985)

Use of early chemotherapy agents began in the 1960s and often consisted of the serial use of single agents. Measurable clinical activity was demonstrated for bleomycin, vinblastine, actinomycin D and minor activity for anthracyclines and classic alkylators. Simple combination therapy, such as vinblastine and bleomycin, demonstrated occasional complete responses, but few durable remissions.

In 1965, Barnett Rosenberg and colleagues[1] at Michigan State University discovered biologic effects of elemental platinum on *Escherichia coli* during experiments using a platinum anode to conduct electricity through bacterial cultures. Dr Rosenberg and his team hypothesized that a platinum compound was disrupting the ability of the *E coli* to divide and went further to identify the platinum species with the most profound effect: *cis*-diaminodichloroplatinum.

[a] Divison of Medical Oncology, Virginia Mason Medical Center, 1100 9th Avenue, Seattle, WA 98101, USA
[b] Divison of Medical Oncology, British Columbia Cancer Agency-Vancouver Cancer Centre, 600 West 10th Avenue, Vancouver, BC, V5Z4E6 Canada
* Corresponding author.
E-mail address: tcconsortiumnichols@gmail.com

Hematol Oncol Clin N Am 25 (2011) 543–556
doi:10.1016/j.hoc.2011.03.011
0889-8588/11/$ – see front matter © 2011 Elsevier Inc. All rights reserved.

hemonc.theclinics.com

The team at Michigan State further speculated that this compound might merit testing in cancer. They performed in vitro experiments with L1210 leukemia cells as well as animal sarcoma models. Ultimately this led to the development of phase I trials of cisplatin in which impressive single-agent activity in patients with testicular cancer was seen.[2] Unfortunately, in these trials, unique toxicity was also identified, including substantial emetogenic potential, nephrotoxicity, neurotoxicity, and ototoxicity.

In 1973, Dr Lawrence Einhorn and Dr John Donohue[3] at Indiana University began the seminal study of cisplatin combination chemotherapy in patients with germ cell tumors. In the original study, patients were treated with cisplatin, vinblastine, and bleomycin (PVB) for 4 cycles of treatment followed by up to 2 years of maintenance therapy. The study also included the incorporation of aggressive postchemotherapy surgery for those who obtained only a partial remission with induction chemotherapy. The results of this Indiana University study changed forever the outlook and approach for patients with testicular cancer. Among the first 47 evaluable patients, 35 (74%) obtained a complete chemotherapy induced remission. An additional 12 patients (26%) obtained partial remission for an overall response rate of 100% and 5 of these 12 underwent aggressive postchemotherapy surgery to be rendered free of disease. Thirty-two patients (68%) obtained in durable remission. These overwhelming results were rapidly confirmed by other institutions in the United States and in Europe.

Subsequent to the initial demonstration of spectacular therapeutic effect of cisplatin combination chemotherapy, efforts turned to improving the tolerability of PVB, and such studies allowed the shaping of current modern therapy. Serial studies at Indiana University allowed two significant changes in the original PVB template. First, a randomized comparison of PVB using the original dose of vinblastine (0.4 mg/kg) to the same cisplatin and bleomycin dose but with a meaningful reduction of the vinblastine dose (0.3 mg/kg) demonstrated therapeutic equivalence and further confirmed the therapeutic punch of PVB in germ cell tumors. As expected, however, there were significant reductions in the myelotoxicity and neurotoxicity associated with the lower doses of vinblastine.[4] Second, a randomized comparison of 4 courses of induction PVB (12 weeks) plus the original maintenance vinblastine schedule (up to 2 years) was compared with induction PVB alone (12 weeks).[5] Again, the arms were therapeutically equivalent and induction therapy without maintenance became the standard approach (as it is today).

In the early 1980s, a new drug, etoposide, began to show activity in recurrent germ cell tumors. The toxicity profile of etoposide was primarily myelotoxicity and, thus, was able to be combined with cisplatin in full doses without overlapping toxicity. Approximately 25% of patients failing PVB responded to single-agent etoposide.[6] Combinations of cisplatin and etoposide resulted in sustained remissions in some patients with recurrent germ cell tumors after PVB. The definitive contribution of etoposide in combination chemotherapy was demonstrated in the randomized comparison of 4 cycles of cisplatin and bleomycin with either vinblastine (PVB) or etoposide (BEP) as primary chemotherapy of disseminated germ cell tumors.[7] The results reported by Dr Stephen Williams and colleagues[7] from Indiana University and the Southeastern Cancer Study Group demonstrated the anticipated decrease in the neurotoxicity and musculoskeletal toxicity attributable to vinblastine. Moreover, PVB and BEP were at least therapeutically equivalent. In a randomized clinical trial in 261 men with disseminated germ cell tumors, etoposide was substituted for the vinblastine in this regimen to compare the efficacy and toxicity of the two treatments. Among 244 patients who could be evaluated for a response, 74% of those receiving PVB and 83% of those receiving BEP became disease-free with or without subsequent surgery but there was no difference in overall survival. Among those 157 patients classified as having high-volume disease, 61% became disease-free with PVB compared with 77% on BEP (P<.05). Among the high–tumor volume patients, BEP was associated with higher overall survival (P = .048). The regimens were similar in terms of myelosuppressive effects and pulmonary toxicity. The etoposide regimen, however, caused substantially fewer paresthesias (P = .02), abdominal cramps (P = .0008), and myalgias (P = .00002).

As a sidelight to these therapeutic advances, careful clinical observations over this time period of rapid discovery of chemotherapy regimens for disseminated germ cell tumors defined the next era of clinical investigations wherein the effective standard regimens were tested and refined. The two categories of observations were development of prognostic indices to define pretreatment expectations of cure with cisplatin-based therapy and careful aggregation of short-term and long-term side-effect profiles to provide a comprehensive impact statement of curative chemotherapy.

ERA OF DEVELOPMENT (1985–2005)

Initial chemotherapy investigations led careful observers to a basic differentiation of patients with disseminated germ cell tumors.[8–10] Even in early studies, it seemed as if there were a group of patients who had a 90% or greater chance of obtaining disease-free status and remaining in that status and a group for whom disease control was considerably less predictable with a 30% to 50% chance of failing to obtain disease-free status. Several institutions developed parochial prognostic systems that defined a good/minimal risk group, a poor/advanced risk group, and sometimes an intermediate-risk or moderate-risk group. This risk discrimination was usually made using readily available clinical parameters, such as anatomic extent of disease, site of primary, seminoma versus nonseminoma, and, in some systems, the degree of elevation of serum markers, such as α-fetoprotein (AFP), human chorionic gronadotropin (hCG), and lactate dehydrogenase (LDH). As can be imagined, these locally developed prognostic systems each had advantages and disadvantages and were variably reliable in predicting outcomes of systemic treatment. Nonetheless, the approximately ability to discriminate a good-risk group from a destined to do less well with standard cisplatin-based chemotherapy sent the field of clinical investigations for disseminated germ cell tumors down the path of testing toxicity reduction strategies in good-risk patients and examining approaches with enhanced therapeutic potential in those patients with predicted poor outcomes.

In good-risk germ cell tumors, the initial questions were aimed at duration of therapy of what was by then standard treatment of disseminated disease—BEP × 4. Investigators at Indiana University and the Southeastern Cancer Study Group performed a randomized clinical trial comparing the standard of 4 cycles of BEP to an experimental arm with the same doses and schedule of chemotherapy but given for 3 rather than 4 cycles.[11] This trial included 184 patients with disseminated germ cell tumors in the Indiana University minimal-risk and moderate-risk class. In the minimal extent category, 106 of 107 patients became disease-free and overall 92% of patients receiving 3 cycles and 92% of patients receiving 4 cycles remained continuously disease-free. Among this group of 184 patients, there was only 1 therapy-related death: a single death related to neutropenic sepsis. The investigators concluded that 3 cycles of BEP was the preferred approach to patients with good-risk disease and the standard of care for good-risk disease changed to this 9-week regimen. These results were confirmed in long-term follow-up of this study.[12] At 10 years, there were no differences in the 118 Indiana University patients receiving either 3 or 4 cycles of BEP. Incorporating serum markers did suggest, however, that patients with hCG greater than 1000 mIU/mL were at higher risk of failure (5/14 deaths) compared with those with hCG less than 1000 mIU/mL (2/104).

In a final attempt to minimize therapy in good-risk patients, investigators at Indiana University and the Eastern Cooperative Oncology Group conducted a randomized trial of 3 cycles of BEP (the new standard for favorable prognosis patients) to 3 cycles of cisplatin and etoposide (EP) in the same dose and schedule as BEP but with the deletion of what was felt to be potentially the most vexing component of the regimen: bleomycin.[13] This trial has defined the floor of minimizing therapy for good-risk disease. Including both Indiana University minimal and moderate disease categories, 178 patients were randomized. There were no clinically significant pulmonary toxicity on either arm and the single therapy-related death was related to sepsis while on BEP. There was a 14% incidence of grade IV neutropenia on the BEP versus 7% on EP. Overall, 94% of patients who received BEP and 88% who received EP achieved a disease-free status with chemotherapy and/or surgery. There was significant difference in treatment failures, however, including persistent carcinoma in postchemotherapy resections of residual disease and relapses from complete remission, which occurred on the arm without bleomycin. Also, a significant negative impact on failure-free (86% vs 69%; $P = .01$) and overall survival (95% vs 86%; $P = .01$) was demonstrated for those receiving EP without bleomycin. The investigators concluded that bleomycin is an essential component of cisplatin combination chemotherapy in patients who receive 3 cycles of treatment for minimal-stage or moderate-stage disseminated germ cell tumors.

Other investigators took a different path trying to refine therapy for good-risk disease based on attempts to reduce the chemotherapy toxicity profile related to cisplatin by substituting carboplatin and reducing the schedule and cumulative dose of bleomycin as well as using attempts to shorten the duration of the traditional 5-day treatments to 3 days. In sum, none of these well-conceived efforts resulted in superior therapeutic profiles or clinically significant improvement in the acute toxicity profile while retaining therapeutic equivalence to BEP $\times$ 3.[14–17]

There have been investigations comparing BEP $\times$ 4 with EP $\times$ 4 and BEP $\times$ 3 with EP $\times$ 4 in favorable prognosis patients to test the relative therapeutic equivalence and comparative toxicities. deWit and colleagues[18] with the European Organisation for Research and Treatment of Cancer (EORTC) conducted a randomized trial of 4 cycles of BEP compared with 4 cycles of EP in favorable prognosis patients. Patients were categorized by the local prognostic system at the time, not the International Germ Cell Consensus Classification (IGCCC), but most patients fell into the Indiana University minimal disease classification; 419 patients were randomized to receive either BEP $\times$ 4 or EP $\times$ 4. Patients received a nonstandard dose of etoposide (120 mg/m^2, days 1, 3, and 5 of the regimen) compared with American BEP (100 mg/m^2 daily $\times$ 5). With treatment, 87% of patients allocated to EP $\times$ 4 achieved complete response compared with 95% of those allocated to BEP $\times$ 4 ($P = .0075$). At 7.3 years' median follow-up, 8 patients in each arm (4%) relapsed. Given the low incidence of unfavorable outcomes, no significant differences could be detected in progression-free or overall survival. In this schedule of 4 cycles of therapy, there were significant differences in neurotoxicity and acute pulmonary toxicity. Two patients on the BEP $\times$ 4 arm died with death attributable to bleomycin. Overall, in this large randomized trial in favorable patients with germ cell tumor, it was concluded that bleomycin was associated with additional toxicity but was an essential component that could not be deleted without sacrificing favorable therapeutic outcomes.

Finally, Culine and colleagues[19] in the French Federation of Cancer Centers Genito-Urinary Group conducted the logical concluding trial in this sequence, which compared the standard therapy for good-risk germ cell tumors, BEP × 3, with the 4-cycle regimen popularized at Memorial Sloan-Kettering, EP × 4. With the exception of deletion of bleomycin in the EP × 4, dose and schedule were American BEP, with bleomycin (30 units, days, 1, 8, and 15) with cisplatin (20 mg/m^2 daily, days 1–5) and etoposide (100 mg/m^2 daily, days 1–5). This trial was powered for equivalence and again the initial prognostic system used was the prevailing regional system and not the IGCCC; 257 eligible patients were randomized and analyzed. There was no statistical difference in obtaining complete remission by arm (BEP ×3:94% vs EP ×4:96%). Twenty patients relapsed (6 on BEP × 3 vs 14 on EP × 4) and 17 died (5 BEP × 3 vs 12 EP × 4). There were no treatment-related deaths. There was no statistical difference in pulmonary toxicity. The trial was not powered to examine event-free survival or overall survival. When these parameters were analyzed by either the prevailing prognostic system at the time of the study or after re-analysis using standardized the IGCCCC, no significant trends favoring BEP × 3 were shown. The authors and most world experts have interpreted this trial as definitive, and the risk of jeopardizing a large group of good-risk patients to what may well be substandard, equitoxic therapy to answer this question statistically was not felt to be merited. The primacy of BEP × 3 as standard therapy for IGCCC good-risk patients was upheld and has now been endorsed by emerging guidelines worldwide.

INTERMEDIATE-PROGNOSIS AND POOR-PROGNOSIS DISEASE

After the demonstration of BEP × 4 as standard therapy for disseminated disease in 1987 and the early recognition of adverse clinical factors associated with relatively poor outcomes, clinical investigation for patients with moderate risk or high risk of failure were steered toward demonstrating approaches with potential increased therapeutic activity. It was recognized that such approaches were likely more toxic, but in young patients facing up to a 50% risk of failure and death, such anticipated toxicity was felt justified.

The initial defining trial in this series stemmed from initial reports in germ cell tumors and in other malignancies that chemotherapy dose intensity was key to improving therapeutic outcome. There was clear-cut evidence in germ cell tumors that less-than-standard cisplatin dose intensity resulted in worse outcomes and it was logical and timely to assume that the dose-intensity curve continued upward and that higher-than-standard dose intensity would result in improved disease control.

This concept led to one of the first large-scale tests of the concept of dose intensity in oncology. Most of the evidence of benefit of high dose intensity in germ cell tumors came from phase II studies or retrospective analysis of dose received. Nichols and colleagues[20] at Indiana University, the Southeastern Cancer Study Group, and the Southwest Oncology Group conducted a randomized trial of standard BEP × 4 (cisplatin 100 mg/m^2/cycle) versus the same schedule and dose of bleomycin and etoposide but with a doubling of the cisplatin dose (200 mg/m^2/cycle) in patients with poor-risk germ cell tumors by the Indiana University classification system; 159 patients were randomized. As expected, the high-dose arm was more toxic, with significantly increased ototoxicity, neurotoxicity, and hematologic toxicity. Despite this, there were only 3 toxic deaths on the high-dose arm compared with 1 toxic death on the standard-dose arm. Two of the 4 deaths were attributed to bleomycin pulmonary toxicity in this 4-course regimen. Despite increased toxicity and chemotherapy delivery, there were no therapeutic differences between the two treatment arms. BEP × 4 remained the standard chemotherapy regimen for intermediate-prognosis and poor-prognosis disease.

The next large-scale attempt to improve therapeutic outcome in patients with poorer prognosis germ cell tumors was the US Intergroup trial comparing standard therapy (BEP × 4) to an experimental arm of etoposide and cisplatin with the substitution of ifosfamide for bleomycin (VIP × 4).[21,22] This concept was based on the impressive single-agent activity of ifosfamide in patients with recurrent or cisplatin-resistant disease and activity of VIP as salvage therapy for those failing BEP[23]; 286 patients with advanced disease by the Indiana University criteria were fully assessable for response and toxicity. There was no difference in favorable response (VIP, 63% and BEP, 60%) and 2-year disease-free survival (VIP, 63% and BEP, 60%) or 2-year overall survival (VIP, 74% and BEP, 71%). Significant pulmonary toxicity was seen in 7 patients on BEP and 6 patients on VIP. The details of the pulmonary toxicity were deemed particularly important in light of the use of bleomycin. Among the 7 patients who received BEP who experienced pulmonary toxicity, 3 experienced difficulty with course 1 (postobstructive pneumonia, pulmonary embolus, and hemorrhage) and, in the 2 survivors of the first course, the patients continued bleomycin throughout the course of treatment. One patient had a diminished diffusion capacity on day 14 of course 2 and bleomycin was discontinued, and 3 patients experienced toxicity with the fourth course and bleomycin was discontinued. Of the 6 patients on VIP who experienced pulmonary toxicity, 4 experienced toxicity with cycle 1 and 1 in conjunction with a febrile neutropenic event. There were 11 treatment-related deaths (5 on VIP and 6 on BEP). For those patients who received VIP, 4 died of sepsis and 1 of intracranial hemorrhage with the second course of treatment. For patients who received BEP, 1 died of pulmonary hemorrhage with the first course (questionably related to treatment), 1 died of respiratory failure (courses 1 and 4), and 3 died of sepsis. Grade 3 or worse toxicity, in particular hematologic toxicity and neurotoxicity, was significantly more common for patients receiving VIP. Based on equivalent therapeutic effect and lesser toxicity, BEP × 4 remained the standard of care for poor-risk patients with germ cell tumor.

The last attempt to improve outcomes in IGCCCC intermediate-risk and poor-risk germ cell tumors was the US intergroup trial comparing BEP × 4 to an experimental arm with BEP × 2 followed by 2 high-dose cycles of chemotherapy with carboplatin, etoposide, and cyclcophosphamide with stem cell support[24]; 219 patients with IGCCC intermediate-risk and poor-risk disease were randomized. The results reported by Motzer and colleagues[24] demonstrated that, as expected, the experimental arm was more toxic. There were no significant differences in therapy-related deaths. Ten patients (5%) died related to therapy: 6 in the high-dose arm and 4 in the standard-dose arm. No patients in either arm died related to bleomycin pulmonary toxicity. In terms of therapeutic outcomes, there was no significant difference in complete response (BEP × 4, 55% and high-dose chemotherapy, 56%). One-year survival was 83% and 2-year survival was 71% with no difference by assigned treatment arms. An exploratory endpoint of the study was to examine the rate of marker decline with therapeutic outcome. Within the subset of patients with unsatisfactory marker decline, patients randomized to high-dose chemotherapy had a statistically significant improvement in outcome whereas patients with satisfactory decline had a superior outcome with standard BEP.

Coordinated efforts in Europe and Australia tested similar concepts. French investigators compared BEP with cisplatin, doxorubicin, and cyclophosphamide alternated with vinblastine and bleomycin (CISC/VB) in intermediate-risk and poor-risk patients.[25] Kaye and colleagues[26] presented the results of a comparison of 6 cycles of BEP/EP to an experimental 6-cycle arm of bleomycin, vincristine, cisplatin/etoposide, ifosfamide, cisplatin, bleomycin (BOP/VIP-B). English investigators developed carboplatin, bleomycin, vincristine, cisplatin/bleomycin, etoposide, cisplatin and this currently is undergoing testing in a phase III trial compared with BEP in poor-risk patients.[27] Grimison and colleages[28] in Australia have explored dose-dense BEP in a phase II trial. The Scandinavian group, Swedish and Norwegian Testicular Cancer Project (SWENOTECA), has invoked an early intensification strategy for the Swedish/Norwegian population based on rate of marker decline or radiographic changes.[29] To date, no therapy has been demonstrated to be therapeutically superior to BEP × 4 and most experimental regimens are demonstrated to be more toxic than BEP. BEP × 4 remains the world standard for intermediate- or poor-prognosis disseminated germ cell tumors.

ERA OF DELIVERY (2005–PRESENT)

One of the major strategies for further improving testis cancer outcomes focuses on improving clinical decision support and consistent delivery of treatment across wide geographies. The underlying hypothesis is that there is a true center effect in play in germ cell tumors and that clinical outcomes, costs, and safety can all be favorably influenced by coordinated care through centers of excellence and experience.

Several lines of evidence support the hypothesis of a center effect. Harding and colleagues[30] in Britain analyzed patient outcomes for a single high-volume center versus low-volume centers. The hazard ratio (HR) for death was higher in the low-volume centers (HR 2.82; CI, 1.53–5.19; $P<.001$). Collette and colleagues[31] report on 360 IGCCCC intermediate-risk and poor-risk disseminated germ cell tumor patients registered in a clinical trial across Europe. There was a significant difference in overall survival between institutions entering fewer than 5 patients into the trial (primarily district general hospitals) and those entering 5 or more patients (mostly university hospitals and cancer centers). An increased HR of death of 1.85 (CI, 1.16–3.03; $P = .01$) was identified for those institutions entering fewer than 5 patients. The number of treatment-related deaths (6% vs 13%) and chemotherapy intensity also favored high-volume centers.

Similar surgical data from Germany strongly suggest that urologic surgical quality in germ cell tumors is higher in patients undergoing primary retroperitoneal lymph node dissection (RPLND) at high-volume centers. Albers and other German colleagues[32] conducted a randomized comparison of primary RPLND versus a single cycle of BEP in patients with clinical stage I nonseminoma. The nature of this trial was that it included many community-based institutions across Germany. There was a relatively high incidence of failures within the retroperitoneum (7/13 failures) as well as 2 scrotal recurrences among 173 patients assigned to primary RPLND. This rate of retroperitoneal failure (4%) is in contrast to the approximately 1% retroperitoneal failure rate seen for primary RPLND at German referral centers and other centers of surgical excellence.

Finally, there is emerging evidence from large population-based studies that centralized oversight and strict guideline adherence can lead to unprecedented outcomes for global management of disseminated germ cell tumors. The University of British Columbia and Oregon share a common setting of centralized management of germ cell tumors and common treatment guidelines. This consortium has reported results on 276 patients with disseminated germ cell tumors, which represent approximately 85% of patients in the State of Oregon and the province of British Columbia over this time frame.[33] Among this group of patients treated between 1998 and 2008, there were 8 deaths related to progressive germ cell tumor (3%). Across IGCCCC risk groups, there were 4 deaths (2%) among 246 IGCCCC good-risk patients, 0 deaths among11 intermediate-risk patients, and 4 deaths (14%) among

29 IGCCCC poor-risk patients. Patients were treated with risk-adapted BEP and appropriate candidates for surgery (eg, those with >1 cm residual disease) had surgery at the provincial or state high-volume center. Salvage therapies included standard but expert surgery and frequent incorporation of high dose chemotherapy and stem cell transplant.

A second similar population-based outcome is seen in the recent report of SWENO-TECA. Sweden and Norway have designated centers of excellence for treatment of germ cell tumors and centrally coordinated treatment guidelines.[29] The treatment protocol included an intensification strategy for those with unfavorable marker decline, but 75% of patients received standard BEP. Outcomes in this centrally managed population-based study were again excellent and exceeded predicted outcomes from IGCCC classification. Among 394 IGCCC good-risk patients, cause-specific survival was 96.3%, 93% among 113 intermediate-risk patients, and 69% among 95 IGCCC poor-risk patients. These 2 population-based studies report outcomes that match or exceed what is seen at single institutions and in clinical trials. The results are demonstrably better than national outcomes for the population as a whole.

For patients with regionally advanced or disseminated seminoma, these 2 groups report similar outcomes. The Oregon/British Columbia group reported on 104 patients with regional or disseminated disease.[34] Three-quarters of patients were treated with primary chemotherapy (almost all received BEP × 3). There were no cancer-related deaths among these 104 patients with regional or disseminated disease. There were 2 treatment-related deaths related to stroke, hyperosmolar coma, and renal failure. SWENOTECA reports similar results.[35] Among 73 patients with stage IIA/IIB seminoma treated with chemotherapy, there were no relapses and no deaths. Six (14%) of 42 patients with stage IIC seminoma disease recurred. Of the 44 patients with disseminated disease (stage III), 4 recurred with 3 deaths. Overall there were 3 cancer deaths among 159 patients with regional/disseminated seminoma treated with primary chemotherapy (2%). EP × 4 was the standard given to almost all patients receiving chemotherapy. Both groups noted high efficacy for IIA/B seminoma treated with primary chemotherapy (aggregated data, 1 relapse among 138 patients) compared with 6 relapses among 48 stage IIA/B seminoma patients treated with primary radiation therapy (13%). A trend over time toward declining percentage of patients with regional seminoma in whom radiation was used as primary management was also noted. Overall, death from seminoma was rare in these centrally managed population-based studies with cause-specific survival in patients with regional or disseminated disease exceeding 98%.

In total, these reports strongly suggest that the remaining low hanging fruit in germ cell tumors seems to be insuring consistent delivery of standard treatment across broad geographies with central coordination of care for all aspects of management and referral of patients for tertiary services, such as postchemotherapy surgery and salvage treatments.

WORK-UP OF DISSEMINATED GERM CELL TUMORS

Work-up of patients with suspected regional or disseminated germ cell tumors is not complicated. The evaluation depends almost entirely on history (including survivorship profile) and physical examination (including examination of the remaining testis), simple laboratory parameters to determine liver and renal function, anatomic imaging and serum hCG, AFP, and LDH. The determination of IGCCC risk relative to marker elevation refers to the stable postorchiectomy markers. Anatomic imaging consists of chest, abdomen, and pelvic CT with intravenous contrast. The routine use of positron emission tomography increases radiation exposure, does not provide additional meaningful clinical information, and is not recommended. Routine imaging of brain or bone is not recommended unless there are clinical concerns regarding these sites or there are widely disseminated, high-volume metastases (IGCCC poor-risk disease).

At times, patients present with symptoms or metastatic disease and have not had an orchiectomy for tissue diagnosis. In this setting, orchiectomy is not mandatory in the pretreatment period if there is a diagnostic elevation of tumor markers (hCG and AFP) in a classic clinical setting or a biopsy of a metastatic sight has established the diagnosis. Chemotherapy is administered first and the testicular primary is removed post-treatment often in conjunction with the postchemotherapy RPLND.

Formal assessment of pulmonary function in all patients is not recommended. In all patients receiving bleomycin, frequent history and physical examination should be performed to elicit symptoms and signs of early pulmonary complications.

The evaluation as outlined provides the substrate to determine the survivorship and treatment plan. Key issues that must be addressed initially are fertility and fertility preservation; physiologic, financial, psychological, and social barriers to effective treatment; patient education; and engagement. For patients without completed families and who desire this option, guidelines and experts recommend consideration of semen analysis and cryopreservation before definitive treatment. Most patients do recover endogenous sperm production to sufficient levels after BEP chemotherapy and many of those who require postchemotherapy surgery are able to have nerve-sparing procedures that allow for antegrade ejaculation.

PRACTICAL DELIVERY OF BEP

Best chemotherapy outcomes in regional and disseminated germ cell tumors depends on timely and safe delivery of standard cisplatin, etoposide, and bleomycin. Doses and schedules of BEP are standardized. There are clinical data suggesting that significant deviations in dose and timing from the well-defined schedule have meaningful negative impacts on outcomes. Also, standard dose and schedule BEP, when given by attentive and experienced chemotherapists with modern supportive care, is remarkably safe with low incidence of intolerable nausea and vomiting, neutropenic fever, and less than 1% incidence of fatal complications of treatment.

Practical Management of Hematologic Complications

In good-risk patients receiving standard BEP, the primary hematologic complication is transient neutropenia. Significant anemia or thrombocytopenia is rare. Neutropenic fever is uncommon and occurs in approximately 15% of cycles in good-risk patients. In patients with more advanced disease or associated poor performance status, the incidence approaches 40% with identical doses and schedules of chemotherapy.

Most centers and most guidelines do not recommend routine prophylactic hematopoietic growth factors in patients with good-risk disease and reserve hematopoietic growth factors for those patients presenting with intermediate-risk or poor-risk disease, those rare patients who present with significantly impaired performance status, those receiving salvage chemotherapy, and those with a history of abdominal/pelvic radiation Those good-risk patients who experience neutropenic fever with initial chemotherapy cycles receive hematopoietic growth factors as secondary prophylaxis. Fossa and colleagues[36] reported the results of a randomized trial of filgrastim prophylaxsis in patients receiving either BEP/EP × 6 or BOP/VIP-B × 6 as primary therapy for intermediate-prognosis and poor-prognosis germ cell tumors.

Treatment with filgrastim was associated with higher dose intensity and schedule adherence. Neutropenic fever occurred in 25 of 128 patients receiving filgrastim and 38 of 129 patients who did not ($P = .052$). Twelve toxic deaths occurred among patients who did not receive filgrastim and 3 toxic deaths among patients who did receive filgrastim. Nine of 12 and 3 of 3 of the toxic deaths were associated with grade IV neutropenia. Overall, there was no difference in failure-free and overall survival associated with the use of filgrastim.

Initiation of chemotherapy should not be delayed based on blood counts. Cycles should start every 21 days without dose attenuation or delay. Holidays or vacations are not suitable reasons to alter the schedule. Nursing colleagues should receive specific instructions regarding treating patients with sometimes astonishing low counts and be reassured that these young patients typically have rapid hematopoietic recovery without initiation of growth factors or dose attenuation or delay.

Management of Chemotherapy-Induced Nausea and Vomiting

BEP combination chemotherapy is highly emetogenic and requires appropriate levels of antiemetic support. Also, delayed nausea and vomiting can be pronounced in this population receiving multiday cisplatin. Optimizing control of both acute and delayed nausea and vomiting is critical to managing fluid balance and keeping patients on schedule. A human substance P/neurokinin 1 receptor antagonist (such as aprepitant) combined with dexamethasone and a 5-hydroxytryptamine3 antagonist (such as ondansetron) is recommended.

Management of Potential Nephrotoxicity

Aggressive prechemotherapy and postchemotherapy hydration is the key to minimizing nephrotoxic consequences of cisplatin-based chemotherapy. If a patient is receiving chemotherapy as an outpatient, at least 1 L of normal saline is given before initiation of cisplatin and 1.5 to 3 additional L after cisplatin each day. Patients should be encouraged to drink liquids aggressively and report significant vomiting immediately. Patients frequently gain a significant amount of water weight over the course of each 5-day session, but this mobilizes rapidly and does not require diuretics for management.

Invariably, patients have some wasting of magnesium, calcium, and potassium over the course of treatment. Rarely is this of clinical consequence. The common practice of adding magnesium to intravenous fluids does not prevent ongoing renal losses and is not recommended.

Management of Potential Bleomycin Complications

Bleomycin is an essential drug for optimal management of testicular cancer and can be given safely in almost all patients. In published experiences of 3 cycles of BEP, deaths from toxicity of any type are rare and in particular it is difficult to find patients in a modern series who have died of bleomycin toxicity. In 4 cycles of BEP, fewer than 1% of patients in large clinical trials are reported to have died from bleomycin pulmonary toxicity. There are some common precautions and ongoing assessments, however, that can help identify early those few patients who may be developing preliminary signs of toxicity. The first challenge is to identify patients who may be at particular risk for bleomycin toxicity. Patients with demonstrable severe lung compromise, patients with significantly reduced renal function, and older patients are at heightened risk. In addition, in good-risk patients, the risk of bleomycin (BEP × 3) must be balanced against the toxicity of the obligate additional course of cisplatin (EP × 4), if bleomycin were deleted, as well as balanced against the potential of losing therapeutic punch by eliminating bleomycin from the regimen. Second, it must be recognized that it is difficult to predict bleomycin lung disease, particularly based on changes in pulmonary function tests.[37] A practical approach to this problem is to reserve EP or VIP for those few good-risk patients who have significant contraindications to bleomycin. All patients who receive bleomycin should be informed of the necessity of reporting pulmonary symptoms, such as a dry cough. Patients should be queried for such symptoms on a regular basis during chemotherapy. Patients should also have a pulmonary examination by the provider with each cycle of therapy to discern if there is an inspiratory lag or the development of dry or Velcro rales. Bleomycin should be discontinued if pneumonitis is suspected. For patients scheduled to receive 3 cycles of BEP in whom bleomycin is discontinued, a fourth cycle of chemotherapy using etoposide and cisplatin should be administered. In patients scheduled to receive 4 cycles of BEP in whom bleomycin is discontinued, VIP may be substituted for BEP in the remaining cycles.

Bleomycin skin changes are common and usually transitory. Bleomycin should not be held or eliminated based on skin streaking, painful nodules on digits, or discoloration.

SUMMARY

The discovery and development of highly curative primary chemotherapy for disseminated germ cell tumor is one of the most storied events in modern medical oncology. Almost 50 years of thoughtful clinical investigations have resulted in a mature and nearly universally accepted combination chemotherapy regimen for patients presenting with or developing regional or disseminated disease. Treatment in these settings with standard BEP can be delivered safely by experienced and attentive chemotherapists and leads to cure rates that exceed 95%. Acute effects of treatment can largely be ameliorated with aggressive supportive care. The full profile of long-term effects and early interventions for potential late effects awaits complete definition. For the foreseeable future, investigative efforts should concentrate on insuring consistent delivery of chemotherapy and applying center-based experience in uncommonly required adjuncts to BEP, such as postchemotherapy surgery and, rarely, salvage treatments. The discovery, development, and delivery of cisplatin combination should serve as a substantial point of pride for clinical investigatiors in cancer and, hopefully, lessons learned in this process can continue to illuminate the process for investigations in other diseases.

REFERENCES

1. Rosenberg B, van Camp L, Krigas T. Inhibition of cell division in Escherichia coli by electrolysis products from a platinum electrode. Nature 1965;205:698–9.
2. Lippman A, Helson C, Helson L, et al. Clinical trials of cis- diamminedichloroplatinum (NSC-119875). Cancer Treat Rep 1973;57:191–200.
3. Einhorn L, Donohue J. Cis-diamminedichloroplatinum, vinblastine, and bleomycin combination chemotherapy in disseminated testicular cancer. Ann Intern Med 1977;87:293–8.
4. Einhorn LH, Williams SD. Chemotherapy of disseminated testicular cancer. Cancer 1980;46:1339–44.
5. Einhorn LH, Williams SD, Troner M, et al. The role of maintenance therapy in disseminated testicular cancer. N Engl J Med 1981;305:727–31.
6. Williams SD, Einhorn LH, Greco FA, et al. VP-16-213 salvage therapy for refractory germinal neoplasms. Cancer 1980;46:2154–8.

7. Williams SD, Birch R, Einhorn LH, et al. Treatment of disseminated germ-cell tumors with cisplatin, bleomycin, and either vinblastine or etoposide. N Engl J Med 1987;316(23):1435–40.
8. Birch R, Williams S, Cone A, et al. Prognostic factors for favorable outcome in disseminated germ cell tumors. J Clin Oncol 1986;4:786–92.
9. Bosl GJ, Geller NL, Cirnncione C, et al. Multivariate analysis of prognostic variables in patients with metastatic testicular cancer. Cancer Res 1983;43:3403–7.
10. International Germ-Cell Cancer Collaborative Group. International Germ-Cell Consensus Classification: a prognostic factor-based staging system for metastatic germ-cell cancers. J Clin Oncol 1997;15:594–603.
11. Einhorn LH, Williams SD, Loehrer PJ, et al. Evaluation of optimal duration of chemotherapy in favorable-prognosis disseminated germ cell tumors: a Southeastern Cancer Study Group protocol. J Clin Oncol 1989;7:387–91.
12. Saxman SB, Finch D, Gonin R, et al. Long-term follow-up of a phase III study of three versus four cycles of bleomycin, etoposide, and cisplatin in favorable-prognosis germ-cell tumors: the Indiana University experience. J Clin Oncol 1998;16:702–6.
13. Loehrer PJ, Johnson D, Elson P, et al. Importance of bleomycin in favorable-prognosis disseminated germ cell tumors: an Eastern Cooperative Oncology Group trial. J Clin Oncol 1995;13:470–6.
14. Bajorin DF, Sarosdy MF, Pfister DG, et al. Randomized trial of etoposide and cisplatin versus etoposide and carboplatin in patients with good-risk germ cell tumors: a multiinstitutional study. J Clin Oncol 1993;11(4):598–606.
15. Horwich A, Sleijfer DT, Fosså SD, et al. Randomized trial of bleomycin, etoposide, and cisplatin compared with bleomycin, etoposide, and carboplatin in good-prognosis metastatic nonseminomatous germ cell cancer: a Multiinstitutional Medical Research Council/European Organization for Research and Treatment of Cancer Trial. J Clin Oncol 1997;15(5):1844–52.
16. Bokemeyer C, Köhrmann O, Tischler J, et al. A randomized trial of cisplatin, etoposide and bleomycin (PEB) versus carboplatin, etoposide and bleomycin (CEB) for patients with 'good-risk' metastatic non-seminomatous germ cell tumors. Ann Oncol 1996;7(10):1015–21.
17. Grimison P, Stockler M, Thomson D, et al. Comparison of two standard chemotherapy regimens for good-prognosis germ cell tumors: updated analysis of a randomized trial. J Natl Cancer Inst 2010;102:1253–62.
18. deWit R, Stoter G, Kaye SB, et al. Importance of bleomycin in combination chemotherapy for good-prognosis testicular nonseminoma: a randomized study of the European organization for research and treatment of cancer genitourinary tract cancer cooperative group. J Clin Oncol 1997;15:1837–43.
19. Culine S, Kerbrat P, Kramar A, et al. Refining the optimal chemotherapy regimen for good-risk metastatic nonseminomatous germ-cell tumors: a randomized trial of the Genito-Urinary Group of the French Federation of Cancer Centers (GETUG T93BP). Ann Oncol 2007;18:917–24.
20. Nichols C, Williams S, Loehrer P, et al. Randomized study of cisplatin dose intensity in advanced germ cell tumors: a Southeastern Cancer Study Group and Southwest Oncology Group protocol. J Clin Oncol 1991;9:1163–72.
21. Nichols CR, Catalano PJ, Crawford ED, et al. Randomized comparison of cisplatin and etoposide and either bleomycin or ifosfamide in treatment of advanced disseminated germ cell tumors: an Eastern Cooperative Oncology Group, Southwest Oncology Group, and Cancer and Leukemia Group B Study. J Clin Oncol 1998;16:1287–93.

22. Hinton S, Catalano PJ, Einhorn LH, et al. Cisplatin, etoposide and either bleomycin or ifosfamide in the treatment of disseminated germ cell tumors: final analysis of an intergroup trial. Cancer 2003;97(8):1869–75.

23. Wheeler BM, Loehrer PJ, Williams SD, et al. Ifosfamide in refractory male germ cell tumors. J Clin Oncol 1986;4:28–34.

24. Motzer RJ, Nichols CR, Margolin KA, et al. Phase III randomized trial of conventional-dose chemotherapy with or without high-dose chemotherapy and autologous hematopoietic stem-cell rescue as first-line treatment for patients with poor-prognosis metastatic germ cell tumors. J Clin Oncol 2007; 25:247–56.

25. Culine S, Kramar A, Théodore C, et al. randomized trial comparing bleomycin/ etoposide/cisplatin with alternating cisplatin/cyclophosphamide/doxorubicin and vinblastine/bleomycin regimens of chemotherapy for patients with intermediate- and poor-risk metastatic nonseminomatous germ cell tumors: Genito-Urinary Group of the French Federation of Cancer Centers Trial T93MP. J Clin Oncol 2008;26(3):421–7.

26. Kaye SB, Mead GM, Fossa S, et al. Intensive induction-sequential chemotherapy with BOP/VIP-B compared with treatment with BEP/EP for poor-prognosis metastatic nonseminomatous germ cell tumor: a Randomized Medical Research Council/European Organization for Research and Treatment of Cancer study. J Clin Oncol 1998;16:692–701.

27. Christian JA, Huddart RA, Norman A, et al. Intensive induction chemotherapy with CBOP/BEP in patients with poor prognosis germ cell tumors. J Clin Oncol 2003;21(5):871–7.

28. Grimison PS, Thomson DB, Stockler M, et al. Accelerated BEP for advanced germ cell tumors: an ongoing multicenter phase I/II trial. American Society of Clinical Oncology Genitourinary Cancers Symposium 2010 [abstract: 258].

29. Olofsson S, Dahl O, Jerkeman M, et al. Individualized intensification of treatment based on tumor marker decline in metastatic nonseminomatous germ cell testicular cancer (NSGCT): a report from the Swedish Norwegian Testicular Cancer Group, SWENOTECA. J Clin Oncol 2009;27(Suppl):15s [abstract: 5015].

30. Harding MJ, Paul J, Gillis CR, et al. Management of malignant teratoma: does referral to a specialist unit matter? Lancet 1993;341(8861):1666.

31. Collette L, Sylvester RJ, Stenning SP, et al. Impact of the treating institution on survival of patients with "poor-prognosis" metastatic nonseminoma. J Natl Cancer Inst 1999;91(10):839–46.

32. Albers P, Siener R, Krege S, et al. Randomized phase III trial comparing retroperitoneal lymph node dissection with one course of bleomycin and etoposide plus cisplatin chemotherapy in the adjuvant treatment of clinical stage I nonseminomatous testicular germ cell tumors: AUO trial AH 01/94 by the German Testicular Cancer Study Group. J Clin Oncol 2008;26(18):2966–72.

33. Kollmannsberger C, Daneshmand S, So A, et al. Management of disseminated nonseminomatous germ cell tumors with risk-based chemotherapy followed by response-guided postchemotherapy surgery. J Clin Oncol 2010; 28(4):537–42.

34. Kollmannsberger C, Tyldesley S, Moore C, et al. Evolution in management of testicular seminoma: population-based outcomes with selective utilization of active therapies. Ann Oncol 2011;22(4):808–14.

35. Tandstad T, Smaaland R, Solberg A, et al. Management of seminomatous testicular cancer: a binational prospective population-based study from the Swedish Norwegian Testicular Cancer Study Group. J Clin Oncol 2011;29:719–25.

36. Fossa SD, Kaye SB, Mead GM, et al. Filgrastim during combination chemotherapy of patients with poor- prognosis metastatic germ cell malignancy. European Organization for Research and Treatment of Cancer, Genito-Urinary Group, and the Medical Research Council Testicular Cancer Working Party, Cambridge, United Kingdom. J Clin Oncol 1998;16:716–24.

37. Houghton BB, Grimison PS, Toner GC, et al. The effect of pulmonary function testing on bleomycin dosing in germ cell tumors [abstract]. J Clin Oncol 2011; 29(Suppl 7):227.

A Review of Second-line Chemotherapy and Prognostic Models for Disseminated Germ Cell Tumors

Martin H. Voss, MD[a,b,c], Darren R. Feldman, MD[a,b,c],
George J. Bosl, MD[a,b,c], Robert J. Motzer, MD[a,b,c],*

KEYWORDS

• Testis cancer • Germ cell neoplasm • Salvage therapy
• Chemotherapy

Most patients who are diagnosed with germ cell tumors (GCT), including those who present with disseminated disease, have an excellent prognosis. At present, approximately 70% to 80% of patients with advanced GCT are cured with first-line cisplatin-based combination chemotherapy and adjunctive surgery.[1–5] Achievement of a complete remission (CR) to such treatment signifies an excellent chance of cure. In less than 10% of these patients, the GCT relapses.[6] However, an estimated 20% to 30% of patients presenting with metastatic GCT are either refractory to or show relapse of the condition after initial treatment.

The development of the International Germ Cell Cancer Collaboration Group (IGCCCG) classification of risk in 1997[7] improved the ability to estimate the risk of failure to first-line chemotherapy. This classification predicts that with standard cisplatin-based chemotherapy, approximately 10% of good-risk, 25% of intermediate-risk, and more than 50% of poor-risk patients will fail such treatment. Although in most malignancies, refractory or relapsed disease that is both not localized and not

Funding support: Supported by the Sidney Kimmel Center for Prostate and Urologic Cancers, New York, NY, USA, and the Craig Tifford Foundation.
[a] Department of Medicine, Memorial Sloan-Kettering Cancer Center, New York, NY, USA
[b] Genitourinary Oncology Service, Department of Medicine, Memorial Sloan-Kettering Cancer Center, New York, NY, USA
[c] Memorial Sloan-Kettering Cancer Center, 1275 York Avenue, New York, NY 10065, USA
* Corresponding author. Memorial Sloan-Kettering Cancer Center, 1275 York Avenue, New York, NY 10065.
E-mail address: motzerr@mskcc.org

Hematol Oncol Clin N Am 25 (2011) 557–576
doi:10.1016/j.hoc.2011.03.007
0889-8588/11/$ – see front matter © 2011 Elsevier Inc. All rights reserved.

amenable to surgical resection is considered incurable, a significant proportion of such patients with GCT can still be cured with either salvage conventional-dose chemotherapy (CDCT) or high-dose chemotherapy (HDCT) plus stem cell rescue with or without adjunctive surgery in the second-line or even third-line setting. A small proportion of patients with relapsed disease that is locally confined may achieve durable remissions with surgical resection alone.[8–10]

Because only a small number of patients require salvage therapy, few large prospective studies have been done to guide management in this setting. Rather, most data are derived from phase 2 trials and retrospective series. The optimal regimen, both for CDCT and HDCT, remains to be determined. Other central questions include (1) how to identify those patients likely to be cured with CDCT, thus avoiding the toxicity of high-dose therapy, and (2) how to identify patients who are unable to achieve cure with CDCT but might be cured with second-line HDCT.

This article reviews reports of initial salvage chemotherapy, including CDCT and HDCT, in patients with disseminated GCT refractory to or relapsing after the standard first-line chemotherapy. It also discusses the prognostic models as well as the salvage approach for special patient populations, such as those with late relapse.

CONVENTIONAL-DOSE CHEMOTHERAPY IN THE SECOND-LINE SETTING

Following seminal work in the 1970s and 1980s that established cisplatin as the essential component for treatment of disseminated disease[11,12] and marked the beginning of the modern era of chemotherapy for GCT, PVB (the combination of cisplatin, vinblastine, and bleomycin) was regarded as the standard of care in the first-line management of advanced GCT. Subsequent investigators identified salvage regimens for the 20% of patients unable to achieve CR and the 10% to 20% of patients in whom the condition relapsed after PVB therapy. In the early 1980s, etoposide was found to have activity in refractory GCT,[13] and subsequently, EP (the combination of etoposide and cisplatin) was shown to exhibit incomplete cross-resistance with PVB,[14,15] and thus became the standard salvage therapy for patients with disease progression after PVB therapy. Durable remissions to salvage therapy with EP, however, remained rare, and investigators continued searching for agents to combine with cisplatin and/or etoposide.

Cisplatin, Ifosfamide, and Vinblastine or Etoposide

In the mid 1980s, ifosfamide was found to have efficacy in patients with refractory GCT.[16,17] One trial using single-agent ifosfamide in heavily pretreated refractory patients reported an objective response rate (RR) of 23%.[17] However, the median duration of the response was short and the median overall survival (OS) was only 3.5 months. Several groups subsequently combined ifosfamide and cisplatin with either etoposide (VIP) or vinblastine (VeIP) to treat refractory disease.[18–23]

Initial reports from American and European groups included mixed populations receiving VIP or VeIP in the second-line, third-line, or later setting.[18,20,24,25] These trials established a 5-day regimen of cisplatin (100 mg/m^2 daily for 5 days) and ifosfamide (1.2 g/m^2 daily for 5 days) with either etoposide (75 mg/m^2 daily for 5 days) or vinblastine (0.11 mg/kg for 2 days) administered every 3 weeks as standard salvage chemotherapy, with CR rates in 25% to 36% of patients and median response durations between 3.5 and 34 months. Nephrotoxicity and myelosuppression were the main toxicities with these regimens.

Building on these reports, investigators evaluated these regimens in the initial salvage setting (**Table 1**).[21–23,26,27] In 1 series, 56 patients with advanced GCT

Table 1
VeIP/VIP for initial salvage therapy for advanced GCT

References	Regimen	Retrospective vs Prospective	No. Evaluable	CR (%)	Durable CR (%)
Pizzocarro et al[21]	VIP[a] or VeIP[a]	Retrospective	36	20 (56)	15 (42)
Farhat et al[26]	VIP[b] or VeIP[b]	Retrospective	54	24 (44)	10 (19)[b]
McCaffrey et al[22]	VIP or VeIP	Retrospective	56	20 (36)	13 (23)
Loehrer et al[23]	VeIP	Prospective	135	67 (50)	32 (24)
Pico et al[27]	VIP or VeIP	Prospective	122	51 (42)	31 (25)

Abbreviation: No, number.
[a] Modified dosing schedule as outlined in text.
[b] Seven of 24 with CR went on to receive consolidative high-dose chemotherapy with stem cell rescue.

resistant to 1 prior cisplatin-containing regimen were treated with 4 cycles of either VIP or VeIP.[22] The reported CR rate was 36%. An additional 15% of patients who did not undergo resection of the residual disease achieved marker-negative partial response (PR). With a median follow-up of 52 months, sustained CRs were seen in 23% of patients and the median OS was 18 months. French investigators from the Institut Gustave Roussy retrospectively reported their experience with second-line VIP/VeIP in 54 patients.[26] The CR rate after VIP/VeIP was 44%, with sustained CR in 19% of treated patients. However, nearly one-third of responders received consolidation with HDCT, making it difficult to interpret the durability of remissions to VIP/VeIP alone. With a 30-month median follow-up, sustained CRs were observed in 63% of those who attained a CR and then received HDCT versus 26% of those with CR without subsequent consolidative treatment. Toxicity profiles were similar for VIP and VeIP; 2 treatment-associated deaths occurred in patients receiving subsequent HDCT. A series from Italy documented 36 patients who failed first-line therapy with either PVB or BEP (a combination of bleomycin, etoposide, cisplatin) and went on to receive second-line treatment with modified versions of VIP or VeIP.[21] In an attempt to reduce renal toxicity, the dosing schedule was altered to avoid simultaneous administration of platinum and ifosfamide; dosages of ifosfamide and etoposide were also slightly reduced, whereas that of cisplatin was increased. The CR rate for all evaluable patients was 56%, and the sustained CR rates were 42%. Remission rates were higher for patients with prior PVB treatment who received modified VIP than for those receiving modified VeIP for progressive disease after prior BEP treatment. This result was not surprising given the known superiority of BEP over PVB in the first-line setting. Renal toxicity was less pronounced than in previous reports of patients receiving heavier pretreatment.

No prospective trial has compared the efficacy of VIP with that of VeIP in the second-line setting. Although PVB was the previous standard first-line regimen for disseminated GCT, VIP had generally been used more frequently for initial salvage because vinblastine was part of PVB. In 1987, a pivotal randomized trial by the Southeastern Cancer Study Group comparing BEP with PVB in the first-line treatment of disseminated GCT demonstrated superiority in the advanced disease subgroup and overall significantly less toxicity for BEP.[3] This study not only established this regimen as the standard of care for first-line treatment but also made VeIP the second-line therapy of choice because vinblastine had been replaced by etoposide in the first-line setting. The first prospective study to exclusively evaluate VeIP in the second-line setting was reported by Loehrer and colleagues[23] in 1998 and included

135 patients who were treated after failing to respond to a cisplatin/etoposide-based first-line regimen, mostly standard BEP (88%). Of 135 assessable patients, 67 (50%) achieved disease-free status; 32 (24%) patients remained in sustained CR with a minimum follow-up of 6 years. In this single-center study, the 2-, 3-, and 7-year survival rates were 38%, 35%, and 32%, respectively.[23] Prospective data for second-line VIP/VeIP are available from the European multicenter randomized phase 3 IT-94 trial,[27] which compared CDCT (VIP or VeIP) with 3 cycles of CDCT consolidated with 1 cycle of HDCT. The VIP/VeIP arm treated 136 patients and yielded a CR rate of 42% with sustained CRs in 26% at a median follow-up of 45 months. The trial's findings comparing CDCT with HDCT are discussed in detail later.

Paclitaxel-Containing Regimen

Early trials of paclitaxel in metastatic GCT were conducted after antitumor activity was seen in other malignancies, including breast and ovarian cancers,[28,29] and the efficacy of this regimen was demonstrated in platinum-refractory ovarian cancer,[30] making paclitaxel an attractive option for salvage therapy for disseminated GCT. Several small phase 2 trials of single-agent paclitaxel were reported. A study from Memorial Sloan-Kettering Cancer Center (MSKCC) treated 31 patients with limited prior therapy (second- and third-line settings) and poor prognostic features, such as incomplete response (IR) to prior therapy (76%) or extragonadal primaries (29%).[31] The results showed an overall response rate (ORR) of 26% including 3 CRs (10%); all responders remained disease free at the time of report. Of 8 patients with treatment response, 3 had primary mediastinal (PM) nonseminomatous (NS) GCT (PMNSGCT). Similarly, a German phase 2 trial treated 24 patients with a median of 7 prior cycles of platinum-containing therapy. The ORR was 25%, including PR in 2 patients who had previously received HDCT and in 1 patient with PMNSGCT. A CR rate of 8% was reported for this trial; the median response duration was 8 months. Additional early-phase trials in more heavily pretreated patients demonstrated slightly lower RRs but confirmed single agent activity for paclitaxel.[32,33]

Following these encouraging results, combination regimens containing paclitaxel were undertaken. Preclinical data showing synergy with cisplatin[34] led to the TIP regimen, which combined paclitaxel, ifosfamide, and cisplatin. Several phase 2 trials evaluated TIP in the initial salvage setting (**Table 2**).[35–37] The original report[38] was a combined phase 1 and 2 study of 30 patients who received 1 prior platinum-containing regimen. In the phase I portion, patients received escalating doses of paclitaxel, with 250 mg/m^2 as a 24-hour continuous infusion established as the maximum tolerated dose for the phase 2 portion of the trial. Paclitaxel was combined with ifosfamide, 6 g/m^2, plus mesna and cisplatin, 100 mg/m^2 per 21-day cycle, each administered over 4 to 5 days after completion of paclitaxel infusion. All patients received prophylactic growth factor support with granulocyte colony-stimulating factor on days 7 to 18. Recognizing earlier reports of low RRs to CDCT salvage therapy in patients with poor-risk features, and hypothesizing that such patients would likely benefit from more aggressive salvage therapy upfront, enrollment was limited to patients with favorable features, requiring all of the following: (1) prior treatment limited to 1 program, or 6 or less prior cycles of cisplatin, (2) gonadal primary site, and (3) best prior response to first-line chemotherapy of CR of any duration or marker-negative PR lasting 6 months or longer. After encouraging results with the first 30 patients, additional subjects were accrued to the phase 2 portion of this trial, and in 2005, the updated analysis of 46 patients with second-line TIP was published.[35] With a median follow-up of nearly 6 years, 32 (70%) of 46 patients achieved CR and 29 (63%) were continuously disease free. Myelosuppression, the major toxicity, was managed with

Table 2
Phase 2 initial salvage therapy with TIP in advanced GCT

References	Drug Doses (Per Cycle)	Selection Criteria	Evaluable	CR (%)	Additional Efficacy Data
Kondagunta et al[35]	Paclitaxel 250 mg/m^2 Ifosfamide 6000 mg/m^2 Cisplatin 100 mg/m^2	First-line salvage in patients with favorable features[a]	46	32 (70)	susCR 63% 2-year PFS 65% 2-year OS 78%
Mead et al[36]	Paclitaxel 175 mg/m^2 Ifosfamide 5000 mg/m^2 Cisplatin 100 mg/m^2	First-line salvage after failure to BEP	43	13 (31)	1-year FFS 38% 1-year OS 70%
Mardiak et al[37]	Paclitaxel 175 mg/m^2 Ifosfamide 6000 mg/m^2 Cisplatin 100 mg/m^2	First-line salvage after failure to cisplatin-based regimens	17	7 (41)	2-year DFS 47% 2-year OS 64%

Abbreviations: DFS, disease-free survival; FFS, failure-free survival; PFS, progression-free survival; susCR, sustained CR (median follow-up 69 mo); TIP, paclitaxel, ifosfamide, and cisplatin.
    [a] Must meet all the following: (1) gonadal primary site, (2) maximum 6 prior cycles of cisplatin (3) CR or PR with negative result for tumor markers after first-line chemotherapy.

growth factor support, whereas nephrotoxicity and neurotoxicity were not more severe than that described with other ifosfamide-based salvage CDCT regimens.

A second phase 2 study of second-line TIP was conducted as a multicenter trial through the British Medical Research Council (MRC).[36] Patients received paclitaxel, 175 mg/m^2; ifosfamide, 5 g/m^2; and cisplatin, 100 mg/m^2 per cycle, without prophylactic growth factor support. A total of 51 patients were included, all had received first-line therapy with BEP, and risk stratification was not part of the eligibility assessment (ie, patients with PMNSGCT as well as those with late relapse were included). The CR rate was 31%. With a median follow-up of 26 months, the 1-year failure-free survival (FFS) and OS were 38% (95% confidence interval [CI], 23%–53%) and 70% (95% CI, 56%–84%), respectively. Less-favorable features in this patient population (compared with those in the MSKCC study) may account for the lower CR rate. However, a subgroup analysis of the MRC trial demonstrated that patients with good-risk features had a CR rate of 35% with 1-year FFS and OS of 43% (95% CI, 23%–63%) and 81% (95% CI, 64%–98%), respectively.[36] Similarly, a small phase 2 trial from Slovakia treated 17 patients after failure to respond to cisplatin-based first-line therapy (mostly BEP [88%]) with 4 to 6 cycles of second-line dose-attenuated TIP (paclitaxel, 175 mg/m^2; ifosfamide, 6 g/m^2; and cisplatin 100 mg/m^2 per cycle). The CR rate, 2-year disease-free survival (DFS), and 2-year OS were 41%, 47% (95% CI, 23%–71%), and 64% (95% CI, 37%–91%), respectively.[37] The investigators identified the lower dose of paclitaxel as the primary reason for the inferior RRs and survival compared with the original report from MSKCC,[35] and this may similarly explain the more modest outcomes to TIP in the MRC study.

On the basis of phase 2 data for TIP and VeIP, a randomized phase 3 trial compared these regimens in the second-line setting, but terminated early because of poor accrual. Hence, both VeIP and TIP continue to be considered standard conventional-dose regimens in the salvage setting, although the single-arm series of TIP suggests this is the more active regimen.

Salvage HDCT

Following success with autologous bone marrow in relapsed hematologic malignancies during the 1970s,[39–44] studies were undertaken in several solid malignancies in the early 1980s.[45–48] This treatment was investigated in GCT because of known chemosensitivity, the dose-response phenomena of individual drugs with synergistic action, the rare occurrence of bone marrow metastasis, and a young patient population with low incidence of significant comorbidities. Characteristics of the drugs chosen for these studies included (1) antitumor activity in conventional doses without evidence that the dose-effect plateau had been reached and (2) myelosuppression, even at high doses, being the dominant adverse effect, a toxicity that could be modulated by autologous bone marrow infusion. In the case of GCT, carboplatin, etoposide, and cyclophosphamide fulfilled these requirements. Carboplatin was chosen over cisplatin because its predominant toxicity is myelosuppression but other adverse effects such as neurotoxicity and nephrotoxicity were not seen. Early phase 1 studies established safety for high-dose carboplatin and etoposide as single agents with and without the use of stem cell rescue.[49–52]

One noteworthy study of HDCT in GCT was a combined phase 1 and 2 trial reported in 1989.[53] The phase 1 portion established a regimen of etoposide, 1200 mg/m^2, and carboplatin, 1500 mg/m^2 per cycle, as the recommended dose. A total of 33 treatment-refractory patients received 1 to 2 cycles of HDCT followed by autologous stem cell rescue. Toxicities were significant, all patients developed severe myelosuppression and 7 treatment-related deaths (21%) were reported. However, the CR rate was 25% despite heavy pretreatment, and a subsequent publication of long-term follow-up (including additional patients treated on this program) reported sustained CR rates of 15%.[54] These results prompted further study of this treatment program in a multi-institutional phase 2 protocol sponsored by the Eastern Cooperative Oncology Group. Similar results were achieved (ORR 44%, CR sustained >1 year 13%, treatment-related deaths 13%).[55] Together, these studies demonstrated that HDCT could be curative, even in the third-line setting. They established the combination of high-dose (HD) carboplatin and etoposide as the basis for subsequent high-dose protocols.

Later efforts focused on confirming activity, increasing the number of patients who achieved durable responses, and reducing toxicity. Better tolerability has largely been achieved through the routine use of growth factor support as well as peripheral blood stem cells in lieu of autologous bone marrow rescue.[56,57] General improvements in supportive care and antibiotics also diminished the toxicity associated with HDCT, and with all the abovementioned measures treatment-related mortality has improved from greater than 20% initially to typically less than 3%.[58–60] Strategies to improve efficacy have included intensification of HD carboplatin/etoposide[56,59] as well as addition of other agents.[61–64] In 2007, an Indiana University group published a retrospective evaluation of 184 patients treated between 1996 and 2004,[59] 73% of whom were in the initial salvage setting. The HD regimen consisted of 2 cycles of carboplatin, 2100 mg/m^2, and etoposide, 2250 mg/m^2, both administered over 3 days and supported by autologous stem cell reinfusion, given in some patients after 1 to 2 cycles of VeIP. After a median follow-up of 4 years, 63% of patients were continuously disease free. PMNSGCTs and late relapses were not included in this trial because of previously observed poor outcomes with HDCT in these subgroups.[59] Other investigators have incorporated additional agents with carboplatin and etoposide into HDCT programs. This incorporation has been tolerable in the case of ifosfamide,[61,64] cyclophosphamide,[62] and paclitaxel[60] but has resulted in excessive toxicity for other combinations such as the addition of thiotepa.[63]

HDCT in the Second-Line Setting

The choice of CDCT versus HDCT is controversial in the initial salvage setting because there are limited data for guidance. A point made in favor of HDCT was its better tolerability in patients with less prior therapy.[65] In 1998, a large single-center series of 150 patients published by Rick and colleagues[64] retrospectively reported a heterogeneous population with respect to the timing of HDCT (first-line treatment vs initial salvage vs later salvage). A program of 3 cycles of CDCT followed by 1 cycle of HD VIP was used. For patients with good-risk Beyer scores (see section on Prognostic Factors),[56] the 2-year OS declined significantly depending on whether HDCT was used as first-line, first-salvage, or subsequent salvage treatment (78%, 66%, and 47%, respectively; $P<.05$). In a retrospective report from the Indiana University, 65 patients who received 2 cycles of HD carboplatin and etoposide with autologous stem cell rescue as initial salvage following relapse after standard cisplatin-based first-line therapy, demonstrated a continuous DFS rate of 57% with or without surgery at a median follow-up of more than 3 years.[66] All patients on this trial had one or more favorable features such as gonadal primary tumor and CR or marker-negative PR to first-line therapy.

Following these encouraging early results, European investigators retrospectively analyzed 193 patients treated with CDCT (119) versus HDCT (74) for first salvage treatment at several centers.[67] A matched-pair analysis between the 2 groups was undertaken using prognostic factors recognized in prior studies,[23,56,68–70] including primary site, response to first-line therapy, relapse-free interval, and tumor marker levels. A total of 38 pairs of patients from both groups were fully matched (all 5 criteria), and an additional 17 pairs were partly matched (4 of 5 criteria including primary site and response to first-line therapy). For these 55 pairs, multivariate analyses examined event-free survival and OS as primary end points. Hazard ratios for OS favoring HDCT ranged between 0.77 and 0.83 (95% CI, 0.60%–0.99%), whereas those for event-free survival showed a trend ranging between 0.72 and 0.84 (95% CI, 0.59%–1.01%). Of note, salvage regimens in the CDCT group contained ifosfamide and etoposide in 36% and 63% of patients, respectively, whereas all patients in the HDCT group were treated with 3 cycles of VIP followed by 1 cycle of HD carboplatin/ifosfamide/etoposide.

The only prospective, randomized study to address the question of the optimal initial salvage approach was the IT-94 trial, a randomized phase 3 trial comparing HDCT with CDCT for second-line therapy. This European multicenter study enrolled 280 patients from 43 institutions in 11 countries between 1994 and 2001.[27] Through 1:1 randomization, the trial compared the efficacy of 4 cycles of CDCT using VIP/VeIP with 3 cycles of the same CDCT followed by 1 cycle of CarboPEC (HDCT using carboplatin [200–550 mg/m^2], etoposide [1800 mg/m^2], and cyclophosphamide [200 mg/kg]) with stem cell rescue in patients who failed first-line cisplatin-based therapy (85% standard BEP or EP regimens). Response to salvage treatment was similar in both groups, with CR rates for CDCT and HDCT of 42% and 43%, respectively; treatment-related mortality was 3% and 7%. With a median follow-up of 45 months, the sustained CR rates were 26% and 35%. No survival benefit was seen for the HDCT arm. This study has recognized the following limitations: (1) only 1 cycle of HDCT was given, whereas 2 to 3 cycles of HDCT are widely accepted as the standard of care; (2) in the HDCT group, only 81% of patients actually proceeded to receive CarboPEC following 3 cycles of CDCT; (3) patients refractory to first-line platinum-containing chemotherapy were excluded; and (4) many centers recruited as few as 1 to 3 patients in the trial, which may have compromised the safety and efficacy of HDCT.

An unplanned subgroup analysis from IT-94 demonstrated that among those patients who achieved a CR to salvage chemotherapy, the 2-year DFS was superior in the HDCT arm. The investigators concluded that future strategies for optimizing HDCT should include multivariate prognostic analyses to identify those patients who were likely to benefit from this approach.[27] A large, more recent international study took this approach. A retrospective analysis of initial salvage chemotherapy in almost 1600 subjects treated at multiple centers worldwide was performed to identify prognostic factors.[71] Approximately equal numbers of patients were treated with CDCT and HDCT. The use of modern first-line and salvage regimens was required for inclusion in the report. On multivariate analysis, prognostic factors that allowed patient stratification into 5 well-defined categories were identified. These data have been further developed and through inclusion of additional patients, have been used to develop a prognostic model for initial salvage therapy regardless of the treatment intensity (see section on Prognostic Models).[72] There was a similar distribution among the 5 prognostic categories for CDCT and HDCT. Despite this, superior progression-free survival (PFS) and OS were seen for HDCT in each category with the exception of OS in the low-risk group.[71] Because of the retrospective nature of this analysis, selection bias is likely a factor behind the favorable outcomes in patients treated with HDCT. A prospective trial comparing sequential HDCT with CDCT as initial salvage is planned.

Choosing second-line therapy for relapsed or recurrent GCT varies. HDCT is considered a standard approach by some investigators, whereas others favor reserving HDCT for the third-line setting to avoid unnecessary toxicity in patients who might potentially be cured with CDCT. The approach at MSKCC is to base initial salvage chemotherapy decisions on prognostic models for CDCT and HDCT.

Prognostic Factors

Although prognostic factors at the initiation of first-line chemotherapy for disseminated GCT are universally accepted, there has previously been no agreement on risk stratification after failure of first-line therapy. Clinical variables that could help predict response to salvage therapy had largely been based on relatively small or single-center retrospective series and early-phase clinical trials. The unresolved question of CDCT versus HDCT has further complicated stratification because prognostic factors had typically been analyzed separately for each entity and could not be readily applied to each other.[73] Lastly, patient populations are heterogeneous as to the extent of prior therapy as well as the first-line and salvage regimens used, making the development of a practical model challenging. Although several groups have systematically applied their findings in selecting patients for subsequent trials and determining whether to opt for CDCT or HDCT,[35,59,60] agreement had not been reached on a universal model until recently.

For CDCT salvage regimens, earlier retrospective series and phase 2 trials identified best response to first-line therapy and location of primary tumor as predictors of response to second- and third-line therapies.[20–23] The authors' group retrospectively reviewed 124 patients who had been treated on 4 prospective trials and failed to achieve a sustained CR, 94 of whom went on to receive second-line therapy. It was determined that response to salvage therapy was significantly enhanced in patients with a prior CR to first-line chemotherapy, testis primary site, normal L-lactate dehydrogenase levels, normal human chorionic gonadotropin (HCG) levels, and 1 site of metastasis.[68] Similarly, a European multicenter retrospective analysis of 164 patients treated in the initial salvage setting reported 3 independent variables of prognostic significance, including progression-free interval, response to induction treatment, and levels of serum markers (HCG and α fetoprotein [AFP]) at relapse.[70] Multivariate analysis from a German report of 60 patients treated with initial salvage chemotherapy identified age less than 35 years, CR to primary treatment, and relapse-free interval greater than 3 months as independent predictors for successful salvage treatment.[74]

For salvage HDCT, several specific variables predictive of a poor outcome have been reported, including pretreatment levels of HCG,[62] PMNSGCT,[75,76] and absolute refractory disease (defined as no marker response to initial treatment).[77] In addition to individual factors, several prognostic models have been developed to help stratify patients in consideration of HDCT. In 1996, Beyer and colleagues[56] retrospectively performed a multivariate analysis of 310 patients treated with at least 1 cycle of salvage HDCT at 4 centers in the United States and Europe. Progressive disease (PD) before HDCT, PMNSGCT, refractory or absolute refractory disease to conventional-dose cisplatin, and HCG levels greater than 1000 U/L were identified as independent adverse prognostic indicators of survival after HDCT. A scoring system based on these risk factors, referred to as the Beyer score,[56] was established to categorize patients as having good (0 points), intermediate (up to 2 points), or poor prognosis (>2 points), with reliable discrimination in regard to RR, proportion of patients in whom the condition relapsed, FFS, and OS (all with $P<.001$). Of note, more than 90% of the patients treated in this European series received a single HDCT course and most were treated with 2 or more regimens before HDCT.

These findings could not be reproduced in a later report from Indiana University evaluating patients with less-extensive prior therapy.[78] Subsequently, investigators from the Indiana University developed a separate prognostic model for HDCT based on 184 patients with testicular GCT treated between 1996 and 2004.[59] Patients with late relapse (>2 years) and PMNSGCT were not included in this analysis because of poor results seen previously in this population.[78] Multivariate analysis identified 3 significant predictors of adverse DFS: (1) IGCCCG poor-risk classification at initial diagnosis, (2) platinum-refractory disease defined as tumor progression within 4 weeks after the most recent cisplatin-based chemotherapy, and (3) receipt of HDCT as third-line or subsequent chemotherapy. Based on these factors, patients were classified into 3 prognostic groups based on their total score (referred to as the Einhorn score). Sustained DFS was approximately 80%, 60%, and 40% for patients with low-, inter-mediate-, and high-risk Einhorn scores, respectively.[59] The Beyer score did not reliably predict DFS in this patient population ($P = .25$).

The authors' group evaluated prognostic factors in a series of 107 patients treated with 2 courses of rapidly recycled (every 14 days) conventional-dose paclitaxel and ifosfamide for stem cell mobilization, followed by 3 cycles of HD carboplatin and eto-poside (TI-CE) plus stem cell support.[60] This HDCT trial targeted patients predicted for a poor prognosis to conventional salvage therapy by requiring at least 1 unfavorable prognostic feature for enrollment, including extragonadal primary site, PD following an IR to first-line chemotherapy, and PD after cisplatin plus ifosfamide–based CDCT salvage. Nearly half of patients (47%) achieved 5-year DFS. Factors predicting unfavorable DFS or OS to TI-CE included mediastinal primary tumor site, HCG levels of 1000 U/mL or more, 2 or more lines of prior therapy, 3 or more metastatic sites, and IGCCCG intermediate- or poor-risk classification at diagnosis.[60] The study also tested both the Einhorn and Beyer prognostic models for their ability to predict DFS. Whereas findings were partially reproduced, the 2 models could not be fully applied because of the differences in eligibility criteria.[60] The lack of complete reproducibility of the Einhorn and Beyer models in the TI-CE series demonstrates the limitations of these prediction rules, each developed in specific patient populations with varying clinical features, prior management, and HDCT regimens.

The International Prognostic Factor Study Group recently presented their prognostic model for initial salvage therapy independent of regimen intensity (**Table 3**).[72] This series comprised a total of 1984 patients from 38 centers throughout 14 countries in Europe and North America. Seven factors were significant for PFS on multivariate analysis, including histology (seminoma vs nonseminoma), primary tumor site (medi-astinal vs retroperitoneal vs gonadal), response to first-line chemotherapy (CR vs PR vs other), progression-free interval after first-line chemotherapy, AFP levels at salvage, HCG levels at salvage, and the presence of nonpulmonary visceral metas-tases. Each factor was assigned a point value, and a sum score was calculated for each patient. Depending on the scores, the patients were divided into 5 risk groups (very low, low, intermediate, high, and very high) with distinct PFS and OS rates regardless of the treatment intensity.[72] The large international and multicenter popu-lation in this study, the strict definition of inclusion criteria and salvage regimen, as well as this model's ability to predict outcomes to both HDCT and CDCT initial salvage approaches allows wider applicability than prior prognostic systems. This scoring system is regarded as the new standard predictive model in the relapsed/refractory setting.

Table 3
International prognostic model for initial salvage therapy in the relapsed/refractory setting

Factors		Points
Primary Site	Gonadal	0
	Retroperitoneal	1
	Mediastinal (NSGCT)	3
Response to 1st line	CR/PR−	0
	PR+/SD	1
	PD	2
Progression-free interval after first line	>3 mo	0
	≤3 mo	1
Serum HCG levels	≤1000 IU/L	0
	>1000 IU/L	1
Serum AFP levels	Normal	0
	≤1000 ng/mL	1
	>1000 ng/mL	2
Liver, bone, or brain metastases	Absent	0
	Present	1

Add points to determine the preliminary score (0–10). Scores of 0, 1–2, 3–4, and ≥5 correspond to categories 0, 1, 2, and 3, respectively.

Add histology points (below) to category score to determine the final risk category.

Histology		
	Seminoma	−1
	NSGCT/mixed	0

Risk Category	Score	2-y PFS (%)	3-y OS (%)
Very low risk	−1	75	77
Low risk	0	51	66
Intermediate risk	1	40	58
High risk	2	26	27
Very high risk	3	6	6

Abbreviations: AFP, alpha fetoprotein; CR, complete response; DFS, disease free survival; FFS, failure free survival; hCG, human chorionic gonadotropin; NSGCT, nonseminomatous germ cell tumor; OS, overall survival; PD, progression of disease; PFS, progression free survival; PR−, partial response with negative markers; PR+, partial response with positive markers; SD, stable disease.

Data from Lorch A, Beyer J, Bascoul-Mollevi C, et al. Prognostic factors in patients with metastatic germ cell tumors who experienced treatment failure with cisplatin-based first-line chemotherapy. J Clin Oncol 2010;28(33):4906–11.

Seminoma

Pure seminoma histology has been associated with a high cure rate because of chemosensitivity. Approximately 90% of patients requiring first-line chemotherapy for disseminated disease are categorized as IGCCCG good risk,[7] and cure rates can exceed 80% to 85%.[79,80] Few of these patients have an IR to initial cisplatin-based chemotherapy or relapse from a CR that requires salvage chemotherapy, and late relapses are rare. Chemotherapy regimens for seminoma have typically mirrored those used in disseminated NSGCT, including in the salvage setting. In fact, most studies of salvage regimens for recurrent disseminated GCT have included some patients with pure seminoma, but most patients in these trials had advanced NSGCT. Only a few retrospective series have specifically studied seminoma in the second-line setting, and these have generally demonstrated favorable results with higher cure rates than what has historically been seen with NSGCT. One report included

24 patients with recurrent seminoma treated with VeIP as initial salvage and demonstrated an 88% CR rate with 54% long-term DFS. Outcome was equally good for patients with primary testicular and extragonadal primary tumors.[81] Similarly, a different retrospective series included 27 patients with seminoma in whom the condition relapsed after prior platinum-based chemotherapy. Overall, this group of patients was more heavily pretreated (15% had received 2 prior regimens). Of the 27 patients, 15 were treated with salvage cisplatin/ifosfamide-based CDCT, whereas 12 received HDCT. The overall CR rate in this series was 56%, with 48% of patients achieving a sustained CR with a median follow-up of 72 months. A total of 8 patients underwent postchemotherapy surgery after salvage treatment. None of the 2 patients with viable seminoma was alive at the time of report, whereas all 6 patients with necrosis remained without evidence of disease.

The superior outcome with seminoma was recognized in a report of the International Prognostic Factor Study Group.[72] The prognostic model, constructed and validated in NSGCT, was applied to a subset of patients with pure seminoma and was able to discern prognostic groups, but demonstrated significantly better survival for each group than what had been seen for patients with NSGCT. Consequently, histology was added to the score, with seminoma coded as −1 and NSGCT as 0. A very-low-risk category was created for patients with seminoma and no adverse factors (sum score −1), with an estimated 3-year PFS and OS of 75.1% and 77%, respectively.[72]

Late Relapse

Late relapse, defined as disease recurrence 2 years or more after successful initial treatment, is seen in 2% to 4% of patients achieving a CR with initial chemotherapy for advanced GCT,[82] that is comprising up to 10% of all relapses in that setting. Late relapse is also seen after management of early-stage disease by surgery, chemotherapy, or radiotherapy, but overall remains uncommon, occurring in only 1% to 4% of patients with GCT who achieve a CR after initial diagnosis.[82–84] It has long been recognized as a poor prognostic indicator for further therapy. Late relapses are more common in patients with NSGCT than those with seminoma,[83] in patients with bulky retroperitoneal adenopathy,[85–87] and in those with teratoma found at the time of postchemotherapy retroperitoneal lymph node dissection.[87–89] Outcome seems particularly poor for patients who previously received cisplatin-containing systemic chemotherapy (vs those who recur many years after surgery, radiation, or carboplatin alone), with 1 report estimating the hazard ratio of death from cancer for this group at 4.0 (95% CI, 1.2%–13.6%; $P = .03$) on multivariate analysis.[90]

Because of an increased incidence of chemotherapy resistance, surgical resection is considered the mainstay of management.[84,89,90] Chemotherapy, however, is attempted in patients with disseminated or unresectable disease. The authors' group has reported durable CR for these patients with the use of paclitaxel-based regimens followed by surgery.[35,82] The previously cited phase 2 trial of second-line TIP included 14 patients with late relapse, all of whom were deemed ineligible for surgery. Of these, 7 (50%) achieved a CR, and all 7 remained in remission at the time of report (median follow-up 51 months).[35]

Cisplatin plus epirubicin has been reported to achieve CR in patients with late-relapse GCT. A phase 2 study of cisplatin plus epirubicin treated 30 patients with a median of 2 prior regimens, most (70%) of whom had a late relapse.[91] The sustained CR rate for patients with late relapse was 29% (follow-up range 28+–48+ months); one-third of these patients with favorable outcome were treated in the second-line setting, the remaining 5 received more extensive prior therapy.

The benefit of HDCT in patients with late relapse is controversial. Two reports on a small number of patients suggested that a subset of patients can achieve complete response with this approach. Of 7 patients, 2 (29%) with late-relapse GCT treated with HDT using the TI-CE regimen achieved long-term DFS.[60] German investigators recently published a secondary analysis of 35 patients with late relapse included in a randomized phase 3 trial of single-cycle HDCT versus sequential HDCT.[92] Of 35 patients, 5 (14%) were disease free at the time of report, 4 of the 5 having received HDCT in the second-line setting.

Teratoma, frequently found in late relapse, is not chemosensitive. The rate of malignant transformation increased in this group.[93,94] Malignant transformation should be suspected if the disease does not respond to cisplatin-based chemotherapy or growth is seen on imaging without increase in levels of disease tumor markers despite cisplatin-based chemotherapy. The isochromosome of chromosome 12, i(12p), is a specific marker of GCT.[95] Identification of i(12p) or excess 12p copy number can be used to establish the clonal origin of malignant transformation. If such disease is localized, outcome is typically more favorable with complete resection.[96] Otherwise, treatment follows the histology paradigm of the secondary somatic malignancy, including chemotherapy, radiation, and/or surgery, as appropriate.[94,97] There are no data supporting the use of HDCT in patients with relapsed GCT comprised exclusively of malignant transformation. Following the above-mentioned treatment paradigm, subjecting patients to the toxicity of such treatment is not warranted, with the exception of the rare case in which the transformed malignancy is sensitive to HDCT.

Surgery in the Salvage Setting

Following cisplatin-based first-line therapy for NSGCT, standard management calls for surgical resection of residual disease when serum tumor marker levels have normalized. Necrotic tissue, fibrosis, teratoma, or viable GCT may be found at the time of surgery. When viable GCT is present, 2 cycles of adjuvant chemotherapy are recommended for the first-line setting.[98] In contrast, the pathologic presence of necrotic tissue, fibrosis, or mature teratoma requires no further therapy because GCT only relapses in 5% to 10% of these patients.

In the salvage setting, pathologic specimens of resected masses after second-line VeIP or VIP chemotherapy demonstrate viable tumor in approximately 50%, teratoma in 40%, and necrosis in only 10%.[98,99] The rate of viable tumor at the time of surgery is significantly higher after salvage chemotherapy than after first-line treatment. Presence of viable tumor in the salvage setting confers a worse prognosis compared with mature teratoma or necrotic tissue,[100] and the risk of relapse despite resection of residual masses is approximately 50% in such cases. In contrast to the first-line setting, there is no established benefit to additional standard-dose chemotherapy in patients who have viable NSGCT in the resected specimen after salvage chemotherapy.

Surgical resection of isolated metastasis in the presence of elevated levels of serum tumor markers is performed in highly select instances. Often referred to as "desperation surgery" or "surgical salvage," this approach has curative potential in patients whose disease is refractory to cisplatin. Patients with a solitary retroperitoneal mass and increased AFP levels alone are the best candidates for this surgery. Resection of all disease seen on imaging studies and normalization of levels of serum tumor markers predict long-term survival.[9] As mentioned earlier, patients with PMNSGCT respond poorly to conventional salvage chemotherapy. In rare cases, surgical resection of residual mediastinal masses in the setting of elevated levels of serum tumor markers can lead to long-term survival.[101]

SUMMARY

Established second-line CDCT regimens are cisplatin/ifosfamide based and include either VeIP or TIP, with sustained CR rates reported in prospective clinical trials ranging from 24–25% with VeIP[23,27] and from 38–63% with TIP.[35–37] Enrollment criteria varied for these studies, and the 2 regimens have never been directly compared. Other investigators routinely consider HDCT in the initial salvage setting and depending on patient selection criteria, have reported sustained CR rates of 40% to 50% for this approach.[59,60,66] HDCT in second-line therapy remains controversial, and prospective data specific to the second-line setting are limited. Direct comparisons of both approaches are sparse. Although retrospective analyses suggest that HDCT may be superior to CDCT,[67,71] this was not confirmed by the 1 randomized prospective trial comparing salvage CDCT with HDCT,[27] a study that is limited by flaws outlined in prior sections of this review. Some investigators, including the authors' group, use a risk-adapted approach to determine salvage strategy, reserving HDCT for those patients at highest risk of failing second-line CDCT. For a more definitive answer regarding the optimal approach to GCT salvage therapy, further prospective studies are needed. The recently developed prognostic model developed by the International Prognostic Factor Study Group for second-line chemotherapy applies to both CDCT and HDCT and should be incorporated into any future investigative efforts.

ACKNOWLEDGMENTS

The authors wish to thank Carol Pearce, MSKCC Department of Medicine, writer/editor, for her contribution to this manuscript.

REFERENCES

1. de Wit R, Stoter G, Sleijfer DT, et al. Four cycles of BEP versus an alternating regime of PVB and BEP in patients with poor-prognosis metastatic testicular non-seminoma; a randomised study of the EORTC Genitourinary Tract Cancer Cooperative Group. Br J Cancer 1995;71(6):1311–4.
2. de Wit R, Stoter G, Sleijfer DT, et al. Four cycles of BEP vs four cycles of VIP in patients with intermediate-prognosis metastatic testicular non-seminoma: a randomized study of the EORTC Genitourinary Tract Cancer Cooperative Group. European Organization for Research and Treatment of Cancer. Br J Cancer 1998;78(6):828–32.
3. Williams SD, Birch R, Einhorn LH, et al. Treatment of disseminated germ-cell tumors with cisplatin, bleomycin, and either vinblastine or etoposide. N Engl J Med 1987;316(23):1435–40.
4. Bosl GJ, Geller NL, Bajorin D, et al. A randomized trial of etoposide + cisplatin versus vinblastine + bleomycin + cisplatin + cyclophosphamide + dactinomycin in patients with good-prognosis germ cell tumors. J Clin Oncol 1988;6(8):1231–8.
5. Culine S, Kerbrat P, Kramar A, et al. Refining the optimal chemotherapy regimen for good-risk metastatic nonseminomatous germ-cell tumors: a randomized trial of the Genito-Urinary Group of the French Federation of Cancer Centers (GETUG T93BP). Ann Oncol 2007;18(5):917–24.
6. Feldman DR, Bosl GJ, Sheinfeld J, et al. Medical treatment of advanced testicular cancer. JAMA 2008;299(6):672–84.
7. International Germ Cell Consensus Classification: a prognostic factor-based staging system for metastatic germ cell cancers International Germ Cell Cancer Collaborative Group. J Clin Oncol 1997;15(2):594–603.

8. Wood DP Jr, Herr HW, Motzer RJ, et al. Surgical resection of solitary metastases after chemotherapy in patients with nonseminomatous germ cell tumors and elevated serum tumor markers. Cancer 1992;70(9):2354–7.

9. Habuchi T, Kamoto T, Hara I, et al. Factors that influence the results of salvage surgery in patients with chemorefractory germ cell carcinomas with elevated tumor markers. Cancer 2003;98(8):1635–42.

10. Kisbenedek L, Bodrogi I, Szeldeli P, et al. Results of salvage retroperitoneal lymphadenectomy (RLA) in the treatment of patients with nonseminomatous germ cell tumours remaining marker positive after inductive chemotherapy. Int Urol Nephrol 1995;27(3):325–9.

11. Einhorn LH, Donohue J. Cis-diamminedichloroplatinum, vinblastine, and bleomycin combination chemotherapy in disseminated testicular cancer. Ann Intern Med 1977;87(3):293–8.

12. Vugrin D, Herr HW, Whitmore WF Jr, et al. VAB-6 combination chemotherapy in disseminated cancer of the testis. Ann Intern Med 1981;95(1):59–61.

13. Williams SD, Einhorn LH, Greco FA, et al. VP-16-213 salvage therapy for refractory germinal neoplasms. Cancer 1980;46(10):2154–8.

14. Hainsworth JD, Williams SD, Einhorn LH, et al. Successful treatment of resistant germinal neoplasms with VP-16 and cisplatin: results of a Southeastern Cancer Study Group trial. J Clin Oncol 1985;3(5):666–71.

15. Bosl GJ, Yagoda A, Whitmore WF Jr, et al. VP-16-213 and cisplatin in the treatment of patients with refractory germ cell tumors. Am J Clin Oncol 1984;7(4): 327–30.

16. Schmoll HJ. The role of ifosfamide in testicular cancer. Semin Oncol 1989; 16(1 Suppl 3):82–95.

17. Wheeler BM, Loehrer PJ, Williams SD, et al. Ifosfamide in refractory male germ cell tumors. J Clin Oncol 1986;4(1):28–34.

18. Loehrer PJ Sr, Lauer R, Roth BJ, et al. Salvage therapy in recurrent germ cell cancer: ifosfamide and cisplatin plus either vinblastine or etoposide. Ann Intern Med 1988;109(7):540–6.

19. Ghosn M, Droz JP, Theodore C, et al. Salvage chemotherapy in refractory germ cell tumors with etoposide (VP-16) plus ifosfamide plus high-dose cisplatin. A VIhP regimen. Cancer 1988;62(1):24–7.

20. Harstrick A, Schmoll HJ, Wilke H, et al. Cisplatin, etoposide, and ifosfamide salvage therapy for refractory or relapsing germ cell carcinoma. J Clin Oncol 1991;9(9):1549–55.

21. Pizzocaro G, Salvioni R, Piva L, et al. Modified cisplatin, etoposide (or vinblastine) and ifosfamide salvage therapy for male germ-cell tumors. Long-term results. Ann Oncol 1992;3(3):211–6.

22. McCaffrey JA, Mazumdar M, Bajorin DF, et al. Ifosfamide- and cisplatin-containing chemotherapy as first-line salvage therapy in germ cell tumors: response and survival. J Clin Oncol 1997;15(7):2559–63.

23. Loehrer PJ, Gonin R, Nichols CR, et al. Vinblastine plus ifosfamide plus cisplatin as initial salvage therapy in recurrent germ cell tumor. J Clin Oncol 1998;16(7): 2500–4.

24. Motzer RJ, Cooper K, Geller NL, et al. The role of ifosfamide plus cisplatin-based chemotherapy as salvage therapy for patients with refractory germ cell tumors. Cancer 1990;66(12):2476–81.

25. Loehrer PJ Sr, Einhorn LH, Williams SD. VP-16 plus ifosfamide plus cisplatin as salvage therapy in refractory germ cell cancer. J Clin Oncol 1986;4(4): 528–36.

26. Farhat F, Culine S, Theodore C, et al. Cisplatin and ifosfamide with either vinblastine or etoposide as salvage therapy for refractory or relapsing germ cell tumor patients: the Institut Gustave Roussy experience. Cancer 1996;77(6):1193–7.
27. Pico JL, Rosti G, Kramar A, et al. A randomised trial of high-dose chemotherapy in the salvage treatment of patients failing first-line platinum chemotherapy for advanced germ cell tumours. Ann Oncol 2005;16(7):1152–9.
28. McGuire WP, Rowinsky EK, Rosenshein NB, et al. Taxol: a unique antineoplastic agent with significant activity in advanced ovarian epithelial neoplasms. Ann Intern Med 1989;111(4):273–9.
29. Reichman BS, Seidman AD, Crown JP, et al. Paclitaxel and recombinant human granulocyte colony-stimulating factor as initial chemotherapy for metastatic breast cancer. J Clin Oncol 1993;11(10):1943–51.
30. Kohn EC, Sarosy G, Bicher A, et al. Dose-intense taxol: high response rate in patients with platinum-resistant recurrent ovarian cancer. J Natl Cancer Inst 1994;86(1):18–24.
31. Motzer RJ, Bajorin DF, Schwartz LH, et al. Phase II trial of paclitaxel shows antitumor activity in patients with previously treated germ cell tumors. J Clin Oncol 1994;12(11):2277–83.
32. Sandler AB, Cristou A, Fox S, et al. A phase II trial of paclitaxel in refractory germ cell tumors. Cancer 1998;82(7):1381–6.
33. Nazario A, Amato RJ, Hutchinson L, et al. Paclitaxel in extensively pretreated nonseminomatous germ cell tumors. Urol Oncol 1995;1(5):184–7.
34. Chou TC, Motzer RJ, Tong Y, et al. Computerized quantitation of synergism and antagonism of taxol, topotecan, and cisplatin against human teratocarcinoma cell growth: a rational approach to clinical protocol design. J Natl Cancer Inst 1994;86(20):1517–24.
35. Kondagunta GV, Bacik J, Donadio A, et al. Combination of paclitaxel, ifosfamide, and cisplatin is an effective second-line therapy for patients with relapsed testicular germ cell tumors. J Clin Oncol 2005;23(27):6549–55.
36. Mead GM, Cullen MH, Huddart R, et al. A phase II trial of TIP (paclitaxel, ifosfamide and cisplatin) given as second-line (post-BEP) salvage chemotherapy for patients with metastatic germ cell cancer: a medical research council trial. Br J Cancer 2005;93(2):178–84.
37. Mardiak J, Salek T, Sycova-Mila Z, et al. Paclitaxel plus ifosfamide and cisplatin in second-line treatment of germ cell tumors: a phase II study. Neoplasma 2005;52(6):497–501.
38. Motzer RJ, Sheinfeld J, Mazumdar M, et al. Paclitaxel, ifosfamide, and cisplatin second-line therapy for patients with relapsed testicular germ cell cancer. J Clin Oncol 2000;18(12):2413–8.
39. Dicke KA, McCredie KB, Stevens EE, et al. Autologous bone marrow transplantation in a case of acute adult leukemia. Transplant Proc 1977;9(1):193–5.
40. Dicke KA, Zander A, Spitzer G, et al. Autologous bone-marrow transplantation in relapsed adult acute leukaemia. Lancet 1979;1(8115):514–7.
41. Graze PR, Gale RP. Autotransplantation for leukemia and solid tumors. Transplant Proc 1978;10(1):177–84.
42. Dicke KA, McCredie KB, Spitzer G, et al. Autologous bone marrow transplantation in patients with adult acute leukemia in relapse. Transplantation 1978;26(3):169–73.
43. Appelbaum FR, Herzig GP, Graw RG, et al. Study of cell dose and storage time on engraftment of cryopreserved autologous bone marrow in a canine model. Transplantation 1978;26(4):245–8.

44. Appelbaum FR, Herzig GP, Ziegler JL, et al. Successful engraftment of cryopre-served autologous bone marrow in patients with malignant lymphoma. Blood 1978;52(1):85–95.
45. Bunn PA Jr, Cohen MH, Ihde DC, et al. Advances in small cell bronchogenic carcinoma. Cancer Treat Rep 1977;61(3):333–42.
46. Spitzer G, Dicke KA, Litam J, et al. High-dose combination chemotherapy with autologous bone marrow transplantation in adult solid tumors. Cancer 1980; 45(12):3075–85.
47. Blijham G, Spitzer G, Litam J, et al. The treatment of advanced testicular carci-noma with high dose chemotherapy and autologous marrow support. Eur J Cancer 1981;17(4):433–41.
48. Fukuda M, Kojima S, Matsumoto K, et al. Autotransplantation of peripheral blood stem cells mobilized by chemotherapy and recombinant human granulocyte colony-stimulating factor in childhood neuroblastoma and non-Hodgkin's lymphoma. Br J Haematol 1992;80(3):327–31.
49. Gore ME, Calvert AH, Smith LE. High dose carboplatin in the treatment of lung cancer and mesothelioma: a phase I dose escalation study. Eur J Cancer Clin Oncol 1987;23(9):1391–7.
50. Lee EJ, Egorin MJ, Van Echo DA, et al. Phase I and pharmacokinetic trial of car-boplatin in refractory adult leukemia. J Natl Cancer Inst 1988;80(2):131–5.
51. Wolff SN, Johnson DH, Hainsworth JD, et al. High-dose VP-16-213 monotherapy for refractory germinal malignancies: a phase II study. J Clin Oncol 1984;2(4): 271–4.
52. Shea TC, Flaherty M, Elias A, et al. A phase I clinical and pharmacokinetic study of carboplatin and autologous bone marrow support. J Clin Oncol 1989;7(5): 651–61.
53. Nichols CR, Tricot G, Williams SD, et al. Dose-intensive chemotherapy in refrac-tory germ cell cancer–a phase I/II trial of high-dose carboplatin and etoposide with autologous bone marrow transplantation. J Clin Oncol 1989;7(7):932–9.
54. Broun ER, Nichols CR, Kneebone P, et al. Long-term outcome of patients with relapsed and refractory germ cell tumors treated with high-dose chemo-therapy and autologous bone marrow rescue. Ann Intern Med 1992;117(2): 124–8.
55. Nichols CR, Andersen J, Lazarus HM, et al. High-dose carboplatin and etopo-side with autologous bone marrow transplantation in refractory germ cell cancer: an Eastern Cooperative Oncology Group protocol. J Clin Oncol 1992; 10(4):558–63.
56. Beyer J, Kramar A, Mandanas R, et al. High-dose chemotherapy as salvage treatment in germ cell tumors: a multivariate analysis of prognostic variables. J Clin Oncol 1996;14(10):2638–45.
57. Beyer J, Schwella N, Zingsem J, et al. Hematopoietic rescue after high-dose chemotherapy using autologous peripheral-blood progenitor cells or bone marrow: a randomized comparison. J Clin Oncol 1995;13(6):1328–35.
58. Kondagunta GV, Motzer RJ. Chemotherapy for advanced germ cell tumors. J Clin Oncol 2006;24(35):5493–502.
59. Einhorn LH, Williams SD, Chamness A, et al. High-dose chemotherapy and stem-cell rescue for metastatic germ-cell tumors. N Engl J Med 2007;357(4): 340–8.
60. Feldman DR, Sheinfeld J, Bajorin DF, et al. TI-CE high-dose chemotherapy for patients with previously treated germ cell tumors: results and prognostic factor analysis. J Clin Oncol 2010;28(10):1706–13.

61. Siegert W, Beyer J, Strohscheer I, et al. High-dose treatment with carboplatin, etoposide, and ifosfamide followed by autologous stem-cell transplantation in relapsed or refractory germ cell cancer: a phase I/II study. The German Testicular Cancer Cooperative Study Group. J Clin Oncol 1994;12(6):1223–31.

62. Motzer RJ, Mazumdar M, Bosl GJ, et al. High-dose carboplatin, etoposide, and cyclophosphamide for patients with refractory germ cell tumors: treatment results and prognostic factors for survival and toxicity. J Clin Oncol 1996; 14(4):1098–105.

63. Rick O, Bokemeyer C, Beyer J, et al. Salvage treatment with paclitaxel, ifosfamide, and cisplatin plus high-dose carboplatin, etoposide, and thiotepa followed by autologous stem-cell rescue in patients with relapsed or refractory germ cell cancer. J Clin Oncol 2001;19(1):81–8.

64. Rick O, Beyer J, Kingreen D, et al. High-dose chemotherapy in germ cell tumours: a large single centre experience. Eur J Cancer 1998;34(12): 1883–8.

65. Motzer RJ, Gulati SC, Crown JP, et al. High-dose chemotherapy and autologous bone marrow rescue for patients with refractory germ cell tumors. Early intervention is better tolerated. Cancer 1992;69(2):550–6.

66. Bhatia S, Abonour R, Porcu P, et al. High-dose chemotherapy as initial salvage chemotherapy in patients with relapsed testicular cancer. J Clin Oncol 2000; 18(19):3346–51.

67. Beyer J, Stenning S, Gerl A, et al. High-dose versus conventional-dose chemotherapy as first-salvage treatment in patients with non-seminomatous germ-cell tumors: a matched-pair analysis. Ann Oncol 2002;13(4):599–605.

68. Motzer RJ, Geller NL, Tan CC, et al. Salvage chemotherapy for patients with germ cell tumors. The Memorial Sloan-Kettering Cancer Center experience (1979–1989). Cancer 1991;67(5):1305–10.

69. Schmoll HJ, Beyer J. Prognostic factors in metastatic germ cell tumors. Semin Oncol 1998;25(2):174–85.

70. Fossa SD, Stenning SP, Gerl A, et al. Prognostic factors in patients progressing after cisplatin-based chemotherapy for malignant non-seminomatous germ cell tumours. Br J Cancer 1999;80(9):1392–9.

71. Lorch A, Mollevi C, Kramar A, et al. Conventional-dose versus high-dose chemotherapy in relapsed or refractory male germ-cell tumors: a retrospective study in 1,594 patients. J Clin Oncol 2010;28(Suppl, abstr 4513):15s.

72. Lorch A, Beyer J, Bascoul-Mollevi C, et al. Prognostic factors in patients with metastatic germ cell tumors who experienced treatment failure with cisplatin-based first-line chemotherapy. J Clin Oncol 2010;28(33):4906–11.

73. Sammler C, Beyer J, Bokemeyer C, et al. Risk factors in germ cell tumour patients with relapse or progressive disease after first-line chemotherapy: evaluation of a prognostic score for survival after high-dose chemotherapy. Eur J Cancer 2008;44(2):237–43.

74. Gerl A, Clemm C, Schmeller N, et al. Prognosis after salvage treatment for unselected male patients with germ cell tumours. Br J Cancer 1995;72(4): 1026–32.

75. Saxman SB, Nichols CR, Einhorn LH. Salvage chemotherapy in patients with extragonadal nonseminomatous germ cell tumors: the Indiana University experience. J Clin Oncol 1994;12(7):1390–3.

76. Broun ER, Nichols CR, Einhorn LH, et al. Salvage therapy with high-dose chemotherapy and autologous bone marrow support in the treatment of primary nonseminomatous mediastinal germ cell tumors. Cancer 1991;68(7):1513–5.

77. Linkesch W, Greinix HT, Hocker P, et al. Longterm follow up of phase I/II trial of ultra-high carboplatin, VP-16, cyclophosphamide with ABMT in refractory or relapsed NSGCT. Proc Am Soc Clin Oncol 1993;12:232.
78. Vaena DA, Abonour R, Einhorn LH. Long-term survival after high-dose salvage chemotherapy for germ cell malignancies with adverse prognostic variables. J Clin Oncol 2003;21(22):4100–4.
79. Mencel PJ, Motzer RJ, Mazumdar M, et al. Advanced seminoma: treatment results, survival, and prognostic factors in 142 patients. J Clin Oncol 1994; 12(1):120–6.
80. Gholam D, Fizazi K, Terrier-Lacombe MJ, et al. Advanced seminoma–treatment results and prognostic factors for survival after first-line, cisplatin-based chemo-therapy and for patients with recurrent disease: a single-institution experience in 145 patients. Cancer 2003;98(4):745–52.
81. Miller KD, Loehrer PJ, Gonin R, et al. Salvage chemotherapy with vinblastine, ifosfamide, and cisplatin in recurrent seminoma. J Clin Oncol 1997;15(4): 1427–31.
82. Ronnen EA, Kondagunta GV, Bacik J, et al. Incidence of late-relapse germ cell tumor and outcome to salvage chemotherapy. J Clin Oncol 2005;23(28): 6999–7004.
83. Oldenburg J, Martin JM, Fossa SD. Late relapses of germ cell malignancies: incidence, management, and prognosis. J Clin Oncol 2006;24(35):5503–11.
84. Baniel J, Foster RS, Gonin R, et al. Late relapse of testicular cancer. J Clin Oncol 1995;13(5):1170–6.
85. Dieckmann KP, Albers P, Classen J, et al. Late relapse of testicular germ cell neoplasms: a descriptive analysis of 122 cases. J Urol 2005;173(3):824–9.
86. Gerl A, Clemm C, Schmeller N, et al. Late relapse of germ cell tumors after cisplatin-based chemotherapy. Ann Oncol 1997;8(1):41–7.
87. Shahidi M, Norman AR, Dearnaley DP, et al. Late recurrence in 1263 men with testicular germ cell tumors. Multivariate analysis of risk factors and implications for management. Cancer 2002;95(3):520–30.
88. Geldart TR, Gale J, McKendrick J, et al. Late relapse of metastatic testicular nonseminomatous germ cell cancer: surgery is needed for cure. BJU Int 2006;98(2):353–8.
89. George DW, Foster RS, Hromas RA, et al. Update on late relapse of germ cell tumor: a clinical and molecular analysis. J Clin Oncol 2003;21(1):113–22.
90. Sharp DS, Carver BS, Eggener SE, et al. Clinical outcome and predictors of survival in late relapse of germ cell tumor. J Clin Oncol 2008;26(34):5524–9.
91. Bedano PM, Brames MJ, Williams SD, et al. Phase II study of cisplatin plus epi-rubicin salvage chemotherapy in refractory germ cell tumors. J Clin Oncol 2006; 24(34):5403–7.
92. Lorch A, Rick O, Wundisch T, et al. High dose chemotherapy as salvage treatment for unresectable late relapse germ cell tumors. J Urol 2010;184(1): 168–73.
93. Korfel A, Fischer L, Foss HD, et al. Testicular germ cell tumor with rhabdomyo-sarcoma successfully treated by disease-adapted chemotherapy including high-dose chemotherapy: case report and review of the literature. Bone Marrow Transplant 2001;28(8):787–9.
94. Donadio AC, Motzer RJ, Bajorin DF, et al. Chemotherapy for teratoma with malignant transformation. J Clin Oncol 2003;21(23):4285–91.
95. Bosl GJ, Motzer RJ. Testicular germ-cell cancer. N Engl J Med 1997;337(4): 242–53.

96. Motzer RJ, Amsterdam A, Prieto V, et al. Teratoma with malignant transformation: diverse malignant histologies arising in men with germ cell tumors. J Urol 1998; 159(1):133–8.

97. El Mesbahi O, Terrier-Lacombe MJ, Rebischung C, et al. Chemotherapy in patients with teratoma with malignant transformation. Eur Urol 2007;51(5): 1306–11 [discussion: 1311–2].

98. Fox EP, Weathers TD, Williams SD, et al. Outcome analysis for patients with persistent nonteratomatous germ cell tumor in postchemotherapy retroperitoneal lymph node dissections. J Clin Oncol 1993;11(7):1294–9.

99. Eggener SE, Carver BS, Loeb S, et al. Pathologic findings and clinical outcome of patients undergoing retroperitoneal lymph node dissection after multiple chemotherapy regimens for metastatic testicular germ cell tumors. Cancer 2007;109(3):528–35.

100. Rick O, Bokemeyer C, Weinknecht S, et al. Residual tumor resection after high-dose chemotherapy in patients with relapsed or refractory germ cell cancer. J Clin Oncol 2004;22(18):3713–9.

101. Vuky J, Bains M, Bacik J, et al. Role of postchemotherapy adjunctive surgery in the management of patients with nonseminoma arising from the mediastinum. J Clin Oncol 2001;19(3):682–8.

Third-Line Chemotherapy and Novel Agents for Metastatic Germ Cell Tumors

Christine M. Veenstra, MD*, David J. Vaughn, MD

KEYWORDS

• Germ cell • Refractory • Testicular • Neoplasm • Cisplatin

Germ cell tumors (GCT) are one of the most curable solid tumors, with a cure-rate of 70% to 80% for patients with metastatic disease who are treated with cisplatin-based combination chemotherapy. Prognosis of patients who do not respond adequately to first-line therapy or who relapse after first-line treatment is poor, with a 20% to 25% cure-rate for those treated with second-line cisplatin-based chemotherapy. High-dose chemotherapy plus autologous peripheral blood stem cell transplant results in durable responses in 30% to 50% of patients with relapsed disease.[1–3] Unfortunately, a subset of patients experience relapse or progression despite salvage chemotherapy, including those with cisplatin-refractory (response or disease stabilization during chemotherapy but disease progression within 4 weeks after cisplatin-based chemotherapy) and those with absolutely cisplatin-refractory disease (progression during cisplatin-based treatment).[4,5] These patients have a very poor prognosis. This review focuses treatment options for patients with multiply-relapsed or cisplatin-refractory disease, and describes the molecular mechanisms of cisplatin resistance, outlines single-agent chemotherapy and combination chemotherapy regimens that are active against GCT in the third-line setting, discusses the use of chemotherapy for the growing teratoma syndrome, outlines novel agents that have been used in to treat GCT, and highlights ongoing clinical trials and future directions in the treatment of refractory GCT.

The authors have nothing to disclose.
Division of Hematology/Oncology, University of Pennsylvania, 16 Penn Tower, 3400 Spruce, Philadelphia, PA 19104, USA
* Corresponding author.
E-mail address: christine.veenstra@uphs.upenn.edu

Hematol Oncol Clin N Am 25 (2011) 577–591
doi:10.1016/j.hoc.2011.03.005
0889-8588/11/$ – see front matter © 2011 Elsevier Inc. All rights reserved.

hemonc.theclinics.com

MOLECULAR MECHANISMS OF CISPLATIN RESISTANCE

Although GCTs generally display exquisite sensitivity to cisplatin, resistance occurs in approximately 20% of patients with metastatic GCT. Resistance to cisplatin can be intrinsic or acquired after repeated exposure to the drug.[6] The molecular mechanisms of cisplatin resistance in GCT arise from a complex series of events that are not yet completely understood. Cisplatin induces apoptosis in sensitive cells by first gaining entry into the cell, then binding with DNA to form DNA adducts. These adducts distort DNA, which is then recognized as damaged, activating the apoptotic cascade. Molecular alterations leading to cisplatin resistance can occur before cisplatin-induced DNA damage occurs, during the process of DNA damage and repair, or after cisplatin-induced DNA damage has occurred (**Fig. 1**). Multiple molecular alterations may exist at various points in the process, leading to cisplatin resistance.[7]

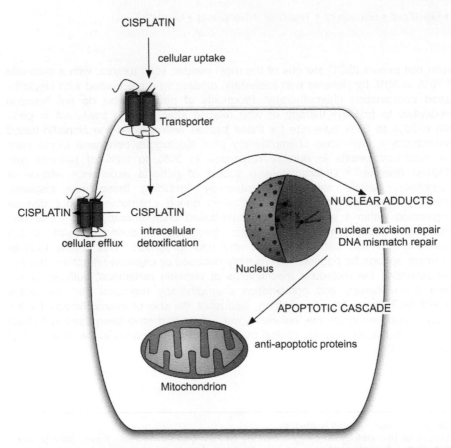

Fig. 1. Molecular mechanisms of cisplatin resistance. Decreased cellular uptake of cisplatin via transporters, increased cellular efflux of cisplatin, or intracellular detoxification by thiols could all lead to cisplatin resistance. Once cisplatin–DNA adducts are formed in the nucleus, mechanisms related to the repair or removal of damaged DNA may contribute to cisplatin resistance. Finally, mechanisms to inhibit apoptosis after initiation of the apoptotic cascade could lead to cisplatin resistance.

Before the occurrence of cisplatin-induced DNA damage, decreased cellular uptake of cisplatin, increased cellular efflux of the drug, or intracellular detoxification of the drug could all potentially lead to resistance. A copper transporter may be involved in the cellular uptake of cisplatin, although little is known about this transporter or its potential for implication in cisplatin resistance.[8,9] Several drug transporters, including the multidrug resistance–associated proteins in the ATP-binding cassette (ABC) transporter family[10,11] and lung resistance–related protein,[12] have been suggested to transport cisplatin out of cells, possibly leading to cisplatin resistance. Studies examining the role of intracellular detoxification of cisplatin by glutathione or metallothionein have had mixed results, with one study suggesting a positive correlation between levels of these thiols and cisplatin resistance in testis tumor cell lines,[13] and a second study finding no correlation between glutathione content and cisplatin resistance in a GCT line or a colon cancer cell line.[14]

Once DNA adducts form, mechanisms related to the repair or removal of damaged DNA may contribute to cisplatin resistance. Nuclear excision repair (NER) is a major pathway for the repair of DNA damaged by cisplatin. GCT cell lines have been shown to have a low intrinsic capacity for nuclear excision repair,[15] perhaps related to low levels of xeroderma pigmentosum group A protein (XPA) or the ERCC1-XPF–specific endonuclease complex. Testis tumor cell lines with low levels of XPA lose their capacity to repair DNA damage, and subsequently regain full NER capacity with the addition of XPA.[16] The reduced NER capacity of GCT might contribute to cisplatin-sensitivity, and perhaps resistant GCT have higher levels of XPA and a more robust NER pathway. However, one study of XPA levels in human samples found no differences between sensitive and resistant tumors and no correlation between XPA protein level and cisplatin sensitivity in three GCT cell lines.[17]

Other factors involved in DNA repair include high mobility group (HMG) proteins, which have been implicated in cisplatin resistance for their role in recognizing cisplatin–DNA adducts and blocking the NER pathway from repairing the damaged DNA.[18] A defective DNA mismatch repair system could lead to failure to recognize DNA damage and subsequent failure to initiate apoptosis. A study of 100 unselected GCT and 11 chemotherapy-resistant GCT found a significantly higher incidence of microsatellite instability (MSI), a marker of defective mismatch repair, in the resistant tumors. Furthermore, the resistant tumors exhibited MSI in several loci.[19] A subsequent study using the same control cohort and 35 cisplatin-resistant GCT found a higher incidence of MSI in the resistant tumors, again in multiple loci. A higher incidence of BRAF V600E mutation was also seen in the resistant tumors compared with controls, and presence of the BRAF mutation was highly correlated with MSI.[20] Although experts had previously postulated that a high level of wild-type p53 in GCT is responsible for cisplatin sensitivity,[21] studies have shown that a high level of p53 does not correlate to chemotherapy sensitivity in GCT, that the inactivation of p53 in a cisplatin-sensitive cell line does not confer resistance, and that the inactivation of p53 is not a common occurrence in resistant GCT.[22,23]

Once the apoptotic cascade has been initiated, mechanisms that inhibit apoptosis could lead to cisplatin resistance. Antiapoptotic proteins such as BAX and BCL-2 have been examined as potential mediators of cisplatin resistance in GCT, but no significant correlation with resistance has emerged.[24] Cisplatin resistance in GCT is likely a multifactorial phenomenon, potentially involving elements of each of the molecular pathways described. Further research, particularly using human tumor samples and clinical correlation, is needed to further clarify this complex issue.

ACTIVE SINGLE AGENTS IN REFRACTORY GCTS

For patients with cisplatin-refractory GCT, additional active agents are used in the third-line or later setting (**Table 1**). Historically, etoposide was the first agent to exhibit activity in GCTs refractory to cisplatin-based chemotherapy.[25] Subsequently, etoposide was incorporated into the first-line combination regimen of bleomycin, etoposide, and cisplatin (BEP).[26] A phase II study of daily oral etoposide in patients with refractory GCT, all of whom had undergone prior etoposide therapy, showed a 14% response rate.[27]

Ifosfamide was first shown to have single-agent activity against refractory GCT in the mid-1980s, with a response rate of approximately 20%.[28,29] Currently, most patients receive ifosfamide as salvage therapy after failure to cure with first-lines regimens such as BEP, or as a component of first-line therapy in poor-risk advanced disease when bleomycin toxicity is a concern.[30]

Paclitaxel showed activity against GCT in patients for whom cisplatin-based chemotherapy failed. Among 31 patients treated, 8 (26%) experienced a major response. None of the patients in the study who had received prior treatment with high-dose chemotherapy experienced a response to paclitaxel.[31] The German Testicular Cancer Study Group reported that 6 of 24 patients with relapsed, mostly cisplatin-refractory GCT (25%) experienced responded to paclitaxel, including 2 who had prior high-dose chemotherapy with stem cell support, although 1 of these patients relapsed again 3 months after treatment with paclitaxel.[32] Including these two trials, five trials of single-agent paclitaxel in cisplatin-refractory GCT have been published. These trials include a total of 98 patients, with a combined response rate of 21%.[31–35]

A single case report exists of the related agent, docetaxel, leading to a durable complete remission when used as a single-agent in the third-line setting in a patient with mediastinal GCT refractory to salvage chemotherapy.[36]

Single-agent gemcitabine has been shown to exhibit activity against refractory GCT in two phase II studies, with response rates of 19%[37] and 15%,[38] respectively. Both studies reported responses in heavily pretreated patients.

In vitro studies of oxaliplatin have shown its activity in cisplatin-resistant nonseminomatous GCT cell lines.[39] A phase II study of single-agent oxaliplatin in patients with heavily pretreated refractory GCT reported a response rate of 13%.[40] A French

Table 1
Studies of active single agents in refractory germ cell tumors

Drug	Author	Number of Patients	Responses	Overall Response Rate (%)
Etoposide	Miller and Einhorn,[27] 1990	21	6 PR, 0 CR	14
Ifosfamide	Wheeler et al,[29] 1986	30	6 PR, 1 CR	23
Paclitaxel	Motzer et al,[31] 1994	31	5 PR, 3 CR	26
	Bokemeyer et al,[33] 1994	10	3 PR, 0 CR	30
	Bokemeyer et al,[32] 1996	24	4 PR, 2 CR	25
	Nazario et al,[34] 1995	15	2 PR, 0 CR	13
	Sandler et al,[35] 1998	18	2 PR, 0 CR	11
Gemcitabine	Bokemeyer et al,[37] 1999	31	6 PR, 0 CR	19
	Einhorn et al,[38] 1999	20	2 PR, 1 CR	15
Oxaliplatin	Kollmannsberger et al,[40] 2002	32	4 PR, 0 CR	13
	Fizazi et al,[41] 2004	8	3 PR, 0 CR	37

Abbreviations: CR, complete response; PR, partial response.

series of eight patients with refractory GCT treated with single-agent oxaliplatin reported a response rate of 37%,[41] although how heavily pretreated these patients were is unclear.

ACTIVE COMBINATION REGIMENS IN REFRACTORY GCTS

Patients with cisplatin-refractory GCTs have been heavily pretreated by the time they receive third-line therapy, but they tend to be young with a preserved performance status, and therefore the tolerability and response rates of doublet and triplet combination regimens have been studied in this setting (**Table 2**). A phase II study by the Eastern Cooperative Oncology Group (ECOG 9897) evaluated the combination of paclitaxel and gemcitabine in 28 patients and showed a 21% response rate, including three complete responses. Complete responses in two of the patients were long-term, with disease-free periods 15+ and 25+ months at study publication.[42]

A retrospective series of 32 patients treated after failure of high-dose salvage chemotherapy showed a 31% response rate, including 4 patients who had complete responses to chemotherapy alone and were continuously disease-free for more than 40 months at study publication. An additional patient underwent two separate resections of cancer after treatment with paclitaxel and gemcitabine, and had been disease-free for more than 63 months at publication. All of the patients in this study had been treated with prior high-dose chemotherapy. Of the 10 patients who had an objective response, 6 had relatively minimal tumor burden at study outset.[43]

Table 2
Studies of active combination regimens in refractory germ cell tumors

Drug Regimen	Author	N (Patients)	Responses	Overall Response Rate (%)
Paclitaxel/ gemcitabine	Hinton et al,[42] 2002	28	3 PR, 3 CR	21
	Einhorn et al,[43] 2007	32	4 PR, 6 CR	31
Gemcitabine/ oxaliplatin	Kollmannsberger et al,[44] 2004	35	13 PR, 3 CR	46
	Pectasides et al,[45] 2004	28	5 PR, 4 CR	32
	De Giorgi et al,[46] 2006	18	2 PR, 1 CR	17
Oxaliplatin/ paclitaxel	Theodore et al,[47] 2008	26	1 PR, 0 CR	4
Cisplatin/epirubicin	Bedano et al,[50] 2006	30	8 PR, 9 CR	57
Oxaliplatin/cisplatin or nedaplatin	Miki et al,[52] 2002	18	7 PR, 2 CR	50
Irinotecan/ oxaliplatin	Pectasides et al,[53] 2004	18	3 PR, 4 CR	40
Irinotecan/ paclitaxel/ oxaliplatin	Shamash et al,[54] 2007	28	15 PR, 5 CR	71
Paclitaxel/cisplatin/ gemcitabine	Nicolai et al,[55] 2009	22 (5 patients treated in third-line setting)	8 PR, 0 CR (0 responses in third-line setting)	36
Gemcitabine/ oxaliplatin/ paclitaxel	Bokemeyer et al,[56] 2008	41	19 PR, 2 CR	51
	Necchi et al,[58] 2008	19	5 PR, 2 CR	36

Abbreviations: CR, complete response; PR, partial response.

The combination of gemcitabine and oxaliplatin has been evaluated in three published phase II studies. A study by the German Testicular Cancer Study Group in 35 patients reported a 46% response rate, including 2 patients who experienced complete remission after chemotherapy alone and 1 who experienced complete remission after surgical resection of residual masses. One of the patients experiencing complete response had absolutely cisplatin-refractory disease, and the other 2 had been previously treated with high-dose chemotherapy. The 3 patients who experienced complete response were disease-free for 16+, 4+, and 12+ months at study publication.[44]

A second study in 28 patients showed a response rate of 32%, including 4 patients who experienced complete responses. Of the patients who experienced complete response, 3 were disease-free at 14+, 19+, and 28+ months at study publication. A fourth patient experienced relapse after complete remission but had subsequent resection of pulmonary nodules followed by a disease-free period exceeding 11 months.[45]

A third, smaller study of 18 patients reported a 17% response rate, including one complete response after chemotherapy alone and two complete responses after post-chemotherapy surgical resection of residual masses. The patients were disease-free after 44+, 20+, and 18+ months.[46]

A phase II study of oxaliplatin and paclitaxel given in the third-line setting included 26 patients and reported two long-term survivors, both of whom underwent postchemotherapy surgical resection of residual masses. High-dose chemotherapy had previously failed in both of these patients.[47] However, whether the patients included were truly refractory to cisplatin is difficult to ascertain from the information reported in the study.[48]

The combination of oxaliplatin and bevacizumab is currently being evaluated in an ongoing phase II trial. Among 16 patients evaluated for serologic response, a preliminary report showed that 3 experienced a complete response and 3 a partial response, and among 10 patients with measurable disease, 1 experienced a partial response and none had a complete response.[49] These results have only been published in abstract format and further information regarding patient characteristics is unavailable.

The combination of cisplatin and the anthracycline epirubicin was administered to 30 patients with refractory GCT. Of these, prior high-dose chemotherapy failed in 4, and 21 experienced late disease relapse after initial cisplatin-based chemotherapy. A 57% overall response rate was reported, with seven long-term complete responses, ranging from 27+ to 48+ months.[50] Two patients for whom prior high-dose chemotherapy failed experienced complete responses with this regimen. Only one patient who had not experienced a late relapse of GCT had a long-term response.

Although single-agent irinotecan did not exhibit significant activity against cisplatin refractory-GCT,[51] doublet regimens combining irinotecan with cisplatin or nedaplatin and oxaliplatin have been studied. A Japanese trial of 18 patients treated with irinotecan and either cisplatin or nedaplatin showed a response rate of 50%.[52] However, no details are given regarding specific previous treatment regimens, and patients who were not heavily pretreated but were defined as cisplatin-refractory for the purpose of this study may actually have retained some sensitivity to cisplatin. The combination of irinotecan and oxaliplatin has been investigated in a phase II trial of 18 patients with refractory GCT, all of whom had received at least two prior cisplatin-based regimens. The response rate was 40%, with four complete responses. Three of the patients with complete response were alive and continuously disease-free for 11+, 14+, and 19+ months.[53]

Three different triplet regimens have been investigated in phase II studies in the third-line setting for refractory GCT. The combination of irinotecan, paclitaxel, and oxaliplatin (IPO) was evaluated in 28 patients. The study included patients with mediastinal primaries who experienced relapsed after only first-line cisplatin-based therapy, and only 4 patients had previously received high-dose chemotherapy. Consolidation therapy with topotecan-based high-dose chemotherapy was given to 12 patients at completion of IPO. A response rate of 71% was reported, with 5 patients experiencing complete response; 32% of patients were progression-free after 14 months of follow-up.[54]

The combination of paclitaxel, cisplatin, and gemcitabine was evaluated in 22 patients with refractory GCT. Although the primary objective of the study was to evaluate this regimen as first-relapse salvage therapy, 5 of the 22 patients received this therapy in the third-line setting. A 36% response rate was reported, with six complete responses.[55] However, none of the 5 patients who entered the study after two previous courses of chemotherapy experienced a response, suggesting that although this regimen may have activity earlier in the treatment course for patients with refractory GCT, it is not likely to be beneficial in the third-line setting.

The most promising triplet regimen has been gemcitabine, oxaliplatin, and paclitaxel, which was administered to 41 heavily pretreated patients, in most of whom prior high-dose chemotherapy failed. The reported response rate was 51%, with two complete responses.[56] At study publication, 17% of patients were continuously disease-free. A recent update of the outcomes of this study, and a previous trial of doublet therapy with gemcitabine and oxaliplatin,[44] was presented in abstract format in 2010.[57] When the studies were originally reported, 26 of 76 patients were alive and disease-free. After a median follow-up of 16 months, the overall long-term survival rate was 6% (2/35) among patients treated with gemcitabine/oxaliplatin, and 20% (8/41) among those treated with gemcitabine/oxaliplatin/paclitaxel. These findings suggest that the triplet combination with paclitaxel achieves higher long-term survival rates than the gemcitabine/oxaliplatin doublet. A randomized trial comparing the two regimens in the third-line setting is needed to confirm this result.

An Italian trial evaluated the use of the triplet regimen in 19 patients with cisplatin-refractory GCT and reported a 36% overall response rate, including two complete remissions.[58] These data were presented in abstract format in 2008, and no further results are currently available.

In sum, combination therapy in the third-line setting can result in significant clinical activity and occasionally long-term disease control, especially when combined with salvage surgery. However, the optimal combination and the benefit of triplet regimens compared with doublet regimens remains to be determined.

DRUG THERAPY FOR GROWING TERATOMA SYNDROME AND TERATOMA WITH MALIGNANT TRANSFORMATION

Growing teratoma syndrome is defined as an enlarging mass during or after chemotherapy for nonseminomatous GCT, with normalization of serum alpha-fetoprotein and human chorionic gonadotropin. Pathology of these tumors shows only mature teratoma.[59] Growing teratoma syndrome occurs in 2% to 7% of patients with nonseminomatous GCTs.[60] Teratomas are resistant to chemotherapy and radiation; therefore, complete surgical resection is the preferred treatment and has been associated with the best long-term outcomes.[61] The development of medical therapy for patients with incurable, inoperable growing teratomas represents an unmet medical need. Anecdotal reports of disease stabilization or response have been reported. Alpha-interferon has been associated with disease stabilization in two case reports.[62,63] All-trans retinoic acid was reported to have activity in a patient with teratoma.[64] A single case report exists of bevacizumab leading to disease stabilization and clinical improvement in growing teratoma syndrome, with extensive disease progression occurring 40 days after treatment with bevacizumab was stopped.[65]

More recently, Vaughn and colleagues[66] reported a case series of three patients with unresectable growing teratoma syndrome treated in a phase I trial of the selective cyclin-independent kinase 4/6 inhibitor PD-0,332,991 (Pfizer). The rationale for this approach was based on the fact that mature teratomas, which are cisplatin-refractory, strongly express the retinoblastoma protein (pRb), suggesting an intact G1/S checkpoint.[67] PD-0,332,991 resulted in prolonged disease stabilization in two patients and a prolonged partial response in a third patient. This agent is currently being studied in a phase II trial of patients with refractory pRb-expressing GCT.

The teratomatous component of a GCT can undergo malignant transformation to a histologic type identical to that of a somatic malignancy. In these rare cases, treatment with systemic chemotherapy specific to the underlying histology may be of benefit. Investigators from Memorial Sloan-Kettering Cancer Center reported on 12 patients with GCT and teratoma with malignant transformation treated with chemotherapy. Four patients with rhabdomyosarcoma histology and one with anaplastic small cell tumor histology were treated with doxorubicin- or ifosfamide-based therapy. One patient with primitive neuroectodermal tumor histology was treated with an intensive regimen of cyclophosphamide, doxorubicin, vincristine, ifosfamide, and etoposide. Two patients with teratoma that transformed into leukemia were treated with standard idarubicin/cytarabine induction chemotherapy. Two patients with adenocarcinoma histology were treated with fluorouracil-based chemotherapy. In this select series, seven patients experienced a major response to chemotherapy, and three were alive and disease-free with combined-modality therapy at publication. Two additional patients underwent chemotherapy after surgical removal of the transformed teratoma; one patient with primitive neuroectodermal tumor was treated with adjuvant combination chemotherapy, and one with rhabdomyosarcoma was treated with adjuvant doxorubicin-based therapy. Both of these patients were alive and disease-free at publication.[68]

More recently, an Italian case series of 48 patients with malignant transformation of GCT was published. Of the 36 patients with metastatic disease, 11 were treated with cisplatin-based GCT therapy combined with surgical resection of disease; 7 are currently alive and disease-free. Three patients were treated with surgery followed by chemotherapy directed at the histology of the malignant transformation. One of these patients relapsed and was treated with salvage chemotherapy for GCT, and another had a bulky abdominal relapse of primitive neuroectodermal tumor (PNET) after BEP therapy and is currently undergoing salvage therapy. All three of these patients are currently alive. The authors concluded that cisplatin-based therapy, both as first-line treatment and as salvage treatment, followed by extensive surgical resection of residual disease, is the most appropriate approach to malignant transformation of GCT. They suggest further investigation of therapies targeted to specific chemosensitive histologies such as rhabdomyosarcoma and PNET. Finally, they developed an international online database to collect new cases of malignant transformation with the hope of facilitating multi-institutional collaboration in the treatment of these rare cancers.[69]

NOVEL AGENTS AND REFRACTORY GCTS

For patients with refractory GCT who are not cured using the currently available treatment options, evaluation of targeted therapies using novel agents has been a particularly interesting area of recent research. Vascular endothelial growth factor (VEGF) has been shown to exhibit significantly higher levels of expression in GCT cells than in non-eoplastic testis cells. Additionally, VEGF appears to be an independent predictor of clinically detectable metastasis in GCT.[70] Therefore, agents that target VEGF have been investigated in refractory GCT.

Thalidomide possesses antiangiogenic properties, presumably from inhibition of the VEGF receptor. Thalidomide was evaluated in 15 patients with refractory GCT, but no complete or partial responses occurred.[71]

Bevacizumab is currently undergoing evaluation in combination with oxaliplatin in refractory GCT, with one partial response seen among 18 patients evaluated thus far.[49] There is a case report of the use of bevacizumab in addition to high-dose ifosfamide, carboplatin, and etoposide (HD-ICE) salvage chemotherapy in a patient with GCT continuously refractory to three lines of standard cisplatin-based chemotherapy. Although the patient had a good serologic response and partial radiologic response lasting 5 months, his disease rapidly progressed and he died 4 months later.[72]

Sunitinib has been studied in a model of human testicular GCTs orthotopically grown in mice, and has been found to exhibit antitumor and antiangiogenic activity in this setting.[73] A phase II trial of single-agent sunitinib in 10 patients with heavily pretreated, refractory GCT reported no objective responses, with all patients developing progressive disease within three cycles of sunitinib.[74] However, a decrease in serum tumor markers was observed to correlate with sunitinib therapy, perhaps implying that pathways inhibited by sunitinib are important in the biology of GCT. A second phase II trial of sunitinib monotherapy in 32 patients with heavily pretreated, refractory GCT has shown two confirmed partial responses and two unconfirmed partial responses, for a total response rate of 12%.[75] The results are reported in abstract format and further information, including the nature of the unconfirmed partial responses, is currently unavailable.

Recently two novel small molecule inhibitors, HP-2 and HP-14, have been shown to inhibit the growth of testicular GCT cells that express VEGF receptor 2 and decrease angiogenic vessel formation in the membranes of fertilized chicken eggs.[76] Thus, other targets in the VEGF pathway may prove important to future advances in the treatment of refractory GCT.

Activating mutations in *KIT* have been found in seminomas and some refractory nonseminomatous GCT.[77–79] There is a case report of a complete response achieved with imatinib in a patient with refractory seminoma.[80] A phase II trial of imatinib therapy in six patients with pretreated, refractory nonseminomatous GCT showed no response.[81] Therefore, imatinib may have a role in refractory seminomas but apparently not in nonseminomatous GCT.

Epidermal growth factor receptor is expressed in nonseminomatous GCT.[78,82] In vitro studies have shown that erlotinib inhibits growth in a line of cisplatin-resistant embryonal carcinoma cells.[83] Therefore, erlotinib is a potentially useful agent to study in refractory GCT.

Although there is a single case report in the literature of a partial response induced by trastuzumab monotherapy in a patient with refractory GCT,[84] two separate studies have shown a very low incidence of HER-2/neu gene amplification by fluorescence in site hybridization, even in GCT samples in which Her-2 neu is detected through

Table 3
Ongoing clinical trials in refractory germ cell tumors

Title of Trial	Principal Investigator	Institution	Recruitment Status	Planned Enrollment	Estimated Completion Date
Everolimus for Patients with Relapsed/Refractory Germ Cell Cancer (RADIT)	Martin H. Fenner, MD	Hannover Medical School, Germany	Recruiting	25	May, 2013
ARQ 197 for Subjects with Relapsed or Refractory Germ Cell Tumors	Darren Feldman, MD	Memorial Sloan-Kettering Cancer Center	This trial closed to accrual after first stage because of ineffectiveness	41	N/A
PD-0,332,991 in Treating Patients with Refractory Solid Tumors	Peter O'Dwyer, MD	Abramson Cancer Center of the University of Pennsylvania	Recruiting	15	N/A
Study of Oxaliplatin Plus Bevacizumab in Germ Cell Tumor Patients	Lawrence Einhorn, MD	Indiana University Cancer Center	Recruiting	28	November, 2013
Alvocidib and Oxaliplatin with or without Fluorouracil and Leucovorin Calcium in Treating Patients with Relapsed or Refractory Germ Cell Tumors	Darren Feldman, MD	Memorial Sloan-Kettering Cancer Center	Recruiting	50	N/A
Sorafenib monotherapy in Inoperable/Recurrent Germ Cell Carcinoma Refractory to Chemotherapy	Iwona Skoneczna, MD	Fondation Wygrajmy Zdrowie, Poland	Recruiting	20	December, 2011
Study of Gemcitabine, Oxaliplatin and Paclitaxel in Patients with Refractory Germ Cell Carcinoma	David Quinn, MD	USC/Norris Comprehensive Cancer Center	Recruiting	20	January, 2010

Data from ClinicalTrials.gov. National Institutes of Health. Available at: http://clinicaltrials.gov. Accessed December 30, 2010.

immunohistochemistry.[85,86] Thus, therapy with trastuzumab is not likely to be beneficial in most patients with refractory GCT.

As more is learned about the molecular mechanisms of cisplatin resistance, the molecular and biologic factors behind late relapse of disease, and the biologic differences in disease between patients who experience response to cisplatin therapy and those who do not, further novel targets may become apparent with resultant development and implementation of effective targeted therapies for cisplatin-refractory GCT.

ONGOING TRIALS AND FUTURE DIRECTIONS

Several clinical trials in refractory GCTs are currently ongoing (Table 3). Relatively small numbers of patients have refractory GCT and they are a heavily pretreated population, which makes the development and testing of new therapeutic agents difficult. First- and second-line therapies for GCT are successful overall, so new agents tend to be tested after two or more lines of chemotherapy have failed, rather than earlier in the treatment regimen. Nevertheless, future research into the molecular mechanisms of cisplatin resistance and the combination of novel agents with chemotherapy agents that have known activity in refractory GCT may yield therapies with improved outcomes for patients with multiply relapsed and cisplatin-refractory disease.

REFERENCES

1. Porcu P, Bhatia S, Sharma M, et al. Results of treatment after relapse from high-dose chemotherapy in germ cell tumors. J Clin Oncol 2000;18(6):1181–6.
2. Kollmannsberger C, Schleucher N, Rick O, et al. Analysis of salvage treatments for germ cell cancer patients who have relapsed after primary high-dose chemotherapy plus autologous stem cell support. Eur J Cancer 2003;39(6):775–82.
3. Einhorn LH. Treatment of testicular cancer: a new and improved model. J Clin Oncol 1990;8(11):1777–81.
4. Kollmannsberger C, Nichols C, Bokemeyer C. Recent advances in management of patients with platinum-refractory testicular germ cell tumors. Cancer 2006; 106(6):1217–26.
5. Kollmannsberger C, Honecker F, Bokemeyer C. Pharmacotherapy of relapsed metastatic testicular cancer. Expert Opin Pharmacother 2008;9(13):2259–72.
6. Piulats JM, Jimenez L, Garcia del Muro X, et al. Molecular mechanisms behind the resistance of cisplatin in germ cell tumours. Clin Transl Oncol 2009;11(12): 780–6.
7. Masters JR, Koberle B. Curing metastatic cancer: lessons from testicular germ-cell tumours. Nat Rev Cancer 2003;3(7):517–25.
8. Ishida S, Lee J, Thiele DJ, et al. Uptake of the anticancer drug cisplatin mediated by the copper transporter Ctr1 in yeast and mammals. Proc Natl Acad Sci U S A 2002;99(22):14298–302.
9. Holzer AK, Howell SB. The internalization and degradation of human copper transporter 1 following cisplatin exposure. Cancer Res 2006;66(22):10944–52.
10. Borst P, Evers R, Wijnholds J. A family of drug transporters: the multidrug resistance-associated proteins. J Natl Cancer Inst 2000;92(16):1295–302.
11. Scheffer GL, Kool M, Hejin M, et al. Specific detection of multidrug resistance proteins MRP1, MRP2, MRP3, MRP5, and MDR3 P-glycoprotein with a panel of monoclonal antibodies. Cancer Res 2000;60(18):5269–77.

12. Scheffer GL, Schroeijers AB, Izquierdo MA, et al. Lung resistance-related protein/ major vault protein and vaults in multidrug-resistant cancer. Curr Opin Oncol 2000;12(6):550–6.
13. Masters JR, Thomas R, Hall AG, et al. Sensitivity of testis tumour cells to chemotherapeutic drugs: role of detoxifying pathways. Eur J Cancer 1996;32A(7):1248–53.
14. Sark MW, Timmer-Bosscha H, Meijer C, et al. Cellular basis for differential sensitivity to cisplatin in human germ cell tumour and colon carcinoma cell lines. Br J Cancer 1995;71(4):684–90.
15. Koberle B, Grimaldi KA, Sunters A, et al. DNA repair capacity and cisplatin sensitivity of human testis tumour cells. Int J Cancer 1997;70(5):551–5.
16. Koberle B, Masters JR, Hartley JA, et al. Defective repair of cisplatin-induced DNA damage caused by reduced XPA protein in testicular germ cell tumours. Curr Biol 1999;9(5):273–6.
17. Honecker F, Mayer F, Stoop H, et al. Xeroderma pigmentosum group a protein and chemotherapy resistance in human germ cell tumors. Lab Invest 2003; 83(10):1489–95.
18. Zamble DB, Mu D, Reardon JT, et al. Repair of cisplatin–DNA adducts by the mammalian excision nuclease. Biochemistry 1996;35(31):10004–13.
19. Mayer F, Gillis AJ, Dinjens W, et al. Microsatellite instability of germ cell tumors is associated with resistance to systemic treatment. Cancer Res 2002;62(10): 2758–60.
20. Honecker F, Wermann H, Mayer F, et al. Microsatellite instability, mismatch repair deficiency, and BRAF mutation in treatment-resistant germ cell tumors. J Clin Oncol 2009;27(13):2129–36.
21. Lutzker SG, Mathew R, Taller DR. A p53 dose-response relationship for sensitivity to DNA damage in isogenic teratocarcinoma cells. Oncogene 2001;20(23):2982–6.
22. Kersemaekers AM, Mayer F, Molier M, et al. Role of P53 and MDM2 in treatment response of human germ cell tumors. J Clin Oncol 2002;20(6):1551–61.
23. Burger H, Nooter K, Boersma AW, et al. Distinct p53-independent apoptotic cell death signalling pathways in testicular germ cell tumour cell lines. Int J Cancer 1999;81(4):620–8.
24. Mayer F, Stoop H, L Scheffer G, et al. Molecular determinants of treatment response in human germ cell tumors. Clin Cancer Res 2003;9(2):767–73.
25. Fitzharris BM, Kaye SB, Saverymuttu S, et al. VP16-213 as a single agent in advanced testicular tumors. Eur J Cancer 1980;16(9):1193–7.
26. Loehrer PJ Sr. Etoposide therapy for testicular cancer. Cancer 1991;67(Suppl 1): 220–4.
27. Miller JC, Einhorn LH. Phase II study of daily oral etoposide in refractory germ cell tumors. Semin Oncol 1990;17(1 Suppl 2):36–9.
28. Scheulen ME, Niederle N, Bremer K, et al. Efficacy of ifosfamide in refractory malignant diseases and uroprotection by mesna: results of a clinical phase II-study with 151 patients. Cancer Treat Rev 1983;10(Suppl A):93–101.
29. Wheeler BM, Loehrer PJ, Williams SD, et al. Ifosfamide in refractory male germ cell tumors. J Clin Oncol 1986;4(1):28–34.
30. Einhorn LH. Ifosfamide in germ cell tumors. Oncology 2003;65(Suppl 2):73–5.
31. Motzer RJ, Bajorin DF, Schwartz LH, et al. Phase II trial of paclitaxel shows antitumor activity in patients with previously treated germ cell tumors. J Clin Oncol 1994;12(11):2277–83.
32. Bokemeyer C, Beyer J, Metzner B, et al. Phase II study of paclitaxel in patients with relapsed or cisplatin-refractory testicular cancer. Ann Oncol 1996;7(1):31–4.

33. Bokemeyer C, Schmoll HJ, Natt F, et al. Preliminary results of a phase I/II trial of paclitaxel in patients with relapsed or cisplatin-refractory testicular cancer. J Cancer Res Clin Oncol 1994;120(12):754–7.
34. Nazario A, Amato R, Hutchinson L, et al. Paclitaxel in extensively pretreated non-seminomatous germ cell tumors. Urol Oncol 1995;1(5):184–7.
35. Sandler AB, Cristou A, Fox S, et al. A phase II trial of paclitaxel in refractory germ cell tumors. Cancer 1998;82(7):1381–6.
36. Berruti A, Saini A, Gorzegno G, et al. Durable complete remission after weekly docetaxel administration in a patient with mediastinal non-seminomatous germ-cell tumor refractory to cisplatin-based chemotherapy. Ann Oncol 2003;14(10):1589–90.
37. Bokemeyer C, Gerl A, Schoffski P, et al. Gemcitabine in patients with relapsed or cisplatin-refractory testicular cancer. J Clin Oncol 1999;17(2):512–6.
38. Einhorn LH, Stender MJ, Williams SD. Phase II trial of gemcitabine in refractory germ cell tumors. J Clin Oncol 1999;17(2):509–11.
39. Dunn TA, Schmoll HJ, Grunwald V, et al. Comparative cytotoxicity of oxaliplatin and cisplatin in non-seminomatous germ cell cancer cell lines. Invest New Drugs 1997;15(2):109–14.
40. Kollmannsberger C, Rick O, Derigs HG, et al. Activity of oxaliplatin in patients with relapsed or cisplatin-refractory germ cell cancer: a study of the German Testicular Cancer Study Group. J Clin Oncol 2002;20(8):2031–7.
41. Fizazi K, Culine S, Chen I. Oxaliplatin in non-seminomatous germ-cell tumors. Ann Oncol 2004;15(8):1295.
42. Hinton S, Catalano P, Einhorn LH, et al. Phase II study of paclitaxel plus gemcitabine in refractory germ cell tumors (E9897): a trial of the Eastern Cooperative Oncology Group. J Clin Oncol 2002;20(7):1859–63.
43. Einhorn LH, Brames MJ, Juliar B, et al. Phase II study of paclitaxel plus gemcitabine salvage chemotherapy for germ cell tumors after progression following high-dose chemotherapy with tandem transplant. J Clin Oncol 2007;25(5):513–6.
44. Kollmannsberger C, Beyer J, Liersch R, et al. Combination chemotherapy with gemcitabine plus oxaliplatin in patients with intensively pretreated or refractory germ cell cancer: a study of the German Testicular Cancer Study Group. J Clin Oncol 2004;22(1):108–14.
45. Pectasides D, Pectasides M, Farmakis D, et al. Gemcitabine and oxaliplatin (GEMOX) in patients with cisplatin-refractory germ cell tumors: a phase II study. Ann Oncol 2004;15(3):493–7.
46. De Giorgi U, Rosti G, Aieta M, et al. Phase II study of oxaliplatin and gemcitabine salvage chemotherapy in patients with cisplatin-refractory nonseminomatous germ cell tumor. Eur Urol 2006;50(5):1032–8 [discussion: 1038–9].
47. Theodore C, Chevreau C, Yataqhene Y, et al. A phase II multicenter study of oxaliplatin in combination with paclitaxel in poor prognosis patients who failed cisplatin-based chemotherapy for germ-cell tumors. Ann Oncol 2008;19(8):1465–9.
48. Necchi A, Nicolai N, Salvioni R. Does oxaliplatin and paclitaxel combination show an activity of some extent in pretreated patients with germ-cell tumors? Reply to the article "A phase II multicenter study of oxaliplatin in combination with paclitaxel in poor prognosis patients who failed cisplatin-based chemotherapy for germ-cell tumors" by C. Theodore et al. (Ann Oncol 2008; doi: 10.1093/annonc/mdn122). Ann Oncol 2008;19(8):1509.
49. Ramasubbaiah J, Brames J, Johnston EL, et al. Phase II study of oxaliplatin (O) and bevacizumab (B) chemotherapy in refractory germ cell tumors (GCT) [abstract]. J Clin Oncol 2010;28(15):e15054.

50. Bedano PM, Brames MJ, Williams SD, et al. Phase II study of cisplatin plus epirubicin salvage chemotherapy in refractory germ cell tumors. J Clin Oncol 2006; 24(34):5403–7.
51. Kollmannsberger C, Rick O, Klaproth H, et al. Irinotecan in patients with relapsed or cisplatin-refractory germ cell cancer: a phase II study of the German Testicular Cancer Study Group. Br J Cancer 2002;87(7):729–32.
52. Miki T, Mizutani Y, Nonomura N, et al. Irinotecan plus cisplatin has substantial antitumor effect as salvage chemotherapy against germ cell tumors. Cancer 2002;95(9):1879–85.
53. Pectasides D, Pectasides M, Farmakis D, et al. Oxaliplatin and irinotecan plus granulocyte-colony stimulating factor as third-line treatment in relapsed or cisplatin-refractory germ-cell tumor patients: a phase II study. Eur Urol 2004; 46(2):216–21.
54. Shamash J, Powles T, Mutsvangwa K, et al. A phase II study using a topoisomerase I-based approach in patients with multiply relapsed germ-cell tumours. Ann Oncol 2007;18(5):925–30.
55. Nicolai N, Necchi A, Gianni L, et al. Long-term results of a combination of paclitaxel, cisplatin and gemcitabine for salvage therapy in male germ-cell tumours. BJU Int 2009;104(3):340–6.
56. Bokemeyer C, Oechsle K, Honecker F, et al. Combination chemotherapy with gemcitabine, oxaliplatin, and paclitaxel in patients with cisplatin-refractory or multiply relapsed germ-cell tumors: a study of the German Testicular Cancer Study Group. Ann Oncol 2008;19(3):448–53.
57. Oeschle K, Kollmannsberger K, Honecker F, et al. Long term outcome in patients with cisplatin-refractory or multiply relapsed germ cell tumors following treatment with gemcitabine and oxaliplatin +/- paclitaxel [abstract]. J Clin Oncol 2010; 28(Suppl 15):4585.
58. Necchi A, Nicolai N, Piva L, et al. Long-term results of a combination of paclitaxel, oxaliplatin and gemcitabine as far rescue in heavily pre-treated male germ-cell tumors (GCT) [abstract]. J Clin Oncol 2008;26(Suppl 15):16036.
59. Logothetis CJ, Samuels ML, Trindade A, et al. The growing teratoma syndrome. Cancer 1982;50(8):1629–35.
60. Andre F, Fizazi K, Culine S, et al. The growing teratoma syndrome: results of therapy and long-term follow-up of 33 patients. Eur J Cancer 2000;36(11): 1389–94.
61. Spiess PE, Kassouf W, Brown GA, et al. Surgical management of growing teratoma syndrome: the M.D. Anderson cancer center experience. J Urol 2007; 177(4):1330–4 [discussion: 1334].
62. van der Gaast A, Kok TC, Splinter TA. Growing teratoma syndrome successfully treated with lymphoblastoid interferon. Eur Urol 1991;19(3):257–8.
63. Ornadel D, Wilson A, Trask C, et al. Remission of recurrent mature teratoma with interferon therapy. J R Soc Med 1995;88(9):533P–4P.
64. Gordon MS, Battiato LA, Finch D, et al. Dramatic response of teratoma-associated non–germ-cell cancer with all-trans retinoic acid in a patient with non-seminomatous germ cell tumor. Am J Clin Oncol 2001;24(3):269–71.
65. Mego M, Reckova M, Sycova-Mila Z, et al. Bevacizumab in a growing teratoma syndrome. Case report. Ann Oncol 2007;18(5):962–3.
66. Vaughn DJ, Flaherty K, Lal P, et al. Treatment of growing teratoma syndrome. N Engl J Med 2009;360(4):423–4.
67. Bartkova J, Lukas C, Sorensen CS, et al. Deregulation of the RB pathway in human testicular germ cell tumours. J Pathol 2003;200(2):149–56.

68. Donadio AC, Motzer RJ, Bajorin DF, et al. Chemotherapy for teratoma with malignant transformation. J Clin Oncol 2003;21(23):4285–91.
69. Necchi A, Colecchia M, Nicolai N, et al. Towards the definition of the best management and prognostic factors of teratoma with malignant transformation: a single-institution case series and new proposal. BJU Int 2011;107(7):1088–94.
70. Fukuda S, Shirahama T, Imazono Y, et al. Expression of vascular endothelial growth factor in patients with testicular germ cell tumors as an indicator of metastatic disease. Cancer 1999;85(6):1323–30.
71. Rick O, Braun T, Siegert W, et al. Activity of thalidomide in patients with platinum-refractory germ-cell tumours. Eur J Cancer 2006;42(12):1775–9.
72. Voigt W, Kegel T, Maher G, et al. Bevacizumab plus high-dose ifosfamide, etoposide and carboplatin (HD-ICE) as third-line salvage chemotherapy induced an unexpected dramatic response in highly platinum refractory germ-cell cancer. Ann Oncol 2006;17(3):531–3.
73. Castillo-Avila W, Piulats JM, Garcia del Muro X, et al. Sunitinib inhibits tumor growth and synergizes with cisplatin in orthotopic models of cisplatin-sensitive and cisplatin-resistant human testicular germ cell tumors. Clin Cancer Res 2009;15(10):3384–95.
74. Feldman DR, Turkula S, Ginsberg MS, et al. Phase II trial of sunitinib in patients with relapsed or refractory germ cell tumors. Invest New Drugs 2010;28(4):523–8.
75. Kollmannsberger C, Oeschle K, Cheng T, et al. Sunitinib in patients with multiply relapsed or cisplatin-refractory germ cell cancer: a CUOG/GTCSG cooperative phase II study [abstract]. J Clin Oncol 2010;28(Suppl 15):4582.
76. Nitzsche B, Gloesenkamp C, Schrader M, et al. Novel compounds with antiangiogenic and antiproliferative potency for growth control of testicular germ cell tumours. Br J Cancer 2010;103(1):18–28.
77. Tian Q, Frierson HF Jr, Krystal GW, et al. Activating c-kit gene mutations in human germ cell tumors. Am J Pathol 1999;154(6):1643–7.
78. Madani A, Kemmer K, Sweeney C, et al. Expression of KIT and epidermal growth factor receptor in chemotherapy refractory non-seminomatous germ-cell tumors. Ann Oncol 2003;14(6):873–80.
79. Kemmer K, Corless CL, Fletcher JA, et al. KIT mutations are common in testicular seminomas. Am J Pathol 2004;164(1):305–13.
80. Pedersini R, Vattemi E, Mazzoleni G, et al. Complete response after treatment with imatinib in pretreated disseminated testicular seminoma with overexpression of c-KIT. Lancet Oncol 2007;8(11):1039–40.
81. Einhorn LH, Brames MJ, Heinrich MC, et al. Phase II study of imatinib mesylate in chemotherapy refractory germ cell tumors expressing KIT. Am J Clin Oncol 2006; 29(1):12–3.
82. Moroni M, Veronese S, Schiavo R, et al. Epidermal growth factor receptor expression and activation in nonseminomatous germ cell tumors. Clin Cancer Res 2001; 7(9):2770–5.
83. Freemantle SJ, Vaseva AV, Ewings KE, et al. Repression of cyclin D1 as a target for germ cell tumors. Int J Oncol 2007;30(2):333–40.
84. Kollmannsberger C, Pressler H, Mayer F, et al. Cisplatin-refractory, HER2/neu-expressing germ-cell cancer: induction of remission by the monoclonal antibody Trastuzumab. Ann Oncol 1999;10(11):1393–4.
85. Soule S, Baldridge L, Kirkpatrick K, et al. HER-2/neu expression in germ cell tumours. J Clin Pathol 2002;55(9):656–8.
86. Mandoky L, Geczi L, Bodrogi I, et al. Clinical relevance of HER-2/neu expression in germ-cell testicular tumors. Anticancer Res 2004;24(4):2219–24.

Role of Postchemotherapy Retroperitoneal Lymph Node Dissection in Advanced Germ Cell Tumors

Carvell T. Nguyen, MD, PhD[a], Andrew J. Stephenson, MD[b],*

KEYWORDS

- Testicular neoplasms • Neoplasms • Germ cell • Embryonal
- Chemotherapy • Retroperitoneum • Lymph node excision
- Neoplasm staging

Testis cancer is the most common malignancy afflicting men between the ages of 15 and 34 years, with 8400 men expected to be diagnosed in the United States in 2010.[1] Most cases (>95%) are germ cell tumors (GCTs), which are broadly divided into seminoma and nonseminoma GCT (NSGCT). Advanced GCT is an example of the importance of multidisciplinary management in the successful treatment of patients. Before the development of cisplatin-based chemotherapy, long-term survival was reported in less than 10% of patients.[2] Long-term cure is now anticipated in 80% to 90%.[3] A recent meta-analysis of 10 trials enrolling a total of 1775 patients with advanced NSGCT reported improved 5-year survival rates for patients with good-risk (94% vs 89%), intermediate-risk (83% vs 75%), and poor-risk disease (71% vs 41%) compared with the original pooled analysis conducted by the International Germ Cell Cancer Collaborative Group (IGCCCG).[3,4] This improved prognosis for patients with advanced GCT is likely caused by better risk stratification and

Financial disclosures: None.

[a] Glickman Urological and Kidney Institute, Cleveland Clinic, 9500 Euclid Avenue, Q10, Cleveland, OH 44195, USA

[b] Center for Urologic Oncology, Glickman Urological & Kidney Institute, Cleveland Clinic, 9500 Euclid Avenue, Desk Q10-1, Cleveland, OH 44195, USA

* Corresponding author.

E-mail address: stephea2@ccf.org

Hematol Oncol Clin N Am 25 (2011) 593–604

doi:10.1016/j.hoc.2011.03.002

hemonc.theclinics.com

risk-appropriate chemotherapy, stage migration, and improved integration of chemotherapy and postchemotherapy surgery (PCS) for resection of residual masses.

For treatment purposes, the distinction between seminoma and NSGCT holds great importance, particularly in the management of residual masses. Compared with NSGCT, seminoma is exquisitely sensitive to cisplatin-based chemotherapy. Thus, residual masses after first-line chemotherapy for seminoma are more likely to show necrosis and less likely to harbor viable GCT elements compared with NSGCT. The risk of teratoma at metastatic sites has a substantial effect on treatment algorithms for NSGCT and necessitates the frequent use of PCS in patients with advanced NSGCT. As discussed later, teratoma is not sensitive to chemotherapy and the outcome of patients with metastatic teratoma is related to the completeness of surgical resection. Although histologically benign, teratoma has unpredictable biology, with a capacity to grow rapidly, undergo malignant transformation, or result in late relapse. The risk of teratoma at metastatic sites is generally not a consideration for advanced seminoma, which has important implications for the management of residual masses after chemotherapy.

Because of the high cure rates anticipated for patients with advanced GCT, numerous clinical trials have been conducted in an attempt to minimize treatment and avoid any unnecessary therapies in an effort to reduce short-term, and particularly long-term, toxicity. One such approach has been to limit the number of patients who receive 2 interventions (double therapy): either surgery or chemotherapy and not both. However, because NSGCTs are usually mixed tumors and teratoma often exists at metastatic sites with other GCT elements, cure often requires chemotherapy to eradicate the chemosensitive components and surgery to remove teratomatous components. It is widely accepted that the successful integration of systemic therapy and PCS is a major contributing factor to the improved cure rates for metastatic GCT seen in the past several decades.

Advances in surgical technique and understanding of retroperitoneal anatomy have reduced the morbidity of RPLND (eg, retrograde ejaculation) while enhancing oncological efficacy. However, postchemotherapy retroperitoneal lymph node dissection (PC-RPLND) can be a challenging undertaking that has historically been associated with higher rates of complications compared with primary RPLND.[5–7] As such, appropriate patient selection and proper surgical technique are critical to optimizing cancer and quality-of-life outcomes following surgery.

The indications and outcomes of PC-RPLND are discussed to determine its role in the contemporary management of advanced GCT. This article focuses primarily on PC-RPLND in the setting of NSGCT, but the limited indications for PCS in advanced seminoma are also discussed.

NSGCT: RATIONALE FOR PC-RPLND

The role of PC-RPLND for residual masses in advanced NSGCT is well established and its rationale is based on several factors. Multiple large series of patients undergoing PC-RPLND for residual masses after first-line chemotherapy have consistently reported evidence of persistent GCT elements in the resected specimens in 50% or more of patients. On average, histopathologic evaluation of resected specimens shows necrosis, teratoma, and viable malignancy (with or without teratoma) in 40%, 45%, and 15% of cases respectively (**Table 1**).[8–20]

The therapeutic benefit of PC-RPLND in cases in which residual masses harbor viable malignancy or teratoma is well documented. Complete resection of viable malignancy (with or without adjuvant chemotherapy) is associated with 5-year survival

Table 1
Histology of postchemotherapy residual masses

	Patients	Necrosis (%)	Viable Malignancy ± Teratoma (%)	Teratoma Only (%)
Steyerberg et al,[19] 1995	556	45	13	42
Carver et a,[9] 2007	504	49	11	39
Hendry et al,[14] 2002	330	25	9	66
Debono et al,[11] 1997	295	25	7	67
Spiess et al,[16] 2006	236	41	17	42
Albers et al,[8] 2004	232	35	31	34
Toner et al,[20] 1990	185	47	16	37
Steyerberg et al,[18] 1998	172	45	13	42
Stenning et al,[17] 1998	153	29	15	55
de Wit et al,[10] 1997	127	35	9	56
Oeschle et al,[47] 2008	121	45	21	34
Sonneveld et al,[15] 1998	113	46	9	45
Gerl et al,[12] 1995	111	47	12	41
Hartmann et al,[60] 1997	109	52	21	27

rates between 45% and 77%.[9,13,16,17,20–25] If not excised, or subject to an inadequate resection, residual viable malignancy within the retroperitoneum will presumably relapse, necessitating second-line (salvage) chemotherapy; however, only a quarter of such relapsing patients experience long-term survival.[26–28]

Although histologically benign, the risk of teratoma within residual masses also mandates complete surgical excision, which is associated with long-term cancer control in 75% to 90% of men.[29] Teratoma is resistant to chemotherapy and radiation therapy and the natural history of unresected teratoma after chemotherapy is unpredictable. It may remain dormant or exhibit slow growth. However, it may also exhibit rapid, expansive, local growth, leading to invasion or impingement of adjacent vital structures. Moreover, a small percentage (typically <10%) of teratomas may undergo malignant transformation to a non-GCT malignancy (eg, rhabdomyosarcoma, primitive neuroectodermal tumor, adenocarcinoma), which is resistant to conventional GCT chemotherapy regimens and is associated with a poor prognosis.[20,29–32] Lastly, unresected teratoma may manifest as late recurrence, which is associated with poor prognosis.[33–35] As with viable malignancy, complete eradication of all residual teratomatous elements following chemotherapy is the best means of optimizing oncological outcomes.[13,15,17,20,29]

The critical role of PC-RPLND in advanced GCT is shown by the results of a recent randomized trial comparing BEPx3 versus EPx4 in 257 men with good-risk, advanced NSGCT. In this trial, the indications for, and technique of, PC-RPLND was not dictated by protocol, and fewer than 50% of study participants underwent PCS for residual masses. Overall, 14 of 20 relapses (70%) and 7 of 14 deaths (50%) occurred in patients who either did not undergo PCS or who relapsed in the retroperitoneum after PC-RPLND (presumably from a limited-template dissection).[36]

Hendry and colleagues[14] analyzed the outcomes of PC-RPLND in 330 and 112 patients after first-line and second-line chemotherapy, respectively. After first-line chemotherapy, patients were more likely to undergo a complete resection, resected specimens were less likely to contain viable malignancy, and the risk of relapse (17% vs 38%) and death (11% vs 44%) was substantially less than after second-line chemotherapy. These results suggest that a potential opportunity to cure patients may be lost if PC-RPLND is not performed following first-line chemotherapy.

Debono and colleagues[11] analyzed the outcomes of 295 patients with NSGCT treated with first-line chemotherapy at Indiana University between 1987 and 1994. Patients with residual masses after chemotherapy who underwent PC-RPLND had excellent relapse-free survival (86%–87%), which approached that of patients who achieved a complete response to chemotherapy alone who were observed without PC-RPLND (92%). However, the former group had a substantially improved relapse-free survival compared with those who were observed after a major (but not complete) response to chemotherapy (74%) and those who had an incomplete surgical resection of residual masses (40%). Taken together, these studies show the potential role of PC-RPLND in reducing the risk of relapse and mortality from GCT.

Besides a therapeutic benefit, resection of residual masses can also provide staging information that can be used to dictate further chemotherapy and/or surveillance protocols. Extent of resection and percentage of viable malignancy in the tissue specimen have been shown to be important prognostic factors in predicting survival.[21] Moreover, the presence of viable malignancy in residual masses suggests the need for more chemotherapy, although its use in this setting is controversial. In a study by Fox and colleagues,[22] 14 of 27 patients (70%) found to have viable malignancy after undergoing PC-RPLND and who were treated with adjuvant chemotherapy were free of recurrence, compared with 0 of 7 patients who were observed. However, a multi-institutional study comprising 238 patients with viable malignancy in PC-RPLND specimens showed that postoperative chemotherapy was associated with improved 5-year progression-free survival (69% vs 52%, $P<.001$) but not overall survival (74% vs 70%, $P = .7$).[21] A confirmatory analysis of 61 patients from the same investigators reported similar findings, with a 15-point improvement in progression-free survival but little difference in overall survival, but the study was not powered for survival analysis.[25] The impact of postoperative chemotherapy in this setting thus remains unclear.

NSGCT: PATIENT SELECTION FOR PC-RPLND

PC-RPLND is generally recommended for patients with NSGCT with significant residual masses (ie, >1 cm) and normal serum tumor markers, because viable malignancy or teratoma is found in residual masses in approximately 15% and 40% of cases, respectively.[37–39] Given that approximately 45% of patients have necrosis, some have argued against the use of PC-RPLND in all patients based on the assumption that those with necrosis do not derive any therapeutic benefit. Although patients with necrosis in resected specimens have a risk of relapse of 10% or less, it is conceivable that such favorable outcomes may be achieved without surgery.[13,17,20,29] However, numerous desperation RPLND series have reported postoperative normalization of serum tumor marker levels even among patients with just necrosis in resected specimens.[40–42] A recent study from Indiana University also reported that 33% of men with necrosis had evidence of molecular changes associated with GCT within stromal cells.[43] These studies suggest that some residual viable GCT elements may be missed on routine histopathologic analysis, indicating a potential therapeutic benefit to PC-RPLND even among patients with necrosis. However, this concept is difficult to prove in the absence of a randomized trial.

The ability to accurately predict tissue histology and identify those men with only necrosis potentially obviates the need for PC-RPLND in select patients. Several clinical factors have been identified as predictors of necrosis in residual masses, including the absence of teratoma in the primary tumor, the percentage reduction in retroperitoneal tumor burden after chemotherapy, and the size of the retroperitoneal mass before and after chemotherapy.[8,18-20,44,45] Nomograms have been developed to predict the presence of necrosis based on these and other factors. Although these nomograms discriminate well between patients with residual GCT versus those with necrosis only, they are associated with a false-negative rate of 20%, and thus cannot be used reliably to dictate therapy.[18,19,46] Furthermore, no imaging modality has proved reliable in the prediction of the histology of residual masses. In a prospective study of 121 patients with residual masses after first-line chemotherapy, the predictive accuracy of positron emission tomography (PET) (56%) for viable malignancy or teratoma was no better than computed tomography (CT) (55%) or postchemotherapy serum tumor markers (56%).[47] Based on these findings, no imaging modality or multiparameter nomogram can be used safely to exclude a man from PC-RPLND who has a residual mass greater than or equal to 1 cm after first-line chemotherapy.

The management of patients with complete serologic and radiographic response is controversial, with some guidelines advocating close observation and others recommending PCS if prechemotherapy mass size is greater than 3 cm.[48-51] Some institutions advocate PC-RPLND in all patients after a complete response to first-line chemotherapy, regardless of the residual mass size, based on the rationale that there are no means to reliably exclude the presence of residual GCT and the risks associated with PC-RPLND are low when performed by experienced surgeons.[20,52] A 1-cm cutpoint is arbitrary and numerous studies have shown that, on average, patients with residual masses 20 mm or smaller have a 30% and 6% incidence of teratoma and viable malignancy, respectively (**Table 2**).[19,20,44,45,52-55] However, 2 studies have reported a low risk of relapse (4%–10%) and 97% to 100% cancer-specific survival

Table 2
Histology of postchemotherapy residual masses 20 mm in size or less

	Patients	Size (mm)	Necrosis (%)	Viable Malignancy ± Teratoma (%)	Teratoma Only (%)
Steyerberg et al,[19] 1995	275	≤20	65	5	30
Steyerberg et al,[19] 1995	162	≤10	72	4	24
Oldenburg et al,[52] 2003	87	≤20	67	7	26
Fossa et al,[44] 1992	78	<20	68	4	29
Fossa et al,[55] 1989	37	≤10	67	3	30
Stephenson et al,[53] 2007	36	≤5	69	6	25
Toner et al,[20] 1990	21	≤15	81	7	12
Stomper et al,[45] 1991	14	≤20	36	14	50

in patients with residual masses less than 1 cm who were observed without PCS.[56,57] The highly select nature of these patients is shown by most being good-risk by IGCCCG criteria, 60% to 76% not having teratoma in the primary tumor, and many having no visible masses after chemotherapy. The median follow-up in 1 of the studies was only 3.8 years, and likely underestimates the risk of relapse and death.[57] In a median follow-up of 15 years in the Indiana University study, half of the relapses occurred in the retroperitoneum. Thus, when deciding on PC-RPLND for small residual masses, the morbidity of PC-RPLND must be balanced with the risks of observation, including chemorefractory relapse and the frequent use of CT imaging in the surveillance of the retroperitoneum. Radiation from CT imaging may be an important cause of secondary malignancies and the safety threshold is exceeded after approximately 7 CT scans; routine CT imaging is not necessary after a full, bilateral template PC-RPLND.[58] Observation is a reasonable strategy for only 25% or less of men with advanced NSGCT. At our institution, observation is restricted to men with IGCCCG good-risk disease, no evidence of teratoma in the primary tumor, no evidence of any residual mass following chemotherapy, and who are anticipated to be compliant with follow-up imaging and testing.

Approximately one-third of patients have residual masses at multiple anatomic sites (the retroperitoneum, chest, and left supraclavicular fossa are the most common) and these patients should undergo resection of all sites of measurable residual disease, because the histology of residual masses at distant sites is similar to that of the retroperitoneum.[20,59–61] Discordant histology between anatomic sites is reported in 22% to 46% of cases. PC-RPLND should be performed before PCS at other sites because the probability of residual disease in the retroperitoneum is highest and RPLND histology is a strong predictor of histology at other sites. Observation of small residual masses at other sites is a reasonable option if the histology of the RPLND specimen indicates necrosis.

CLASSIFICATION OF PC-RPLND

A keen grasp of retroperitoneal anatomy as well as an appreciation of the tissue effects of chemotherapy are critical to the proper performance of PC-RPLND to maximize oncological efficacy and minimize morbidity. As discussed earlier, the strongest predictor of survival for patients with viable cancer after chemotherapy is complete eradication of all residual disease. The rate of retroperitoneal recurrence (<2%) is exceedingly low after an adequate (ie, bilateral template) RPLND.[62] In contrast, an inadequate dissection that leaves residual disease behind invariably leads to relapse and portends a poor prognosis, with a cancer-specific mortality of up to 80% for such patients.[22]

Compared with primary RPLND for low-stage disease, PC-RPLND has generally been associated with a higher risk of morbidity, caused by tissue effects, decreased pulmonary, renal, and hematological reserves, as well as a higher volume of disease in patients with GCTs treated with chemotherapy.[6] Complications can be classified as intraoperative (injury to adjacent viscera or great vessels), postoperative (ileus-related and bleomycin-related pulmonary dysfunction), and late (ejaculatory dysfunction, small bowel obstruction, and lymphocele). Furthermore, the increased difficulty of performing PC-RPLND is evident from data showing greater operative times, blood loss, and transfusion rates.[7]

Some investigators have gone further by making a distinction between standard and nonstandard PC-RPLND, presumably to facilitate perioperative planning and patient counseling regarding the higher cancer-specific mortality observed and/or the potential for increased morbidity. Standard PC-RPLND is that performed in the setting of residual masses with normalization of serum tumor markers after first-line chemotherapy. Nonstandard PC-RPLND refers to surgery performed in several high-risk clinical scenarios: in patients who have received second-line or third-line chemotherapy; in those with late relapse after previous primary RPLND and/or chemotherapy; in those with advanced seminoma; and those with cisplatin-refractory disease marked by rising serum tumor markers after second-line or third-line chemotherapy (referred to as desperation PC-RPLND). Surgery in such settings can be a challenging endeavor and potentially more morbid than standard PC-RPLND.

The overall data do not seem to support such a conclusion. Mosharafa and colleagues[63] reviewed their experience with PC-RPLND in patients with advanced seminoma and NSGCT, and reported perioperative complications in 25% and 20% ($P = .3$), respectively. We recently reviewed the perioperative outcomes of patients treated by RPLND at our institution and were unable to show a significant difference in overall complication rates between patients who had undergone RPLND after first-line chemotherapy and those patients who had PC-RPLND after second-line chemotherapy, for advanced seminoma, for late recurrence, or after previous RPLND.[7] These results reflect the experience at high-volume academic centers and may not be representative of the outcomes observed at low-volume academic centers or community hospitals.

RPLND After Second-line Chemotherapy

Patients who fail first-line chemotherapy but eventually achieve normalization of serum tumor markers following second-line chemotherapy should undergo resection of residual masses because the incidence of viable malignancy in residual masses is substantially higher (>50%) compared with after first-line chemotherapy, whereas the rates of necrosis (26%) and teratoma (21%) are lower. A complete resection of residual disease is less likely after second-line chemotherapy (56%–72%) compared with first-line chemotherapy (85%).[11,13,17,22,64] Accordingly, survival in this population is generally poor, with 5-year rates ranging from 44% to 61%.[13,17,22,24]

Desperation PC-RPLND

Patients who show progression of disease despite multiple rounds of chemotherapy invariably have poor survival. However, surgery may have therapeutic benefit in a select number of patients who have residual disease limited to the retroperitoneum. Desperation PC-RPLND performed in these circumstances can result in long-term survival in up to 57% of patients.[40–42,65,66]

PC-RPLND for Advanced Seminoma

PC-RPLND has less of a role in the management of patients with seminoma with residual masses for several reasons. First, half of these residual masses undergo spontaneous resolution in a median time of 13 to 18 months.[67,68] Second, unlike NSGCT, residual masses in advanced seminoma rarely contain teratoma. Third, seminoma is exquisitely sensitive to cisplatin-based chemotherapy and only 10% of residual masses contain viable malignancy.[67–71] Lastly, chemotherapy for seminoma induces an intense desmoplastic response in the retroperitoneum, rendering surgical dissection extremely difficult, because of loss of natural tissue planes, and sometimes infeasible.[63] Complete resection of residual masses after first-line chemotherapy in advanced seminoma is reported in 58% to 74% of cases compared with more than 85% for NSGCT.[67–71]

Based on these findings, observation is the preferred management for residual masses in patients with advanced seminoma. The exception is patients who have discrete masses greater than 3 cm in size, because 27% to 38% of these contain viable malignancy, compared with 0% to 4% for those less than 3 cm.[67–70] Recently, PET with fludeoxyglucose F 18 (FDG-PET) imaging was investigated as an adjunct to CT imaging in patients with residual masses larger than 3 cm in size in a prospectively study.[67] A positive FDG-PET for masses larger than 3 cm shows a sensitivity of 80% and specificity of 100% for viable seminoma. Therefore, patients with masses larger than 3 cm that are positive on FDG-PET scan should undergo PC-RPLND, whereas masses less than 3 cm, or those that are PET negative, should be managed expectantly.

SUMMARY

The mainstay of treatment of advanced stage GCT is cisplatin-based chemotherapy followed by complete surgical resection of all residual masses. Because it is the most common anatomic site for metastatic spread and chemorefractory disease, control of the retroperitoneum with PC-RPLND is essential in patients with residual masses. Long-term survival is anticipated in approximately two-thirds of patients who undergo a complete resection of viable malignancy and 85% or more of patients with residual teratoma are cured. Even in high-risk settings such as after second-line chemotherapy, chemorefractory disease, and late relapse, a substantial proportion of patients can be cured with appropriate application of PC-RPLND, which can be performed with acceptable morbidity. PC-RPLND in the absence of a residual mass is controversial but there is a rationale for the practice. A critical component to the successful treatment of patients with advanced GCT is the appropriate integration of chemotherapy and PCS. It is recommended that these patients have treatment plans developed at high-volume academic centers and that PC-RPLND be performed by surgeons with extensive experience with this procedure.

REFERENCES

1. SEER Stat Fact Sheets: Testis, 2010. Available at: http://www.seer.cancer.gov/statfacts/html/testis.html. Accessed March 11, 2011.
2. Einhorn LH. Treatment of testicular cancer: a new and improved model. J Clin Oncol 1990;8:1777–81.
3. International Germ Cell Consensus Classification: a prognostic factor-based staging system for metastatic germ cell cancers. International Germ Cell Cancer Collaborative Group. J Clin Oncol 1997;15:594–603.
4. van Dijk MR, Steyerberg EW, Habbema JD. Survival of non-seminomatous germ cell cancer patients according to the IGCC classification: an update based on meta-analysis. Eur J Cancer 2006;42:820–6.
5. Baniel J, Foster RS, Rowland RG, et al. Complications of post-chemotherapy retroperitoneal lymph node dissection. J Urol 1995;153:976–80.
6. Baniel J, Sella A. Complications of retroperitoneal lymph node dissection in testicular cancer: primary and post-chemotherapy. Semin Surg Oncol 1999;17:263–7.
7. Subramanian VS, Nguyen CT, Stephenson AJ, et al. Complications of open primary and post-chemotherapy retroperitoneal lymph node dissection for testicular cancer. Urol Oncol 2010;28:504–9.
8. Albers P, Weissbach L, Krege S, et al. Prediction of necrosis after chemotherapy of advanced germ cell tumors: results of a prospective multicenter trial of the German Testicular Cancer Study Group. J Urol 2004;171:1835–8.

9. Carver BS, Serio AM, Bajorin D, et al. Improved clinical outcome in recent years for men with metastatic nonseminomatous germ cell tumors. J Clin Oncol 2007; 25:5603–8.

10. de Wit R, Stoter G, Kaye SB, et al. Importance of bleomycin in combination chemotherapy for good-prognosis testicular nonseminoma: a randomized study of the European Organization for Research and Treatment of Cancer Genitourinary Tract Cancer Cooperative Group. J Clin Oncol 1997;15:1837–43.

11. Debono DJ, Heilman DK, Einhorn LH, et al. Decision analysis for avoiding post-chemotherapy surgery in patients with disseminated nonseminomatous germ cell tumors. J Clin Oncol 1997;15:1455–64.

12. Gerl A, Clemm C, Schmeller N, et al. Outcome analysis after post-chemotherapy surgery in patients with non-seminomatous germ cell tumours. Ann Oncol 1995;6: 483–8.

13. Hartmann JT, Schmoll HJ, Kuczyk MA, et al. Postchemotherapy resections of residual masses from metastatic non-seminomatous testicular germ cell tumors. Ann Oncol 1997;8:531–8.

14. Hendry WF, Norman AR, Dearnaley DP, et al. Metastatic nonseminomatous germ cell tumors of the testis: results of elective and salvage surgery for patients with residual retroperitoneal masses. Cancer 2002;94:1668–76.

15. Sonneveld DJ, Sleijfer DT, Koops HS, et al. Mature teratoma identified after post-chemotherapy surgery in patients with disseminated nonseminomatous testicular germ cell tumors: a plea for an aggressive surgical approach. Cancer 1998;82: 1343–51.

16. Spiess PE, Brown GA, Pisters LL, et al. Viable malignant germ cell tumor in the postchemotherapy retroperitoneal lymph node dissection specimen: can it be predicted using clinical parameters? Cancer 2006;107:1503–10.

17. Stenning SP, Parkinson MC, Fisher C, et al. Postchemotherapy residual masses in germ cell tumor patients: content, clinical features, and prognosis. Medical Research Council Testicular Tumour Working Party. Cancer 1998;83:1409–19.

18. Steyerberg EW, Gerl A, Fossa SD, et al. Validity of predictions of residual retroperitoneal mass histology in nonseminomatous testicular cancer. J Clin Oncol 1998; 16:269–74.

19. Steyerberg EW, Keizer HJ, Fossa SD, et al. Prediction of residual retroperitoneal mass histology after chemotherapy for metastatic nonseminomatous germ cell tumor: multivariate analysis of individual patient data from six study groups. J Clin Oncol 1995;13:1177–87.

20. Toner GC, Panicek DM, Heelan RT, et al. Adjunctive surgery after chemotherapy for nonseminomatous germ cell tumors: recommendations for patient selection. J Clin Oncol 1990;8:1683–94.

21. Fizazi K, Tjulandin S, Salvioni R, et al. Viable malignant cells after primary chemotherapy for disseminated nonseminomatous germ cell tumors: prognostic factors and role of postsurgery chemotherapy–results from an international study group. J Clin Oncol 2001;19:2647–57.

22. Fox EP, Weathers TD, Williams SD, et al. Outcome analysis for patients with persistent nonteratomatous germ cell tumor in postchemotherapy retroperitoneal lymph node dissections. J Clin Oncol 1993;11:1294–9.

23. Gerl A, Clemm C, Kohl P, et al. Testicular tumor after cisplatin-based chemotherapy for germ cell malignancy. Eur Urol 1994;25:216–9.

24. Donohue JP, Leviovitch I, Foster RS, et al. Integration of surgery and systemic therapy: results and principles of integration. Semin Urol Oncol 1998;16: 65–71.

25. Fizazi K, Oldenburg J, Dunant A, et al. Assessing prognosis and optimizing treatment in patients with postchemotherapy viable nonseminomatous germ-cell tumors (NSGCT): results of the sCR2 international study. Ann Oncol 2008;19: 259–64.

26. Kondagunta GV, Bacik J, Donadio A, et al. Combination of paclitaxel, ifosfamide, and cisplatin is an effective second-line therapy for patients with relapsed testicular germ cell tumors. J Clin Oncol 2005;23:6549–55.

27. Loehrer PJ Sr, Einhorn LH, Williams SD. VP-16 plus ifosfamide plus cisplatin as salvage therapy in refractory germ cell cancer. J Clin Oncol 1986;4: 528–36.

28. McCaffrey JA, Mazumdar M, Bajorin DF, et al. Ifosfamide- and cisplatin-containing chemotherapy as first-line salvage therapy in germ cell tumors: response and survival. J Clin Oncol 1997;15:2559–63.

29. Carver BS, Shayegan B, Serio A, et al. Long-term clinical outcome after postchemotherapy retroperitoneal lymph node dissection in men with residual teratoma. J Clin Oncol 2007;25:1033–7.

30. Little JS Jr, Foster RS, Ulbright TM, et al. Unusual neoplasms detected in testis cancer patients undergoing post-chemotherapy retroperitoneal lymphadenectomy. J Urol 1994;152:1144–9.

31. Ahmed T, Bosl GJ, Hajdu SI. Teratoma with malignant transformation in germ cell tumors in men. Cancer 1985;56:860–3.

32. Motzer RJ, Amsterdam A, Prieto V, et al. Teratoma with malignant transformation: diverse malignant histologies arising in men with germ cell tumors. J Urol 1998; 159:133–8.

33. Baniel J, Foster RS, Gonin R, et al. Late relapse of testicular cancer. J Clin Oncol 1995;13:1170–6.

34. George DW, Foster RS, Hromas RA, et al. Update on late relapse of germ cell tumor: a clinical and molecular analysis. J Clin Oncol 2003;21:113–22.

35. Sharp DS, Carver BS, Eggener SE, et al. Clinical outcome and predictors of survival in late relapse of germ cell tumor. J Clin Oncol 2008;26:5524–9.

36. Culine S, Kerbrat P, Kramar A, et al. Refining the optimal chemotherapy regimen for good-risk metastatic nonseminomatous germ-cell tumors: a randomized trial of the Genito-Urinary Group of the French Federation of Cancer Centers (GETUG T93BP). Ann Oncol 2007;18(5):917–24.

37. Albers P, Siener R, Krege S, et al. Randomized phase III trial comparing retroperitoneal lymph node dissection with one course of bleomycin and etoposide plus cisplatin chemotherapy in the adjuvant treatment of clinical stage I nonseminomatous testicular germ cell tumors: AUO trial AH 01/94 by the German Testicular Cancer Study Group. J Clin Oncol 2008;26:2966–72.

38. Krege S, Beyer J, Souchon R, et al. European consensus conference on diagnosis and treatment of germ cell cancer: a report of the second meeting of the European Germ Cell Cancer Consensus group (EGCCCG): Part I. Eur Urol 2008;53:478–96.

39. Schmoll HJ, Jordan K. Current treatment of high risk testis cancer. Eur J Cancer 2009;45(Suppl 1):433–5.

40. Beck SD, Foster RS, Bihrle R, et al. Outcome analysis for patients with elevated serum tumor markers at postchemotherapy retroperitoneal lymph node dissection. J Clin Oncol 2005;23:6149–56.

41. Eastham JA, Wilson TG, Russell C, et al. Surgical resection in patients with nonseminomatous germ cell tumor who fail to normalize serum tumor markers after chemotherapy. Urology 1994;43:74–80.

42. Wood DP Jr, Herr HW, Motzer RJ, et al. Surgical resection of solitary metastases after chemotherapy in patients with nonseminomatous germ cell tumors and elevated serum tumor markers. Cancer 1992;70:2354–7.

43. Cheng L, Zhang S, Wang M, et al. Molecular genetic evidence supporting the neoplastic nature of stromal cells in 'fibrosis' after chemotherapy for testicular germ cell tumours. J Pathol 2007;213:65–71.

44. Fossa SD, Qvist H, Stenwig AE, et al. Is postchemotherapy retroperitoneal surgery necessary in patients with nonseminomatous testicular cancer and minimal residual tumor masses? J Clin Oncol 1992;10:569–73.

45. Stomper PC, Kalish LA, Garnick MB, et al. CT and pathologic predictive features of residual mass histologic findings after chemotherapy for nonseminomatous germ cell tumors: can residual malignancy or teratoma be excluded? Radiology 1991;180:711–4.

46. Vergouwe Y, Steyerberg EW, Foster RS, et al. Validation of a prediction model and its predictors for the histology of residual masses in nonseminomatous testicular cancer. J Urol 2001;165:84–8 [discussion: 88].

47. Oechsle K, Hartmann M, Brenner W, et al. [18F]Fluorodeoxyglucose positron emission tomography in nonseminomatous germ cell tumors after chemotherapy: the German Multicenter Positron Emission Tomography Study Group. J Clin Oncol 2008;26:5930–5.

48. Albers P, Albrecht W, Algaba F, et al. Guidelines on testicular cancer. Eur Urol 2005;48:885–94.

49. Krege S, Beyer J, Souchon R, et al. European consensus conference on diagnosis and treatment of germ cell cancer: a report of the second meeting of the European Germ Cell Cancer Consensus Group (EGCCCG): Part II. Eur Urol 2008;53:497–513.

50. Schmoll HJ, Jordan K, Huddart R, et al. Testicular non-seminoma: ESMO clinical recommendations for diagnosis, treatment and follow-up. Ann Oncol 2009;20: iv89–96.

51. Motzer RJ, Bolger GB, Boston B, et al. Testicular cancer. Clinical practice guidelines in oncology. J Natl Compr Canc Netw 2006;4:1038–58.

52. Oldenburg J, Alfsen GC, Lien HH, et al. Postchemotherapy retroperitoneal surgery remains necessary in patients with nonseminomatous testicular cancer and minimal residual tumor masses. J Clin Oncol 2003;21:3310–7.

53. Stephenson AJ, Bosl GJ, Motzer RJ, et al. Nonrandomized comparison of primary chemotherapy and retroperitoneal lymph node dissection for clinical stage IIA and IIB nonseminomatous germ cell testicular cancer. J Clin Oncol 2007;25: 5597–602.

54. Beck SD, Foster RS, Bihrle R, et al. Teratoma in the orchiectomy specimen and volume of metastasis are predictors of retroperitoneal teratoma in post-chemotherapy nonseminomatous testis cancer. J Urol 2002;168:1402–4.

55. Fossa SD, Ous S, Lien HH, et al. Post-chemotherapy lymph node histology in radiologically normal patients with metastatic nonseminomatous testicular cancer. J Urol 1989;141:557–9.

56. Ehrlich Y, Brames MJ, Beck SD, et al. Long-term follow-up of cisplatin combination chemotherapy in patients with disseminated nonseminomatous germ cell tumors: is a postchemotherapy retroperitoneal lymph node dissection needed after complete remission? J Clin Oncol 2010;28:531–6.

57. Kollmannsberger C, Daneshmand S, So A, et al. Management of disseminated nonseminomatous germ cell tumors with risk-based chemotherapy followed by response-guided postchemotherapy surgery. J Clin Oncol 2010;28:537–42.

58. Brenner DJ, Hall EJ. Computed tomography–an increasing source of radiation exposure. N Engl J Med 2007;357:2277–84.

59. Gerl A, Clemm C, Schmeller N, et al. Sequential resection of residual abdominal and thoracic masses after chemotherapy for metastatic non-seminomatous germ cell tumours. Br J Cancer 1994;70:960–5.

60. Hartmann JT, Candelaria M, Kuczyk MA, et al. Comparison of histological results from the resection of residual masses at different sites after chemotherapy for metastatic non-seminomatous germ cell tumours. Eur J Cancer 1997;33:843–7.

61. McGuire MS, Rabbani F, Mohseni H, et al. The role of thoracotomy in managing postchemotherapy residual thoracic masses in patients with nonseminomatous germ cell tumours. BJU Int 2003;91:469–73.

62. Carver BS, Shayegan B, Eggener S, et al. Incidence of metastatic nonseminomatous germ cell tumor outside the boundaries of a modified postchemotherapy retroperitoneal lymph node dissection. J Clin Oncol 2007;25:4365–9.

63. Mosharafa AA, Foster RS, Leibovich BC, et al. Is post-chemotherapy resection of seminomatous elements associated with higher acute morbidity? J Urol 2003; 169:2126–8.

64. Eggener SE, Carver BS, Loeb S, et al. Pathologic findings and clinical outcome of patients undergoing retroperitoneal lymph node dissection after multiple chemotherapy regimens for metastatic testicular germ cell tumors. Cancer 2007;109: 528–35.

65. Albers P, Ganz A, Hannig E, et al. Salvage surgery of chemorefractory germ cell tumors with elevated tumor markers. J Urol 2000;164:381–4.

66. Murphy BR, Breeden ES, Donohue JP, et al. Surgical salvage of chemorefractory germ cell tumors. J Clin Oncol 1993;11:324–9.

67. De Santis M, Becherer A, Bokemeyer C, et al. 2-18fluoro-deoxy-D-glucose positron emission tomography is a reliable predictor for viable tumor in postchemotherapy seminoma: an update of the prospective multicentric SEMPET trial. J Clin Oncol 2004;22:1034–9.

68. Flechon A, Bompas E, Biron P, et al. Management of post-chemotherapy residual masses in advanced seminoma. J Urol 2002;168:1975–9.

69. Herr HW, Sheinfeld J, Puc HS, et al. Surgery for a post-chemotherapy residual mass in seminoma. J Urol 1997;157:860–2.

70. Puc HS, Heelan R, Mazumdar M, et al. Management of residual mass in advanced seminoma: results and recommendations from the Memorial Sloan-Kettering Cancer Center. J Clin Oncol 1996;14:454–60.

71. Ravi R, Ong J, Oliver RT, et al. The management of residual masses after chemotherapy in metastatic seminoma. BJU Int 1999;83:649–53.

Treatment of Brain Metastases from Germ Cell Tumors

Karin Oechsle, MD, Carsten Bokemeyer, MD*

KEYWORDS

- Germ cell tumor • Brain metastases • Cerebral metastases
- Chemotherapy • Radiotherapy • Surgery

Brain metastases are rare in germ cell tumors, occurring in fewer than 1% of all patients and in approximately 10% of patients with advanced metastatic disease.[1] Patients presenting with cerebral metastases are classified as "poor prognosis" according to the International Germ Cell Consensus classification (IGCCCG). The overall survival of this risk category is only approximately 50%, in contrast to the high rates of long-term survival of 80% to 90% in patients without metastases to organs other than the lungs.[2] In patients with primary brain metastases, the prognosis may even be worse, with only 30% to 35% of patients achieving long-term survival compared with the overall group of "poor risk" patients.[2,3]

Single cases of patients with brain metastases who had experienced long-term survival after combined modality treatment were reported in the early 1980s,[4–6] but large systematic analyses or prospectively conducted trials on the optimal management of adult patients with brain metastases of germ cell tumors, including chemotherapy, radiotherapy, and surgery, are still lacking. Today, treatment recommendations for adult patients with cerebral metastases of germ cell tumors are mainly based on retrospective case series, subanalyses of clinical studies, and expert opinion.[7]

CHARACTERISTICS OF PATIENTS WITH CEREBRAL METASTASES AT FIRST DIAGNOSIS OF METASTATIC DISEASE

One of the first case series of patients with brain metastases from germ cell cancer reported the presence of synchronous lung metastases in each of the 10 reported patients and β-human chorionic gonadotropin (β-HCG) higher than 40,000 U/L in 70% of patients.[6] Further cohort studies repeatedly showed synchronous lung

The authors have nothing to disclose.
Department of Oncology/Hematology/Bone Marrow Transplantation/Pneumology, University Medical Center Eppendorf, Martinistr. 52, 20246 Hamburg, Germany
* Corresponding author.
E-mail address: c.bokemeyer@uke.uni-hamburg.de

Hematol Oncol Clin N Am 25 (2011) 605–613
doi:10.1016/j.hoc.2011.03.012
0889-8588/11/$ – see front matter © 2011 Elsevier Inc. All rights reserved.

metastases in 90% to 100% of patients with brain metastases and extremely elevated serum levels of β-HCG in 50% to 90% of those patients.[8–12] Of patients with brain metastases, 30% to 90% present with additional metastases to other organs. No cases with isolated cerebral metastases at primary diagnosis without evidence of metastases in other locations have been reported so far. The primary site of germ cell cancer in patients with brain metastases at first diagnosis was extragonadal in 15% to 20%, a relatively high proportion. The histology was nonseminoma in 90% to 99% of cases. Pure seminoma is rarely found in patients with brain metastasis. Nonseminomatous histologies were mainly malignant teratoma in 20% to 50%, embryonal carcinoma in 20% to 30%, and choriocarcinoma in 15% to 30%.[8–12] Choriocarcinoma has been reported to be associated with a particularly poor prognosis independent of the treatment strategy.[8,9,13] However, multivariable analysis of the IGCCCG had not shown a prognostic impact of different nonseminomatous histology subtypes in general.[2]

In the previously reported series, patients with brain metastases at primary diagnosis presented with single brain metastases in 40% to 50% and without neurologic symptoms in 40% to 70%.[8–12] Metastases were frequently diagnosed through extended upfront staging investigations. Two analyses have shown a significantly better prognosis for patients with a single brain metastasis. Among 56 patients with brain involvement at first detection of metastatic disease, 2-year survival was 76% for those with a single brain lesion versus 38% for those with multiple brain tumors ($P = .023$).[9] In a second study of 44 patients with brain metastases discovered either at initial diagnosis or at relapse after chemotherapy, those with a single brain lesion had a higher overall survival (44% vs 9%; $P<.02$).[8]

BRAIN METASTASES IN RELAPSED GERM CELL TUMORS

Relapses with isolated brain metastases within a few months after successful completion of platinum-based chemotherapy for metastatic germ cell cancer have been reported in 13 patients from four case reports in the 1990s, resulting in a frequency of 0.1% to 2%. These cases have suggested a correlation between the presence of primary lung metastases and nonseminomatous histology, mainly embryonal carcinoma, with the occurrence of an isolated cerebral relapse after chemotherapy.[14–17] However, two cases with pure seminomatous histology and isolated cerebral relapse have also been reported.[15]

In 2007, Azar and colleagues[18] presented a series of five patients with isolated cerebral relapse after initial cisplatin-based chemotherapy who all had components of embryonal carcinoma and pulmonary metastases at primary diagnoses. The investigators discussed an incomplete penetration of cytostatic drugs through the blood–brain barrier as the reason for isolated cerebral relapse after chemotherapy.

In this article's authors' own analysis of patients experiencing relapse with brain metastases after primary high-dose chemotherapy, all 13 patients with isolated cerebral relapse had initially presented with lung metastases and highly elevated β-HCG levels. In addition, all patients with cerebral plus systemic relapse had presented with primary lung metastases and highly elevated β-HCG levels at initial diagnosis. In total, cerebral metastases have been detected in 25% of the whole cohort of "poor prognosis" patients who had relapsed after primary high-dose chemotherapy.[11]

In contrast to other locations, where de novo metastases at relapse had occurred in only 6% to 16%, 73% of patients relapsing with brain metastases had no evidence of cerebral metastases before chemotherapy.[11,19] The high rate of patients with cerebral relapse after high-dose chemotherapy is in marked contrast to publications on conventional-dose chemotherapy postulating an incidence of only 2% for all metastatic stages.[15] This finding could either be attributed to a different tumor biology in patients with advanced metastatic disease or more likely to an increased extracerebral efficacy of high-dose chemotherapy in a "poor risk" population while the effect of chemotherapy in the cerebrum still remains limited.

Comparing the prognosis of patients presenting with brain metastases at primary diagnosis to those developing brain metastases during or shortly after adequate cisplatin-based chemotherapy, the latter patients have considerably worse outcomes. In one analysis of a cohort of patients with brain metastases, the occurrence of brain metastases at initial diagnoses was a statistically significant positive prognostic factor among patients presenting with brain metastases at any point during their disease. The proportion surviving at least 2 years was 33% in patients with brain metastases at initial diagnosis compared with 5% in those who developed brain metastases during or after first-line chemotherapy.[8] Other studies indicated 2-year or longer survival rates of approximately 30% to 50% in patients with primary brain metastases and 10% to 30% in those with brain metastases at first relapse.[9,11,20,21]

PROGNOSTIC IMPACT OF BRAIN METASTASES

Patients presenting with nonpulmonary visceral metastases at initial diagnosis are classified as poor-risk patients according to IGCCCG. Within this poor-risk group, patients with brain metastases have the poorest 5-year survival rate (33%) in the multivariate analysis of the IGCCCG compared with 35% for those with bone metastases and 49% for those with liver metastases.[2] This finding is strengthened by an explorative analysis of prognostic subgroups within the poor-risk patients, showing that nonabdominal, nonpulmonary organ metastases, which mainly represent brain and bone involvement, are associated with an especially poor prognosis, with a 2-year progression-free survival rate of only 36%.[22] In another study analyzing prognostic factors in patients with extragonadal germ cell tumors, brain metastases only occurred in patients with nonseminomatous histology and were correlated with an inferior prognosis in multivariate analysis, with 5-year overall survival rates of 25% compared with 53% in patients without brain metastases.[23]

In previous prognostic models for patients experiencing progression or relapse after cisplatin-based chemotherapy, brain metastases did not have a prognostic impact on patient survival.[24,25] A recent analysis of the International Prognostic Factors Study Group, including approximately 2000 patients after failure of cisplatin-based chemotherapy, showed that the presence of liver, bone, or brain metastases represent relevant prognostic factors in addition to the location of primary tumor, the response to prior chemotherapy, and tumor marker levels.[26]

DIAGNOSTIC PROCEDURES FOR DETECTION OF BRAIN METASTASES

Clinical data on the optimal diagnostic strategies for detection of brain metastases are rare and prospective trials on the impact of diagnostic procedures are missing. Today, international consensus guidelines on diagnostics in patients with germ cell tumors recommend CT scans of the cerebrum only in patients with advanced metastatic disease or neurologic symptoms at primary diagnosis.[27] Taking into account the earlier-outlined analyses on characteristics of patients with brain metastases, CT or MRI scans of the brain are especially indicated in patients presenting with pulmonary metastases and highly elevated β-HCG levels at primary diagnosis, irrespective of the presence of neurologic symptoms.[8–11] No standardized recommendation for diagnostic procedures in patients experiencing relapse after cisplatin-based chemotherapy have been defined so far, but according to the limited number of retro-spective analyses presented earlier, CT scan might be indicated in patients relapsing with pulmonary metastases and high β-HCG levels, especially after primary high-dose chemotherapy.[11] In patients with lung metastases at primary diagnosis and a histology of embryonal carcinoma, clinicians should be aware of the risk of an isolated cerebral relapse after successful cisplatin-based chemotherapy, and CT scans should be per-formed immediately at the first appearance of neurologic symptoms.[11-19] Another indication may be the search for the relapse site in patients with elevated tumor markers and no sign of peripheral metastases.

CHEMOTHERAPY IN PATIENTS WITH BRAIN METASTASES

Penetration of cytostatic agents through the blood–brain barrier is of fundamental rele-vance for the treatment of intracerebral metastases. Cisplatin, the most important chemotherapeutic agent in germ cell cancer, poorly penetrates the blood–brain barrier, but in patients with intracerebral metastases or after cerebral irradiation, significant levels of cisplatin of 50% to 150% of the serum area under the curve are found in the cerebrospinal fluid.[6,20] In addition, relevant intracerebral concentrations after intravenous application in patients with brain metastases have been shown for etoposide and bleomycin, but not for vinblastine.[20,28] Carboplatin and etoposide seem to penetrate the blood–brain barrier even in patients without previous irradiation.[21]

Prospective clinical trials are lacking that evaluate treatment strategies involving chemotherapy in adult patients with brain metastases from germ cell tumors. However, various retrospective case series are available. An overview of these retro-spective analyses investigating different treatment strategies based on cisplatin-containing chemotherapy in patients with brain metastases at initial diagnosis is presented in **Table 1**. In these case series, all patients underwent cisplatin-based combination chemotherapy and 30% to 60% of patients underwent additional radio-therapy or surgery, resulting in long-term survival rates ranging from 30% to 80%. Long-term survival of more than 2 years was achieved in 30% to 55% of patients after standard-dose and 60% to 80% after high-dose chemotherapy.[8-13,29-31] The large variability in long-term outcome might be caused by the varying numbers of patients included and the heterogeneous treatment strategies, but in summary these data suggest higher overall survival rates in patients treated with primary high-dose chemotherapy.[10,11] In one case series, 6 of 11 patients received intrathecal chemo-therapy with methotrexate in combination with systemic chemotherapy, but an impact on patient outcomes could not be concluded because of the limited number of patients.[30] Therefore, intrathecal chemotherapy is not part of the recommended treat-ment approach (unless, perhaps, meningiosis is present).

Data on patients with brain metastases at first relapse after cisplatin-based chemo-therapy data are even rarer. The largest study by Fossa and colleagues[9] included 83 patients presenting with cerebral metastases after a median period of 9 months. Of these patients, 41% received another course of systemic chemotherapy, 11% received additional intrathecal chemotherapy, 69% radiotherapy, and 29% surgery, resulting in a 5-year overall survival rate of 12% in patients with cerebral and systemic relapse, but of 39% in patients with isolated cerebral relapse.

In the authors' own study on 22 patients with cerebral relapse after primary high-dose chemotherapy, 78% of patients underwent another course of systemic chemotherapy combined with other treatment modalities in 74% of cases, resulting in a long-term survival rate of 26%.[11] Other case reports with smaller numbers of

Table 1
Analyses and reports on chemotherapy in patients with primary brain metastases from germ cell tumors

Authors	N	Chemotherapy Regimen	Additional Treatment	Outcome
Bokemeyer et al[8]	18	PEB, PVB	± RTX, ± surgery	OS>2 y: 33 %
Boyle et al[12]	13	Cisplatin-based CTX	Surgery: 1 patient, RTX: 3 patients	OS>2 y: 38%
Fossa et al[9]	56	Cisplatin-based CTX	Surgery: 10 patients, RTX: 36 patients	OS>5 y: 45 %
Gremmer et al[29]	10	Cisplatin-based CTX	RTX: 5 patients	OS>4 y: 50%
Kollmannsberger et al[10]	22	High-dose VIP	Surgery + RTX: 2 patients Surgery: 1 patient RTX: 10 patients	OS>2 y: 81 %
Mahalati et al[30]	11	PEB or POMB/ACE	Surgery + RTX: 4 patients RTX: 1 patient	OS: 36%; (3+, 12+, 34, 47 mo)
Nonomura et al[31]	10	PEB/PVB	Surgery + RTS: 2 patients RTX: 8 patients	OS>3 y: 50%
Oechsle et al[11]	50	High-dose VIP/TaxVIP	Surgery: 8 patients, RTX 20 patients	OS>2 y: 60%
Salvati et al[13]	15	Cisplatin-based CTX	Surgery: 15 patients, RTX: 15 patients	Median OS, 37.7 mo; OS>5 y: 53%

Abbreviations: CTX, chemotherapy; N, number of patients; OS, overall survival; PEB, cisplatin, etoposide, and bleomycin; POMB/ACE, cisplatin, vincristine, methotrexate, bleomycin, actinomycin-D, cyclophosphamide, etoposide, and intrathecal methotrexate; PVB, cisplatin, vinblastine, and bleomycin; RTX, radiotherapy; TaxVIP, paclitaxel, cisplatin, etoposide, and ifosfamide; VIP, cisplatin, etoposide, and ifosfamide.

patients reported long-term survival rates of 10% to 20% in patients with relapsed germ cell tumors and cerebral metastases after treatment with conventional-dose chemotherapy plus additional treatment modilities.[29,31]

SURGERY IN PATIENTS WITH BRAIN METASTASES

The impact of neurosurgery on patient outcomes and the optimal time for neurosurgical therapy in patients with brain metastases of metastatic germ cell tumors have not been evaluated in prospective clinical trials. Currently, neurosurgery is performed after completion of chemotherapy in some centers, but whether neurosurgical treatment should be performed as secondary resection after chemotherapy or immediately after initial diagnosis before chemotherapy to prevent cerebral complications remains unclear. In addition, data are insufficient to clarify the efficacy of secondary surgery compared with secondary radiotherapy, or the combination of both methods after completion of chemotherapy.

The number of patients who underwent secondary surgery is small in all published retrospective series. A univariate analysis showed a significant impact of neurosurgery in addition to chemotherapy in patients with primary brain metastases with 2-year survival rates of 80% in 10 patients who underwent additional neurosurgery compared with 48% in 46 patients without neurosurgery. However, in 9 of these patients, neurosurgery had to be performed within 1 week after primary diagnosis because of severe neurologic symptoms, and not after completion of chemotherapy. In patients with cerebral metastases at relapse, the positive impact of neurosurgery was also significant, with a 40% 2-year survival rate in patients with surgery compared with 4% in patients who had no additional surgery.[9] However, a true comparison is not possible because only patients with operable brain lesions underwent resections and these series are biased by this fact. In other words, presence of an inoperable brain lesion probably has adverse prognostic implications.

RADIOTHERAPY IN PATIENTS WITH BRAIN METASTASES

Systematic data on the impact of radiotherapy alone or in combination with chemotherapy or surgery are also sparse. In a multivariate analysis, radiotherapy failed to show a positive impact on the outcome of patients with primary brain metastases with a 2-year overall survival rate of 53% versus 54% for chemotherapy with or without surgery without radiotherapy, but showed a significant 2-year survival benefit in patients with brain metastases at relapse of 18% versus 8% ($P = .042$).[9] In another analysis that did not discriminate between patients with brain metastases at initial diagnosis and at relapse, the 2-year survival rate was significantly higher (32% vs 0%; $P<.03$) in patients who underwent chemotherapy plus radiotherapy with or without additional surgery, compared with patients treated with either chemotherapy or radiotherapy alone.[8]

In an analysis evaluating 11 patients who received whole-brain irradiation because of brain metastases from germ cell tumors, only 3 survived for more than 12 months. All 11 patients had a single brain metastasis and were treated with additional surgery and whole-brain irradiation. One patient died from cerebral hemorrhage after whole-brain irradiation at a dose of 8 Gy.[32] Delayed toxicities of whole-brain irradiation in patients with germ cell tumors were reported in a cohort of five patients who developed symptoms of progressive multifocal leukoencephalopathy after a median of 72 months after irradiation. Treatment with surgery or steroids had only modest efficacy, and this long-term toxicity resulted in significant debility in all five patients, and death in three.[33]

MULTIMODAL TREATMENT

Based on all previously published data on treatment strategies for patients with brain metastases from germ cell tumors, multimodal treatment approaches seem to be more effective than strategies using chemotherapy, radiotherapy, or surgery alone. However, the optimal combination and sequence of treatment strategies remains unclear. Previous studies also showed different outcomes for patients with single versus multiple brain metastases and for patients with brain metastases at primary diagnosis versus those developing brain metastases during or after first-line chemotherapy, respectively. Therefore, the optimal combination and sequence of treatment strategies might be different for these subgroups. This problem has been highlighted in the German Registry Study of nearly 200 patients with brain metastases of germ cell tumor at primary diagnosis, isolated cerebral relapse, or intra- plus extracerebral recurrences. Estimated 2-year progression-free and overall survival rates were 45% and 57% in patients with primary brain metastases, 39% and 44% in patients with isolated cerebral relapse, and 26% and 26% in patients with intra- plus extracerebral recurrences, respectively ($P<.001$). Chemotherapy alone was a negative prognostic factor in all subgroups, whereas local treatment strategies, radiotherapy, or neurosurgery, without systemic chemotherapy, presented negative prognostic factors only in patients with brain metastases at relapse despite extracerebral disease.[34] Nevertheless, local treatment strategies alone cannot be considered an adequate treatment strategy in patients with brain metastases at primary diagnosis, because brain metastases nearly always occur in patients with advanced disease at primary diagnosis requiring intensive systemic chemotherapy. Therefore, current international guidelines recommend systemic chemotherapy for all patients with brain metastases at primary diagnosis.[7,35]

Although the European consensus conference on diagnosis and treatment of germ cell cancer considers the impact of radiotherapy unclear,[7] the National Comprehensive Cancer Network (NCCN) recommends radiotherapy after completion of combination chemotherapy in all patients with brain metastases.[35] The impact of surgery remains unclear in all international guidelines and is "recommended if clinically indicated" or "might be considered in patients with solitary brain metastases."[7,35] Based on currently available data, surgery seems to be indicated for patients with resectable single brain metastases in addition to chemotherapy. Additional whole-brain irradiation after completion of cisplatin-based chemotherapy might be considered in patients with multiple brain metastases and should be performed in patients experiencing only partial cerebral remission after chemotherapy.

SUMMARY

Patients with brain metastases should undergo multimodal treatment strategies, including cisplatin-based combination chemotherapy plus at least one local treatment, radiotherapy, or surgery. The optimal combination and sequence of systemic and local treatment strategies remain unclear, especially when taking into account the different subgroups of patients with primary or secondary brain metastases and single or multiple brain metastases and isolated cerebral or systemic plus cerebral relapse, respectively. For further clarification, large international databases should be initiated, because prospectively conducted randomized trials might be unrealistic considering the low overall incidence of brain metastases in patients with germ cell tumors.

Meanwhile, patients with brain metastases from germ cell tumors should be referred to specialized centers with a high level of multidisciplinary competence. Diagnostic procedures in patients with germ cell tumors should include CT or MRI scans of the brain in the presence of advanced disease, especially when lung metastases or extremely high β-HCG-levels are present. Furthermore, physicians caring for patients with germ cell tumors should be aware of the risk of isolated cerebral relapses after cisplatin-based chemotherapy.

REFERENCES

1. Williams SD, Einhorn LH. Brain metastases in disseminated germinal neoplasms: incidence and clinical course. Cancer 1979;44:1514–6.
2. International germ cell consensus classification: a prognostic factor-based staging system for metastatic germ cell cancers. International Germ Cell Cancer Collaborative Group. J Clin Oncol 1997;15:594–603.
3. Spears WT, Morphis JG 2nd, Lester SG, et al. Brain metastases and testicular tumors: long-term survival. Int J Radiat Oncol Biol Phys 1992;22:17–22.
4. Logothetis CJ, Samuels ML, Trindade A. The management of brain metastases in germ cell tumors. Cancer 1982;49:12–8.
5. Raghavan D, Mackintosh JF, Fox RM, et al. Improved survival after brain metastases in non-seminomatous germ cell tumours with combined modality treatment. Br J Urol 1987;60:364–7.

6. Rustin GJ, Newlands ES, Bagshawe KD, et al. Successful management of metastatic and primary germ cell tumors in the brain. Cancer 1986;57:2108–13.
7. Krege S, Beyer J, Souchon R, et al. European consensus conference on diagnosis and treatment of germ cell cancer: a report of the second meeting of the European Germ Cell Cancer Consensus Group (EGCCCG): part II. Eur Urol 2008;53:497–513.
8. Bokemeyer C, Nowak P, Haupt A, et al. Treatment of brain metastases in patients with testicular cancer. J Clin Oncol 1997;15:1449–54.
9. Fossa SD, Bokemeyer C, Gerl A, et al. Treatment outcome of patients with brain metastases from malignant germ cell tumors. Cancer 1999;85:988–97.
10. Kollmannsberger C, Nichols C, Bamberg M, et al. First-line high-dose chemotherapy +/- radiation therapy in patients with metastatic germ-cell cancer and brain metastases. Ann Oncol 2000;11:553–9.
11. Oechsle K, Kollmannsberger C, Honecker F, et al. Cerebral metastases in non-seminomatous germ cell tumour patients undergoing primary high-dose chemotherapy. Eur J Cancer 2008;44:1663–9.
12. Boyle HJ, Droz J, Jouanneau E, et al. Management of brain metastases from germ cell tumors. J Clin Oncol 2008;26(15s):16076.
13. Salvati M, Piccirilli M, Raco A, et al. Brain metastasis from non-seminomatous germ cell tumors of the testis: indications for aggressive treatment. Neurosurg Rev 2006;29:130–7.
14. Gerl A, Clemm C, Kohl P, et al. Central nervous system as sanctuary site of relapse in patients treated with chemotherapy for metastatic testicular cancer. Clin Exp Metastasis 1994;12:226–30.
15. Raina V, Singh SP, Kamble N, et al. Brain metastasis as the site of relapse in germ cell tumor of testis. Cancer 1993;72:2182–5.
16. Cohn DA, Stuart-Harris R. Isolated central nervous system relapse of non-seminomatous germ cell tumour of the testis. A case report and review of the literature. Oncology 2001;61:184–8.
17. Crabb SJ, McKendrick JJ, Mead GM. Brain as sanctuary site of relapse in germ cell cancer patients previously treated with chemotherapy. Clin Oncol (R Coll Radiol) 2002;14:287–93.
18. Azar JM, Einhorn LH, Schneider BP. Is the blood-brain barrier relevant in metastatic germ cell tumors? Int J Radiat Oncol Biol Phys 2007;69:163–6.
19. Oechsle K, Lorch A, Honecker F, et al. Patterns of relapse after chemotherapy in patients with high-risk non-seminomatous germ cell tumor. Oncology 2010;78: 47–53.
20. Ginsberg S, Kirshner J, Reich S, et al. Systemic chemotherapy for a primary germ cell tumor of the brain: a pharmacokinetic study. Cancer Treat Rep 1981;65:477–83.
21. Balmaceda C, Heller G, Rosenblum, et al. Chemotherapy without irradiation - a novel approach for newly diagnosed CNS germ-cell tumors: results of an international cooperative trial. J Clin Oncol 1996;14:2908–15.
22. Kollmannsberger C, Nichols C, Meisner C, et al. Identification of prognostic subgroups among patients with metastatic 'IGCCCG poor-prognosis' germ-cell cancer: an explorative analysis using cart modeling. Ann Oncol 2000;11:1115–20.
23. Hartmann JT, Nichols CR, Droz JP, et al. Prognostic variables for response and outcome in patients with extragonadal germ-cell tumors. Ann Oncol 2002;13: 1017–28.
24. Fosså SD, Stenning SP, Gerl A, et al. Prognostic factors in patients progressing after cisplatin-based chemotherapy for malignant non-seminomatous germ cell tumours. Br J Cancer 1999;80:1392–9.

25. Beyer J, Kramar A, Mandanas R, et al. High-dose chemotherapy as salvage treatment in germ cell tumors: a multivariate analysis of prognostic variables. J Clin Oncol 1996;14:2638–45.
26. International Prognostic Factors Study Group, Lorch A, Beyer J, et al. Prognostic factors in patients with metastatic germ cell tumors who experienced treatment failure with cisplatin-based first-line chemotherapy. J Clin Oncol 2010;28: 4906–11.
27. Krege S, Beyer J, Souchon R, et al. European consensus conference on diagnosis and treatment of germ cell cancer: a report of the second meeting of the European Germ Cell Cancer Consensus group (EGCCCG): part I. Eur Urol 2008;53:478–96.
28. Stewart OJ, Richard M, Hugenholtz H, et al. VP-16 (VP) and VM-26 (VM) penetration into human brain tumors (BT). Proc Am Assoc Cancer Res 1983;24:133.
29. Gremmer R, Schröder ML, Bokkel ten Huinink WW, et al. Successful management of brain metastases from malignant germ cell tumors with standard induction chemotherapy. J Neurooncol 2008;90:335–9.
30. Mahalati K, Bilen CY, Ozen H, et al. The management of brain metastasis in non-seminomatous germ cell tumours. BJU Int 1999;83:457–61.
31. Nonomura N, Nagahara A, Oka D, et al. Brain metastases from testicular germ cell tumors: a retrospective analysis. Int J Urol 2009;16:887–93.
32. Lutterbach J, Spetzger U, Bartelt S, et al. Malignant germ cell tumors metastatic to the brain: a model for a curable neoplasm? The Freiburg experience and a review of the literature. J Neurooncol 2002;58:147–56.
33. Doyle DM, Einhorn LH. Delayed effects of whole brain radiotherapy in germ cell tumor patients with central nervous system metastases. Int J Radiat Oncol Biol Phys 2008;70:1361–4.
34. Hartmann JT, Bamberg M, Albers P, et al. Multidisciplinary treatment and prognosis of patients with central nervous system metastases from testicular germ cell tumor origin [abstract]. Proc Am Soc Clin Oncol 2003;22:400 [abstract: 1607].
35. NCCN Clinical Practice Guidelines in Oncology: Testicular Cancer. Version 1, 2011. Available at: http://www.nccn.org/professionals/physician_gls/f_guidelines.asp. Accessed April 9, 2011.

Late Relapse of Germ Cell Tumors

Jan Oldenburg, MD, PhD[a,b,*], Anja Lorch, MD[c],
Sophie D. Fosså, MD, PhD[d,e]

KEYWORDS

• Germ cell tumors • Late relapse • Seminoma • Clinical stage

INCIDENCE

Late relapses of malignant germ cell tumors (MGCTs) represent, as per definition, recurrences at least 2 years after treatment discontinuation and apparently complete remission. Despite this clear definition, varying criteria are applied in publications on patients with late relapse.

Some authorities include only recurrences after chemotherapy[1–3] or require the histologic finding of an MGCT, that is, no teratoma only.[3] Further, inclusion of patients with prior relapses affects incidence, treatment, and prognosis of the assessed cohort.[2] In this review, the authors refer to late relapse according to the earlier-mentioned definition and, thereby, include late relapse among clinical stage (CS) I patients after surveillance as well as among those in whom relapse occurs after multi-modal treatment, as long as the treatment led to the status of no evidence of disease (NED) for at least 2 years.

Around 1% to 6% of patients with testicular cancer (TC) experience a late relapse.[4] Patients with an extragonadal germ cell tumor (EGGCT) have probably an increased risk,[5] but this finding has not been corroborated. Reports on the incidence of late relapses require the number of primarily treated patients, a number usually unknown to referral centers, which have published the largest series on these rare conditions.

In a pooled analysis comprising roughly 3700 patients with nonseminoma and 2200 patients with seminoma, late relapses were reported in 119 (3.2%) patients with non-seminoma and in 31 (1.4%) of those with seminoma, ($P<.0001$).[4]

This project was supported financially by the Norwegian Radium Hospital Foundation.
Disclosure of conflict: The authors have no conflicts of interests.
[a] Department of Oncology, The Norwegian Radium Hospital, Oslo, Norway
[b] Buskerud University College, Institute of Health, Drammen, Norway
[c] Department of Oncology, Marburg University Clinic, Marburg, Germany
[d] Department of Clinical Cancer Research, The Norwegian Radium Hospital, Oslo, Norway
[e] University of Oslo, Oslo, Norway
* Corresponding author. Department of Oncology, Oslo University Hospital, The Norwegian Radium Hospital, Oslo, Norway.
E-mail address: jan.oldenburg@medisin.uio.no

Hematol Oncol Clin N Am 25 (2011) 615–626
doi:10.1016/j.hoc.2011.03.006
0889-8588/11/$ – see front matter © 2011 Elsevier Inc. All rights reserved.

The most frequent site of late relapse in both patients with seminoma and nonsemi-noma is the retroperitoneal space (>50%), with correspondingly reduced recurrence rates among patients who underwent a retroperitoneal lymph node dissection (RPLND) or abdominal radiotherapy. The chest is the next frequent site of relapse (25%–30% of patients), that is, the lungs in nonseminoma and mediastinal lymph nodes in seminoma. Initial treatment, histology, and CS are associated with the late-relapse risk. However, several yet unidentified factors of cancer and the host obscure the personalized risk prediction and preclude identification of patients benefiting from prolonged follow-up schedules.

SEMINOMA CS I

Approximately 80% of patients with seminoma present with clinical stage (CS) I disease, that is, no clinically detectable cancer outside the testicle. Disease-specific survival rate approaches 100%, independent of which the following 3 management strategies are applied: adjuvant radiotherapy, surveillance, or adjuvant carboplatin.[6] In prospective reports, the overall crude relapse rate was 1.4% to 6.9% after radiotherapy,[6,7] 15.2% to 19.3% during surveillance,[6,8,9] and 0% to 8.6% after carbo-platin (either 1 or 2 cycles).[6,10–12] The adjusted hazard ratio for late relapse is between 0.25% to 1% from the fourth to the sixth posttreatment year, and only sporadic late relapses are reported after more than 6 years.[13]

Most survivors of contemporary seminoma stage I have received adjuvant radio-therapy to para-aortic and ipsilateral pelvic lymph nodes because this has been the treatment standard during the last 50 to 60 years. After a median observation time of 9.7 years, 16 of 272 patients (5.8%) irradiated at the Princess Margaret Hospital experienced a relapse from 2 to 12 years.[14] Irradiation of para-aortic lymph nodes as compared with that of dogleg fields renders the pelvis a more frequent site of early and probably also late relapses.[7] Therefore, repeated imaging during follow-up is mandated.[15] Magnetic resonance imaging (MRI) or, in lean patients, ultrasonographic examinations of the iliac region might be used in an effort to reduce the carcinogenic side effects of computed tomographic (CT) scanning.

Surveillance is the treatment standard in Europe and avoids overtreatment of roughly 80% of the patients who do not harbor micrometastases. A strict follow-up schedule should ensure early detection of metastases, and prompt radiotherapy or chemotherapy cures almost all relapsing patients. The frequency of follow-up controls and CT imaging of the retroperitoneum varies between different institutions but, in general, intervals increase after 2 to 3 years.[15] Compliance, critical to the success of this strategy,[16] might be substantially weakened by the patient's perception of an unsatisfactory affective relationship with the clinician as reported by the Royal Marsden Hospital group.[17] Poor compliance to the follow-up schedule might result in detection of relapses first at advanced stages, and the authors recommend discus-sing the responsibility of adherence to the follow-up schedule in detail with the patients and, if possible, with their partners or parents present. A disadvantage of this otherwise so compelling concept is the requirement of repeated CT scans with cumulative radiation doses, increasing the risk of second cancers.[18] However, MRI may provide an acceptable alternative.

A meta-analysis demonstrated invasion of the rete testis and tumor size larger than 4 cm to confer a higher risk of relapse, but these data have not yet been validated prospectively.[9] Of 638 patients with CS I seminoma managed by surveillance, 38 of 121 relapses (31%) occurred later than 2 years, including 6 patients in whom relapse occurred after 6 years, the latest relapse being detected after 12 years.[9] The Princess

Margaret Hospital reported that among 203 men with CS I seminoma managed by surveillance, the actuarial risk of experiencing a relapse more than 5 years after orchiectomy was 4%.[19]

Oliver and colleagues[20] have investigated carboplatin as an adjuvant treatment of CS I seminoma since the 1980s. A single dose of carboplatin (area under the curve of 7) has been tested in a randomized noninferiority trial against radiotherapy with no significant difference in 3-year relapse-free survival (95.9% and 94.8%, respectively).[11] In concordance with surveillance series, systemic carboplatin left the retroperitoneum as the most frequent site of relapse, with the latest one occurring after 50 months. However, the median follow-up of 4 years is too short to conclude about the true risk of late relapse or long-term efficacy of salvage multiagent chemotherapy. Powles and colleagues[12] recently published long-term results after adjuvant carboplatin treatment of 199 patients with seminoma. Of these patients, 4 developed a late relapse between 2 and 4 years after primary treatment. One patient had liver metastases, 1 had lung metastases, and 2 had their disease confined to retroperitoneal lymph nodes. All patients were salvaged by cisplatin-based chemotherapy. However, the findings of contralateral testicular seminoma in 5 patients (2.5%) were remarkable, especially because a reduced incidence of contralateral TC after carboplatin administration versus radiotherapy (0.54% vs 1.96%) represented an intriguing finding in the European Organization for Research and Treatment of Cancer trial.[11] Probably, a postponed development rather than an eradication of carcinoma in situ explains these clinical observations.[12] There is no indication for carboplatin delaying the growth of metastases as well. Extended long-term results are, however, necessary to rule out this potential effect, which might lead to an increase in late-relapsing seminoma.

SEMINOMA CS GREATER THAN I

In case of CS II (infradiaphragmatic lymph node metastases only), radiotherapy, chemotherapy, or both is usually applied, and 5-year specific survival approaches 100%.[6] A prospective German trial on radiotherapy comprising 66 patients with CS IIA and 21 with CS IIB reported 4 relapses after 70 months of median follow-up. In 2 patients with CS IIA, relapse occurred at 33 and 40 months after radiotherapy, whereas relapse occurred at 17 months for both patients with CS IIB.[21] In the Princess Margaret Hospital series, relapse beyond 3 years occurred in none of the 79 patients with CS IIA-B treated with radiotherapy after a median follow-up of 8.5 years.[22]

Radiotherapy for advanced seminoma CS II and CS III bulky (>5 cm) retroperitoneal disease may lead to relapses in more than 50% of patients,[23] and 3 to 4 cycles of cisplatin-based chemotherapy have become the treatment of choice.[6,24] Patients with large diaphragmatic or supradiaphragmatic metastases, that is, CS IIC or CS III, should receive cisplatin-based chemotherapy.[24,25]

Residual postchemotherapy (PC) seminoma masses are of less concern than nonseminomatous ones. First, masses of size less than 3 cm do not usually contain viable tumor, and teratoma is exceedingly rare in patients with seminoma.[26–28] Second, positron emission tomography (PET) helps to appreciate the viability of larger lesions.[27,29] Third, progression of residual seminoma masses occurs early after chemotherapy,[27] and late relapses are extremely rare in these patients.[5,30]

NONSEMINOMA CS I

Roughly, two-thirds of patients with nonseminoma are diagnosed with CS I, whereas only one-third of the reported late relapses in patients with nonseminoma occurred in these patients.[4] The cancer-specific survival rate approaches 100% irrespective of the postorchiectomy treatment strategy, that is, surveillance, cisplatin-based chemotherapy, or RPLND.[31] Kollmannsberger and colleagues[31] pursue surveillance in most patients, also in those with lymphovascular invasion (LVI), which is the most important predictor for occult metastases. Relapse occurred in only 7 of 223 patients (3%) after surveillance beyond 2 years. All relapses were in long-term remission after chemotherapy with or without RPLND. Only 17 of 223 patients (8%) required surgery postorchiectomy. Disease-specific survival was 100% after a median follow-up of 52 months (3–136 months) without the need of second-line chemotherapy for any patient. The elegance of this approach lies in obviation of any postorchiectomy therapy in nearly 75% of patients.

In a prospective randomized study, the German Testicular Cancer Group demonstrated a reduced risk of relapse after 1 course of bleomycin, etoposide, and cisplatin (BEP) when compared with primary RPLND.[32] After a median observation time of 4.7 years, relapses occurred in 2 patients among those treated with 1 course of adjuvant BEP as opposed to 13 patients in the RPLND group (2-year recurrence-free survival rates 99.4% and 92.4%, respectively). Of the 2 patients in whom relapse occurred after BEP, 1 was cured at 15 months with 3 courses of BEP, whereas the other patient underwent RPLND for the removal of a marker-negative retroperitoneal teratoma recurrence at 5 months. Cisplatin-based chemotherapy cured all 15 patients with recurrences after RPLND with or without additional surgery. Some investigators cautioned against generalization of these findings because the staging was insufficient (5 of 141 patients with CS I had pathologic stage IIB [lesions larger than 2 cm], and one had pathologic stage IIC [>5 cm] at RPLND). Further, a high risk of retroperitoneal or even scrotal relapses after RPLND indicates suboptimal surgery. Nevertheless, these findings might reflect outcomes for minor hospitals better than superior reports by highly specialized centers of excellence.

Tandstad and colleagues[33] showed that 1 course of BEP reduces the risk of relapse by 90% among patients with CS I, whereas an additional second course of BEP virtually eliminated recurrences. The investigators recommend 1 course of BEP as a standard treatment in patients with CS I with vascular invasion to minimize the risk of relapses, whereas low-risk patients, that is, those without vascular invasion, should be managed by surveillance. For conclusions on the risk of late relapses, however, the median observation time of 5.2 years is too short, especially because some micrometastases might be delayed in their development and not eradicated by only 1 cycle of BEP.

All 3 treatment strategies seem reasonable in CS nonseminoma I. Primary RPLND is the only approach to eradicate retroperitoneal teratoma, which might advance first after many years of apparent NED.

NONSEMINOMA CS GREATER THAN I

Although only one-third of patients with nonseminoma are diagnosed with metastases, that is, CS greater than I, most late relapses are found in these patients. Treatment in patients with metastasis usually consists of cisplatin-based chemotherapy with or without surgery. However, low stage II may be managed by primary RPLND only.[34,35] The Indiana University Hospital group reported no benefit of adjuvant chemotherapy after RPLND in these patients.[34] In patients with elevated tumor markers or with CS IIB, the Memorial Sloan-Kettering Cancer Center group shifted treatment strategy from primary RPLND to primary chemotherapy and PC-RPLND and reported an increase of 5-year progression-free survival from 79% to 98%.[36]

Residual PC masses comprise complete necrosis, teratoma, or vital MGCT in 40% to 60%, 45% to 25%, and 5% to 20%, respectively. The issue whether minimal residual lesions should be removed is a controversial issue. Among 87 patients with residual retroperitoneal masses of 2 cm or larger operated at the Norwegian Radium Hospital, 29 (33%) had teratoma (27%) or vital nonteratomatous MGCT (6%).[37] Furthermore, 5 of 6 patients with vital nonteratomatous MGCT had lesions of 1 cm or smaller. The clinical significance of small lesions has recently been challenged by the outcome of 302 patients with minimal residual lesions of 1 cm or smaller who had been followed-up only. The experts from Indiana University reported on a retrospective analysis of 141 patients with nonseminoma who were observed for median 15.5 years after achieving a serologic and radiographic complete remission to cisplatin-based chemotherapy only.[38] The calculated 15-year disease-specific survival was 97%. Of the 12 patients in whom relapse had occurred, 5 had late recurrences after 3 to 13 years, and all could be cured. No teratoma was found at late relapse. Two patients were cured from yolk sac tumor in the retroperitoneum and in the neck by surgery only, whereas 2 patients received preoperative chemotherapy and 1 patient underwent postsurgical radiotherapy for sarcoma in the femur.

Kollmannsberger and colleagues[39] reported a disease-specific survival of 100% in 161 patients who achieved a complete remission defined as no residual masses larger than 1 cm after cisplatin-based chemotherapy for patients with disseminated nonseminoma. Surgery was not done in these patients, and within 52 months median observation time, relapse occurred in 10 patients, in 2 of them beyond 2 years. These 2 patients and further 6 of the 10 relapses were cured by RPLND only for retroperitoneal teratoma.

The retroperitoneal space is the most common site of relapse, and there is no doubt that resection of lymph nodes containing MGCT, also of normal-sized ones, reduces the risk of late relapse. Furthermore, RPLND reduces the need of repeated CT scanning during follow-up and reduces, thereby, the risk of radiation-induced second cancers.

Resections of lesions larger than 1 cm by RPLND is considered treatment standard and templates as compared with full bilateral RPLND are increasingly applied, especially for small nodal left-sided metastases. The optimal template is another controversial issue, and in-depth discussion of this question is beyond the scope of this review. Principally, the aim of template resection, that is, removal of all metastatic lymph nodes within specified anatomic regions, has to be balanced against complications, first, dry ejaculation caused by damage to sympathetic nerves. Templates are designed to include the lymph nodes likely to harbor metastatic disease. Inevitably, some affected lymph nodes lie outside of such templates, and Carver and colleagues[40] have assessed the prevalence of extratemplate metastases in men with residual retroperitoneal masses depending on the boundaries of the applied template. In 7% to 32% of 269 patients with residual affected lymph nodes containing teratoma and/or viable MGCT, pathologic lymph nodes were identified outside of the assessed templates. Even in patients with small residual lesions, that is, smaller than 1 cm and 1 to 2 cm, this incidence was 8% and 18%, respectively. Beck and colleagues,[41] on the other hand, reported on 100 patients with nonseminoma with normalized tumor markers after chemotherapy undergoing unilateral template RPLND at Indiana University from 1991 to 2004. After a median observation time of 32 months, 4 cases of relapse occurred, all of them localized outside the boundaries of a full bilateral template. Thereby, the investigators concluded that a full bilateral RPLND does not seem to be necessary in such patients.

Heidenreich and colleagues[42] retrospectively reviewed the outcome in 152 patients who underwent PC-RPLND. Of these, 54 and 98 patients underwent a radical template resection and a modified template resection, respectively. After a mean observation time of 39 months, 1 patient had an in-field relapse after modified

PC-RPLND, and 7 patients developed recurrences outside the boundaries of a full bilateral PC-RPLND. This observation in combination with preserved antegrade ejaculation in 85% and 25% of patients undergoing modified and bilateral PC-RPLND, respectively, led the investigators to the conclusion that modified PC-RPLND suffices for patients with well-defined masses.

However, the risk of dry ejaculation depends on both the extent of template resection and tumor. For fair risk-interpretation, one should keep in mind that residual masses removed by bilateral RPLND were double as large as those removed by modified template resection, 10.9 cm versus 4.5 cm, respectively. Preservation of sympathetic nerves is possible despite large retroperitoneal masses as indicated by a proportion as high as 79% of patients with antegrade ejaculation after bilateral PC-RPLND.[43]

The apparent contradiction between the approaches of aggressive surgery, that is, resection of minimal PC lymph nodes and full bilateral RPLND, respectively, versus arguments for observation and template RPLND, respectively, relies largely on different end-points: histopathology of excised tissues versus occurrence of relapse. Evidently, only few retroperitoneal lymph nodes with microscopic MGCT do progress. However, there are no biomarkers reliably predicting an increased risk of relapse.

Nevertheless, relapses may occur as late as 3 decades after primary treatment limiting the conclusive power of the studies mentioned earlier. In the authors' view, the only way to come to a valid recommendation is by thorough studies on the risk of late relapses to determine which end-point will be more relevant in the long term.

Histopathologic findings of removed retroperitoneal tissue do not necessarily represent lesions at other localizations. Removal of residual PC masses from extraretroperitoneal sites is strongly recommended in patients with teratoma and/or vital tumor.[44]

DETECTION OF LATE RELAPSE AND DIFFERENTIAL DIAGNOSIS

Back pain and abdominal tumor are typical symptoms of relapse in patients with TC.[5,45] Both patients and their general practitioners should be informed about the risk of late relapses to minimize the patient's and doctor's delay. Routine follow-up examinations may reveal late relapses by elevated tumor markers, radiological abnormalities, or palpable masses. The data whether detection of late relapse in patients with asymptomatic TC versus symptomatic TC is associated with survival are equivocal. In the series of George and colleagues[46] and Sharp and colleagues,[47] symptoms at late relapse were associated with decreased chances of survival (hazard ratio, 3.8; 95% confidence interval (CI), 1.3–11.3 and hazard ratio, 4.9; 95% CI, 1.6–15.2, respectively). On the other hand, a German and a Norwegian study did not find such association.[5,45] Despite inconclusive data, however, it seems reasonable to assume asymptomatic patients to represent earlier-detected and a less-advanced disease with a better prognosis. Duration and frequency of follow-up is an important issue. Late relapses may occur even decades after primary treatment, and lifelong follow-up is desirable. However, there are several problems to this strategy: a limited capacity of some cancer centers because controls should take place at least annually because of possibly abrupt onset,[48] presumably falling compliance after decades of event-free survival, and the fear to induce second cancers by abdominal CT scanning in patients who did not undergo bilateral RPLND.[18] Clinicians, who do not have the opportunity to offer lifelong follow-up to all their patients with MGCT, might consider prioritizing the following patients: those with previous relapse after chemotherapy, those with primary EGGCT, and possibly those with high amounts of metastatic teratoma.

When suspecting a late MGCT relapse, the following alternative conditions require consideration: metastases from a new contralateral TC, a new primary EGGCT, a somatic transformation of teratoma, or a new non–germ cell malignancy. The differentiation between transformed teratoma and a new non-MGCT primary requires an expert pathologist who should base the diagnosis on a representative presalvage biopsy and a comparison with previous specimens. The achievement of a representative presalvage biopsy is important because the choice of appropriate treatment depends on it.

PET, based on an increased uptake of substances such as fluorodeoxyglucose F 18 into fast-growing tissues, is unreliable with respect to detection of slow-growing late relapses and is definitely no substitute for biopsies. However, PET might help to localize the site of relapse in patients with rising tumor markers without visible lesions on radiography or CT. In this setting, PET scans yielded a localization of marker-only relapses in 12 of 23 patients.[49]

HISTOPATHOLOGY OF LATE RELAPSES

Teratoma is the most frequently encountered histologic element in patients with MGCT with late relapses.[50] The fluid of cystic teratoma may contain α-fetoprotein and/or human chorionic gonadotropin, sometimes leaking into the serum, such that slightly elevated serum tumor markers do not always prove presence of nonteratomatous MGCT.[4] The histologic diagnosis of teratoma is usually straightforward but can be challenging in case of somatic differentiation, which had been identified by Michael and colleagues[50] in 23% of 91 patients with MGCT with late relapse. The most common types of these rare neoplasms comprise different sarcoma subtypes, adenocarcinoma, and undifferentiated cancer.[50] In case of uncertainty, presence of isochromosome 12p proves germ cell tumor clonality.[46]

Yolk sac tumor is found in up to 50% of patients with late relapse, but atypical appearance with glandular, parietal, clear cell, or hepatoid pattern may cause misclassification.[50] Virtually initially encountered histologic types occur at late relapse, including shift from seminoma to nonseminoma and, more seldom, vice versa.[5,50]

TREATMENT AND SURVIVAL

Optimal treatment for the individual patient requires careful evaluation and planning by an experienced interdisciplinary team of urological surgeons, oncologists, pathologists, and radiologists and possibly also vascular surgeons, thoracic surgeons, orthopedic surgeons, and neurosurgeons. Survival of patients with poor prognosis increases by treatment in high-volume centers.[51] Most probably, this rationale applies also to patients with a late relapse.

A representative presalvage biopsy directs treatment of patients with late-relapsing marker-negative MGCT. One might consider late relapses of MGCT to represent 2 different entities: teratoma only or viable nonteratomatous nonseminomatous germ cell tumor (including somatic transformation). Survival approaches 100% in cases of single-site teratoma, and the effect of the primary histology, that is, seminoma versus nonseminoma, on survival is low (**Fig. 1**).[5] Teratoma must be removed surgically, and preoperative or postoperative chemotherapy and/or radiotherapy confers no benefit to a complete resection.[1]

Conventional-dose chemotherapy with paclitaxel, ifosfamide, and cisplatin in combination with removal of residual lesions may result in long-term remission rates of 50% or more.[3,47,52,53] However, not all patients in previous reports had metastatic disease at initial presentation and many of those patients had never received any chemotherapy before their late relapse. Chemotherapy-naive patients with relapses have a better prognosis than those who had been pretreated with chemotherapy.[3,47,54]

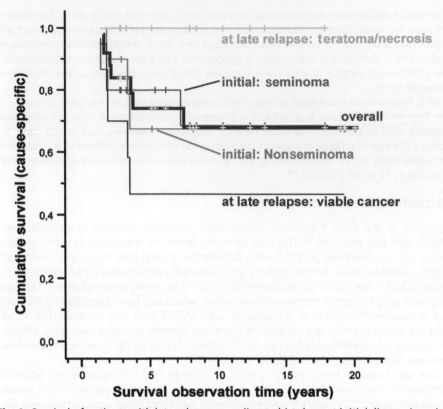

Fig. 1. Survival of patients with late relapse according to histology at initial diagnosis and at late relapse. (*Reproduced from* Oldenburg J, Alfsen GC, Waehre H, et al. Late recurrences of germ cell malignancies: a population-based experience over three decades. Br J Cancer 2006;94:826; with permission.)

Lorch and colleagues[54,55] evaluated the activity of high-dose chemotherapy (HDCT) in 34 patients with unresectable late-relapse MGCT on an intention-to-treat basis within a prospective randomized multicenter phase 3 trial of single versus sequential HDCT. All patients had failed standard-dose cisplatin-based first-line treatment of metastatic MGCT, standard-dose cisplatin-based salvage treatment, or both, and 88% had multifocal disease. Only 83% of the patients proceeded to HDCT and were scheduled for subsequent surgical removal of residual lesions whenever possible. The remaining patients progressed or died before HDCT could be given. The rate of vital MGCT in operated patients was 67%, with a low frequency of teratoma and absence of malignant transformation.[47] Despite a response rate of 63% to HDCT and removal of residual lesions in 43% of patients, the progression-free survival after 6 years was only 15%. Patients unsuitable for surgery with only partial response to HDCT succumbed to their MGCT. The small sample size precluded evaluation of prognostic factors. However, patients in whom relapse occurred after salvage chemotherapy had a poorer outcome than those in whom relapse occurred after first-line chemotherapy, possibly because of a high incidence of microsatellite instability and mutations in cell signaling pathways.[56]

In addition, identification of viable cancer seemed to be an adverse prognostic factor for long-term progression-free survival even in completely resected patients.

Despite the poor prognosis of these patients, HDCT and surgery yielded long-term survival in 17% of patients. Notably, 1 patient achieved an ongoing complete remission after HDCT alone without any surgery. The finding of chemosensitivity in a subset of patients with late relapse was corroborated by recent results of application of TI-CE (paclitaxel plus ifosfamide followed by high-dose carboplatin plus etoposide with stem-cell support), which rendered 2 of 7 patients with late relapse after cisplatin-based chemotherapy continuously free from disease.[57,58]

Despite recent progress in salvage chemotherapy, surgery is still the most important part of treatment in patients with late-relapsing TC and increases the chances of cure.[1,2,45,46] Even patients with chemorefractory germ cell tumors have a chance to be cured by salvage "desperation" surgery.[57] Conceivably, incomplete resection of viable residual tumor portends a poor prognosis as mirrored by a 5-year cancer-specific survival of 39% as opposed to 77% in patients with complete resection.[47] Enhanced experience with late relapses combined with increased vigilance toward early detection might have contributed to improving cure rates as reported by the following first investigators on late-relapse studies during the last decades: 1995 (Baniel), 26%[1]; 1997 (Gerl), 36%[2]; 2002 (Shahidi), 69%[30]; 2003 (George), 47%[46]; 2005 (Dieckmann), 63%[45]; 2006 (Oldenburg), 68%[5]; and 2008 (Sharp), 60%.[47] Most of these series on late relapse are reported by high-volume cancer centers with supremely experienced surgeons. Nevertheless, survival remains less than 75%, and the chances of cure should not be spoiled by exploratory operations. Repeated operations, because of incomplete resection of viable tumor, are technically very challenging and should be avoided by ensuring that only surgeons with particular expertise operate on patients with relapses in the first place.[59]

SUMMARY

Patients with MGCT suspected to have a late relapse depend on referral to dedicated experts for proper diagnosis and treatment. This policy provides the best chances of cure and enables collection of data, which increase our knowledge about these rare tumors. Long-term reports on the incidence of late relapse among patients with MGCT help to adjust follow-up strategies and define efficacy of primary treatment.

REFERENCES

1. Baniel J, Foster RS, Gonin R, et al. Late relapse of testicular cancer. J Clin Oncol 1995;13:1170–6.
2. Gerl A, Clemm C, Schmeller N, et al. Late relapse of germ cell tumors after cisplatin-based chemotherapy. Ann Oncol 1997;8:41–7.
3. Ronnen EA, Kondagunta GV, Bacik J, et al. Incidence of late-relapse germ cell tumor and outcome to salvage chemotherapy. J Clin Oncol 2005;23:6999–7004.
4. Oldenburg J, Martin JM, Fossa SD. Late relapses of germ cell malignancies: incidence, management, and prognosis. J Clin Oncol 2006;24:5503–11.
5. Oldenburg J, Alfsen GC, Waehre H, et al. Late recurrences of germ cell malignancies: a population-based experience over three decades. Br J Cancer 2006;94:820–7.
6. Kollmannsberger C, Tyldesley S, Moore C, et al. Evolution in management of testicular seminoma: population-based outcomes with selective utilization of active therapies. Ann Oncol 2011;22(4):808–14.
7. Fossa SD, Horwich A, Russell JM, et al. Optimal planning target volume for stage I testicular seminoma: a Medical Research Council randomized trial.

Medical Research Council Testicular Tumor Working Group. J Clin Oncol 1999; 17:1146.

8. von der Maase H, Specht L, Jacobsen GK, et al. Surveillance following orchidectomy for stage I seminoma of the testis. Eur J Cancer 1993;29A:1931–4.

9. Warde P, Specht L, Horwich A, et al. Prognostic factors for relapse in stage I seminoma managed by surveillance: a pooled analysis. J Clin Oncol 2002;20: 4448–52.

10. Dieckmann KP, Bruggeboes B, Pichlmeier U, et al. Adjuvant treatment of clinical stage I seminoma: is a single course of carboplatin sufficient? Urology 2000;55: 102–6.

11. Oliver RTD, Mason MD, Mead GM, et al. Radiotherapy versus single-dose carboplatin in adjuvant treatment of stage I seminoma: a randomised trial. Lancet 2005; 366:293–300.

12. Powles T, Robinson D, Shamash J, et al. The long-term risks of adjuvant carboplatin treatment for stage I seminoma of the testis. Ann Oncol 2008;19:443–7.

13. Martin JM, Panzarella T, Zwahlen DR, et al. Evidence-based guidelines for following stage 1 seminoma. Cancer 2007;109:2248–56.

14. Warde P, Gospodarowicz M. Adjuvant carboplatin in stage I seminoma. Lancet 2005;366:267–8.

15. van As NJ, Gilbert DC, Money-Kyrle J, et al. Evidence-based pragmatic guidelines for the follow-up of testicular cancer: optimising the detection of relapse. Br J Cancer 2008;98:1894–902.

16. Groll RJ, Warde P, Jewett MA. A comprehensive systematic review of testicular germ cell tumor surveillance. Crit Rev Oncol Hematol 2007;64:182–97.

17. Moynihan C, Norman AR, Barbachano Y, et al. Prospective study of factors predicting adherence to medical advice in men with testicular cancer. J Clin Oncol 2009;27:2144–50.

18. Tarin TV, Sonn G, Shinghal R. Estimating the risk of cancer associated with imaging related radiation during surveillance for stage I testicular cancer using computerized tomography. J Urol 2009;181(2):627–32.

19. Chung P, Parker C, Panzarella T, et al. Surveillance in stage I testicular seminoma—risk of late relapse. Can J Urol 2002;9:1637–40.

20. Oliver RT, Lore S, Ong J. Alternatives to radiotherapy in the management of seminoma. Br J Urol 1990;65:61–7.

21. Classen J, Schmidberger H, Meisner C, et al. Radiotherapy for stages IIA/B testicular seminoma: final report of a prospective multicenter clinical trial. J Clin Oncol 2003;21:1101–6.

22. Chung PW, Gospodarowicz MK, Panzarella T, et al. Stage II testicular seminoma: patterns of recurrence and outcome of treatment. Eur Urol 2004;45:754–9.

23. Warde P, Gospodarowicz M, Panzarella T, et al. Management of stage II seminoma. J Clin Oncol 1998;16:290–4.

24. Krege S, Beyer J, Souchon R, et al. European consensus conference on diagnosis and treatment of germ cell cancer: a report of the second meeting of the European Germ Cell Cancer Consensus Group (EGCCCG): part II. Eur Urol 2008;53:497–513.

25. Mead GM, Stenning SP, Cook P, et al. International Germ Cell Consensus Classification: a prognostic factor-based staging system for metastatic germ cell cancers. International Germ Cell Cancer Collaborative Group. J Clin Oncol 1997;15:594–603.

26. Herr HW, Sheinfeld J, Puc HS, et al. Surgery for a post-chemotherapy residual mass in seminoma. J Urol 1997;157:860–2.

27. Flechon A, Bompas E, Biron P, et al. Management of post-chemotherapy residual masses in advanced seminoma. J Urol 2002;168:1975–9.
28. Quek ML, Simma-Chiang V, Stein JP, et al. Postchemotherapy residual masses in advanced seminoma: current management and outcomes. Expert Rev Anticancer Ther 2005;5:869–74.
29. De Santis M, Becherer A, Bokemeyer C, et al. 2-18fluoro-deoxy-D-glucose positron emission tomography is a reliable predictor for viable tumor in postchemotherapy seminoma: an update of the prospective multicentric SEMPET trial. J Clin Oncol 2004;22:1034–9.
30. Shahidi M, Norman AR, Dearnaley DP, et al. Late recurrence in 1263 men with testicular germ cell tumors. Multivariate analysis of risk factors and implications for management. Cancer 2002;95:520–30.
31. Kollmannsberger C, Moore C, Chi KN, et al. Non-risk-adapted surveillance for patients with stage I nonseminomatous testicular germ-cell tumors: diminishing treatment-related morbidity while maintaining efficacy. Ann Oncol 2010;21: 1296–301.
32. Albers P, Siener R, Krege S, et al. Randomized phase III trial comparing retroperitoneal lymph node dissection with one course of bleomycin and etoposide plus cisplatin chemotherapy in the adjuvant treatment of clinical stage I nonseminomatous testicular germ cell tumors: AUO trial AH 01/94 by the German Testicular Cancer Study Group. J Clin Oncol 2008;26(18):2966–72.
33. Tandstad T, Dahl O, Cohn-Cedermark G, et al. Risk-adapted treatment in clinical stage I nonseminomatous germ cell testicular cancer: the SWENOTECA management program. J Clin Oncol 2009;27:2122–8.
34. Donohue JP, Thornhill JA, Foster RS, et al. Clinical stage B non-seminomatous germ-cell testis cancer: the Indiana University experience (1965–1989) using routine primary retroperitoneal lymph-node dissection. Eur J Cancer 1995;31: 1599–604.
35. Eggener SE, Carver BS, Sharp DS, et al. Incidence of disease outside modified retroperitoneal lymph node dissection templates in clinical stage I or IIA nonseminomatous germ cell testicular cancer. J Urol 2007;177:937–42.
36. Stephenson AJ, Bosl GJ, Motzer RJ, et al. Nonrandomized comparison of primary chemotherapy and retroperitoneal lymph node dissection for clinical stage IIA and IIB nonseminomatous germ cell testicular cancer. J Clin Oncol 2007;25: 5597–602.
37. Oldenburg J, Alfsen GC, Lien HH, et al. Postchemotherapy retroperitoneal surgery remains necessary in patients with nonseminomatous testicular cancer and minimal residual tumor masses. J Clin Oncol 2003;21:3310–7.
38. Ehrlich Y, Brames MJ, Beck SDW, et al. Long-term follow-up of cisplatin combination chemotherapy in patients with disseminated nonseminomatous germ cell tumors: is a postchemotherapy retroperitoneal lymph node dissection needed after complete remission? J Clin Oncol 2010;28:531–6.
39. Kollmannsberger C, Daneshmand S, So A, et al. Management of disseminated nonseminomatous germ cell tumors with risk-based chemotherapy followed by response-guided postchemotherapy surgery. J Clin Oncol 2010;28:537–42.
40. Carver BS, Shayegan B, Eggener S, et al. Incidence of metastatic nonseminomatous germ cell tumor outside the boundaries of a modified postchemotherapy retroperitoneal lymph node dissection. J Clin Oncol 2007;25:4365–9.
41. Beck SD, Foster RS, Bihrle R, et al. Is full bilateral retroperitoneal lymph node dissection always necessary for postchemotherapy residual tumor? Cancer 2007;110:1235–40.

42. Heidenreich A, Pfister D, Witthuhn R, et al. Postchemotherapy retroperitoneal lymph node dissection in advanced testicular cancer: radical or modified template resection. Eur Urol 2008;55(1):217–24.

43. Pettus JA, Carver BS, Masterson T, et al. Preservation of ejaculation in patients undergoing nerve-sparing postchemotherapy retroperitoneal lymph node dissection for metastatic testicular cancer. Urology 2009;73(2):328–31.

44. McGuire MS, Rabbani F, Mohseni H, et al. The role of thoracotomy in managing postchemotherapy residual thoracic masses in patients with nonseminomatous germ cell tumours. BJU Int 2003;91:469–73.

45. Dieckmann KP, Albers P, Classen J, et al. Late relapse of testicular germ cell neoplasms: a descriptive analysis of 122 cases. J Urol 2005;173:824–9.

46. George DW, Foster RS, Hromas RA, et al. Update on late relapse of germ cell tumor: a clinical and molecular analysis. J Clin Oncol 2003;21:113–22.

47. Sharp DS, Carver BS, Eggener SE, et al. Clinical outcome and predictors of survival in late relapse of germ cell tumor. J Clin Oncol 2008;26:5524–9.

48. Pezaro CJ, Mallesara G, Toner GC. Late relapsing stage I nonseminoma. J Clin Oncol 2008;26:5647–8.

49. Hain SF, O'Doherty MJ, Timothy AR, et al. Fluorodeoxyglucose positron emission tomography in the evaluation of germ cell tumours at relapse. Br J Cancer 2000; 83:863–9.

50. Michael H, Lucia J, Foster RS, et al. The pathology of late recurrence of testicular germ cell tumors. Am J Surg Pathol 2000;24:257–73.

51. Collette L, Sylvester RJ, Stenning SP, et al. Impact of the treating institution on survival of patients with "poor-prognosis" metastatic nonseminoma. European Organization for Research and Treatment of Cancer Genito-Urinary Tract Cancer Collaborative Group and the Medical Research Council Testicular Cancer Working Party. J Natl Cancer Inst 1999;91:839–46.

52. Motzer RJ, Sheinfeld J, Mazumdar M, et al. Paclitaxel, ifosfamide, and cisplatin second-line therapy for patients with relapsed testicular germ cell cancer. J Clin Oncol 2000;18:2413–8.

53. Kondagunta GV, Bacik J, Donadio A, et al. Combination of paclitaxel, ifosfamide, and cisplatin is an effective second-line therapy for patients with relapsed testicular germ cell tumors. J Clin Oncol 2005;23:6549–55.

54. Lorch A, Rick O, Wundisch T, et al. High dose chemotherapy as salvage treatment for unresectable late relapse germ cell tumors. J Urol 2010;184:168–73.

55. Lorch A, Kollmannsberger C, Hartmann JT, et al. Single versus sequential high-dose chemotherapy in patients with relapsed or refractory germ cell tumors: a prospective randomized multicenter trial of the German Testicular Cancer Study Group. J Clin Oncol 2007;25:2778–84.

56. Mayer F, Wermann H, Albers P, et al. Histopathological and molecular features of late relapses in non-seminomas. BJU Int 2011;107(6):936–43.

57. Feldman DR, Sheinfeld J, Bajorin DF, et al. TI-CE high-dose chemotherapy for patients with previously treated germ cell tumors: results and prognostic factor analysis. J Clin Oncol 2010;28:1706–13.

58. Murphy BR, Breeden ES, Donohue JP, et al. Surgical salvage of chemorefractory germ-cell tumors. J Clin Oncol 1993;11:324–9.

59. Heidenreich A, Ohlmann C, Hegele A, et al. Repeat retroperitoneal lymphadenectomy in advanced testicular cancer. Eur Urol 2005;47:64–71.

Testicular Cancer Survivorship

Timothy Gilligan, MD

KEYWORDS

- Testicular cancer • Germ cell tumors • Survivorship
- Late effects • Complications

The enormous progress in the treatment of testicular cancer that occurred during the second half of the 20th century has had the happy result that there are many more survivors of testicular cancer. Given their young age at diagnosis, the survivors have long life expectancies; so the number of survivors of testicular cancer is high despite the low incidence of the disease. In the United States, mortality from testicular cancer has declined from 0.74 to 0.22 per 100,000 men, whereas the incidence has increased from 3.73 to 5.85 per 100,000 men. Increasing incidence paired with declining mortality results in increasing prevalence, and thus, the number of 5-year survivors increased from 116,130 in 2000 to 156,418 in 2007, and the number of 10-year survivors increased from 84,024 to 119,511.[1,2] A growing number of men in the population have been treated for testicular cancer and are experiencing the consequences of that treatment.

Over the past few decades and particularly in this century, research into the short- and long-term effects of the treatments of testicular cancer has grown rapidly, and now there exists a much greater body of data to help counsel patients about the risks and side effects of these treatments. In the future, however, survivors would benefit from better prophylactic and therapeutic interventions to prevent or ameliorate the complications of treatment. Achieving that goal will require high-quality research and collaboration among different treatment centers and disciplines.

Issues affecting survivors of testicular cancer vary depending on the treatment given, but they include an increased risk of death from several causes and an increased risk of cardiovascular disease, second cancers, hypogonadism, infertility, peripheral neuropathy, hearing loss, Raynaud phenomenon, and diminished pulmonary and renal function.[3]

LIFE EXPECTANCY

Compared with the general population, survivors of testicular cancer suffer increased mortality from several broad disease categories. A Norwegian analysis of patients with

Late Effects Clinic, Taussig Cancer Institute, Cleveland Clinic, 9500 Euclid Avenue, R35, Cleveland, OH 44195, USA
E-mail address: gilligt@ccf.org

Hematol Oncol Clin N Am 25 (2011) 627–639
doi:10.1016/j.hoc.2011.03.010
0889-8588/11/$ – see front matter © 2011 Elsevier Inc. All rights reserved.

hemonc.theclinics.com

testicular cancer who survived at least 1 year after diagnosis reported that increased mortality was observed from cardiovascular disease (standardized mortality ratio [SMR], 1.2; 95% confidence interval [CI], 1.0–1.5), benign gastrointestinal disorders (SMR, 2.1; 95% CI, 1.1–3.5), and non–germ cell cancers (SMR, 2.0; 95% CI, 1.7–2.4).[4] Most of these patients have been treated with radiotherapy, chemotherapy, or both. Similarly, a US study of 477 men treated with radiotherapy for stage I or II seminoma between 1951 and 1999 reported an increased overall mortality (SMR, 1.59; 99% CI, 1.21–2.04) among the 453 who never had disease relapse compared with the general population.[5] In this group of patients, both cardiac-specific mortality (SMR, 1.61; 99% CI, 1.21–2.24) and cancer-specific mortality (SMR, 1.91; 99% CI, 1.14–2.98) were elevated compared to the age- and sex-matched general population. In this study, statistically significant increases in mortality only became apparent after 15 years of follow-up.

The largest study of long-term survival reported an analysis of non-cancer mortality in 38,907 survivors diagnosed between 1943 and 2001 who were included in the North American and European population-based cancer registries.[6] Overall, there was a 6% increase in non-cancer deaths compared with the general population (SMR, 1.06; 95% CI, 1.02–1.10). Broken down by cause of death, mortality was higher for infections (SMR, 1.28; 95% CI, 1.12–1.47) and digestive disease (SMR, 1.44; 95% CI, 1.26–1.64). However, the increased mortality seemed to be limited to certain subgroups on further analysis. The SMR for all noncancer deaths was 1.05 (95% CI, 0.93–1.17) for those treated with surgery only, 1.00 (95% CI, 0.91–1.09) for those treated with radiotherapy, 1.26 (95% CI, 1.05–1.49) for those who received chemotherapy, and 1.65 (95% CI, 1.18–2.24) for those who received both radiotherapy and chemotherapy. The increased mortality from digestive disease was limited to those treated with radiotherapy (SMR, 1.61; 95% CI, 1.21–2.10), whereas the risk of death from infectious disease was limited to those who received chemotherapy (SMR, 2.48; 95% CI, 1.64–3.58). Increased mortality from cardiovascular disease was seen in men younger than 35 years who were treated with radiotherapy (SMR, 1.70; 95% CI, 1.21–2.31) and those who received chemotherapy as part of their treatment regardless of their age at diagnosis (SMR, 1.44; 95% CI, 1.06–1.91). Men treated with chemotherapy also had an increased risk of death from respiratory diseases (SMR, 2.66; 95% CI, 1.21–5.04), most likely because of bleomycin and cisplatin toxicity.[7]

CARDIOVASCULAR DISEASE
Cardiovascular Risk Factors

In addition to the studies mentioned earlier that documented increased mortality from cardiovascular disease in the survivors of testicular cancer after treatment with radiotherapy or chemotherapy, numerous reports have investigated the cardiovascular disease risk factors and cardiovascular events in the survivors of testicular cancer. Early investigations of cardiovascular complications of the treatment of testicular cancer revealed that serum cholesterol increased after cisplatin-based chemotherapy for germ cell tumors.[8,9] Subsequent investigations have documented hyperlipidemia and other components of the metabolic syndrome in the survivors of testicular cancer. A Norwegian study of 1289 survivors of testicular cancer reported that 11 years after treatment, chemotherapeutically treated patients had higher systolic and diastolic blood pressure and an increased risk of hypertension (odds ratio, 2.4; 95% CI, 1.4–4.0) compared with those treated with surgery alone.[10] Compared with healthy controls, those receiving either radiotherapy or chemotherapy had an increased risk of hypertension. An analysis of 62 patients treated with chemotherapy at least 10 years previously compared with 40 patients treated with orchiectomy alone and with similarly long follow-up reported that the patients treated with chemotherapy had higher blood pressure, total cholesterol, and triglyceride levels.[11] A subsequent study of 86 chemotherapeutically treated patients, 44 patients with stage I disease treated with orchiectomy only, and 47 healthy controls reported that the total cholesterol and total cholesterol/high-density lipoprotein (HDL) cholesterol ratio were elevated in patients treated with chemotherapy compared with the controls.[12] Moreover, the incidence of metabolic syndrome was higher in patients treated with chemotherapy (26%, $P = .017$) and also in those with stage I disease (36%, (36%, $P = .002$) compared with the controls (9%).

One of the many Norwegian studies in this area compared 140 patients treated with surgery alone, 231 who received infradiaphragmatic radiotherapy, and 218 treated with chemotherapy.[13] Patients treated with radiotherapy had elevated C-reactive protein and soluble CD40 ligand, whereas those treated with chemotherapy had lower HDL cholesterol and a higher prevalence of metabolic syndrome. These findings suggested that radiotherapy resulted in chronic inflammation and endothelial dysfunction, whereas chemotherapy resulted in increased risk factors for atherosclerosis. In contrast, Dutch investigators had previously reported that, compared with healthy controls and survivors treated with orchiectomy alone, chemotherapeutically treated patients with testicular cancer had higher levels of C-reactive protein and von Willebrand factor and other plasma markers of inflammation and endothelial stimulation.[14] Supporting the relevance of these findings, a Norwegian study of 586 survivors of testicular cancer found that those with higher C-reactive protein levels ($\geq$1.5 mg/L) had a 2.79 times higher risk of cardiovascular disease compared with the survivors with lower levels (95% CI, 1.22–6.34).[15] In a different study, carotid artery intima-media thickness and plasma von Willebrand factor increased in patients with testicular cancer after chemotherapy compared with pre-chemotherapy values,[16] supporting a causative role for chemotherapy.

A 2010 Norwegian study of 990 patients with testicular cancer treated between 1980 and 1994 reported that compared with age-matched controls, patients with testicular cancer were more likely to be using lipid-lowering medication regardless of whether they had received chemotherapy.[17] Patients treated with radiotherapy and/or chemotherapy were more likely than controls to be using antihypertensive medications, but patients treated with surgery alone were not. Men treated with radiotherapy were also more likely to be taking medication for diabetes.

Although the strongest evidence regarding elevated risk factors for cardiovascular disease points to chemotherapy and radiotherapy as the contributing causes, hypogonadism after orchiectomy may also contribute. Among the survivors of testicular cancer, hypogonadism has been documented in about 10% after surgical treatment alone and 13% to 26% after chemotherapy or radiotherapy.[18–20] In turn, there is compelling evidence that hypogonadism may be a risk factor for cardiovascular disease. A group studying the survivors of testicular cancer found that hypogonadism was associated with a higher body mass index, higher systolic and diastolic blood pressure (140/90 vs 130/85, $P<.016$), and cardiovascular events.[19,21] Moreover, numerous studies have reported that hypogonadism is associated with metabolic syndrome, both generally and in survivors of testicular cancer specifically.[12,22–25] In support of this association, androgen deprivation has been shown to result rapidly in increased insulin resistance before any changes in body mass index.[26] If hypogonadism leads to the development of metabolic syndrome, it would explain part of the increased risk of cardiovascular morbidity and mortality in patients with testicular cancer.

Cardiovascular Events

The literature documenting that the survivors of testicular cancer have increased risk factors for cardiovascular disease is paralleled by numerous studies reporting an increased incidence of cardiovascular events.[11,17,21,27] Dutch investigators reported a 7.1 observed-to-expected ratio for cardiac events among 87 ten-year survivors who had received chemotherapy,[11] whereas British researchers reported a more than 2-fold increased risk of cardiovascular events in a study of 992 ten-year survivors of testicular cancer after radiotherapy, chemotherapy, or both.[21]

A much larger Dutch study of 2512 five-year survivors treated between 1965 and 1995 reported an increased incidence of cardiovascular events (standardized incidence ratio [SIR], 1.17; 95% CI, 1.04–1.31) compared with men in the general population matched for age and calendar period, although the difference was only seen if angina pectoris and myocardial infarction (MI) in the same person were counted as separate events.[27] Moreover, although the risk of MI was roughly doubled among young survivors of nonseminoma , it was reduced by 50% among survivors of nonseminoma aged 55 years or older, and there was no significant change in the risk of MI among patients with seminoma of any age. Broken down by treatment, a significantly increased incidence of MI was seen only among survivors who had been treated with both radiotherapy and chemotherapy (SIR, 2.06; 95% CI, 1.17–3.35), although a clinically significant increased incidence was also reported after chemotherapy alone (SIR, 1.46; 95% CI, 0.91–2.21). In this study, radiotherapy was only associated with an increased risk of MI if mediastinal irradiation was included. Among men treated with surgery alone, there was no increased risk of MI (SIR, 0.95).

The 2010 Norwegian study of 990 survivors discussed earlier reported that in addition to increased risk factors for cardiovascular events, the incidence of coronary artery disease and atherosclerotic disease events was higher after chemotherapy and/or radiotherapy, although not all the differences were statistically significant.[17] Compared with survivors treated with surgery alone, diagnosis with coronary artery disease was more common in patients treated with radiotherapy and chemotherapy (hazard ratio [HR], 5.3; 95% CI, 1.5–18.5), whereas the risk of cardiovascular events was higher after radiotherapy (HR, 2.3; 95%, CI 1.04–5.3), chemotherapy (HR, 2.6; 95% CI, 1.1–5.9), or both (HR, 4.8; 95% CI, 1.6–14.4). The risk of coronary artery disease was nonsignificantly increased after radiotherapy alone (HR, 2.1; 95% CI, 0.78–5.5) and chemotherapy alone (HR, 2.6; 95% CI, 0.96–6.9).

Prevention

As discussed earlier, risk factors for cardiovascular disease as well as cardiovascular morbidity and mortality are all increased in the survivors of testicular cancer or at least within certain subgroups of these men. Chemotherapy and radiotherapy have both been implicated as contributing to this risk. Hypogonadism because of the underlying cancer and/or orchiectomy may also contribute. Risk modification has proved highly effective for cardiovascular disease, although not specifically among the survivors of testicular cancer. Because these men are at elevated risk of cardiovascular disease, it is logical to be rigorous about following the standard preventive guidelines addressing screening for and treating conditions and behaviors associated with cardiovascular disease, including hypertension, hyperlipidemia, diabetes mellitus, and cigarette smoking. Regular aerobic exercise, a healthy diet, and maintenance of a healthy body weight are also logical recommendations, although there are little data to guide such advice in this patient population. Research is needed regarding whether the standard guidelines should be modified, intensified, or initiated at a younger age for the survivors of testicular cancer based on their increased risk.[3]

SECOND MALIGNANCIES

It is well documented that the survivors of testicular cancer face an increased risk of second cancers, including second primary germ cell tumors in the contralateral testis and non–germ cell malignancies. The risk of contralateral germ cell tumors may be reduced by chemotherapy, whereas the much more dangerous problem of second non–germ cell cancers seems to result from treatment with radiotherapy and chemotherapy.

Second Primary Germ Cell Tumors

The increased risk of a second primary contralateral testis germ cell tumor is well established. A population-based study of 29,515 US men diagnosed with testicular cancer reported that the 15-year cumulative risk was 2.5% (95% CI, 1.7–2.1), including a 0.6% risk of having synchronous tumors and a 1.9% risk of diagnosis with a metachronous tumor. Of 462 contralateral tumors, 62% were metachronous and 38% were synchronous.[28] The median time to diagnosis of the second cancer was 5 years, and the risk of death from it was 0.3%. Risk factors for a contralateral cancer included an initial cancer that was pure seminoma and age below 30 years at diagnosis of the first cancer. Several smaller contemporary studies have reported roughly similar results.[29–31] Because of the increased risk of developing a second germ cell tumor, the survivors of testicular cancer are often advised to perform a regular self-examination of their remaining testis.

Secondary contralateral testis germ cell tumors have a better prognosis than primary testicular cancers but represent a problem nonetheless because of the impact of bilateral orchiectomy on fertility, sex hormone levels, and body image. Testosterone replacement therapy can effectively treat hypogonadism, and sperm banking before treatment often provides a way to make procreation possible.

Secondary Non–Germ Cell Cancers

Non–germ cell cancers represent a much bigger threat to the long-term health of the survivors of testicular cancer who have been treated with radiotherapy and/or chemotherapy.[4,5,32–46] Numerous studies have linked both the treatment modalities to an increased risk of cancer and cancer-related mortality, but there is no strong evidence of an increased risk among men treated with surgery alone (orchiectomy with or without retroperitoneal lymph node dissection [RPLND]). Thus, the risk seems to derive primarily from the treatment rather than from an inherent predisposition to develop malignancies. A population-based cancer registry study of more than 29,000 survivors of testicular cancer reported that a survival analysis of the 621 who developed a second cancer with known stage revealed that cancer-specific and over-all survival were similar among these men and controls matched for a cancer site, stage, year of diagnosis, and age.[47]

The 2 biggest studies of non–germ cell cancers in the survivors of testicular cancer evaluated 2 largely overlapping population-based data sets. The first studied 40,576 men in the US and Nordic cancer registries and reported that a man diagnosed with testicular cancer at 35 years of age had twice the risk of being diagnosed with a second non–germ cell solid tumor over the subsequent 10 years compared with men of the same age in the general population (relative risk [RR], 1.9; 95% CI, 1.8–2.1).[39] Forty years after diagnosis, his risk of being diagnosed with a second cancer was 36% if the testicular cancer was seminoma and 31% if it was nonseminoma, compared with 23% for a man in the general population. There were 13 and 8 additional cancers diagnosed per 100 men treated for seminoma and nonseminoma, respectively. The RR for second cancer was similar for radiotherapy alone (RR, 2.0; 95% CI, 1.9–2.2) and chemotherapy alone (RR, 1.8; 95% CI, 1.3–2.5) and was highest among men who had received both (RR, 2.9; 95% CI, 1.9–4.2). Significantly increased risks were reported for melanoma and for cancers of the pleura, esophagus, lung, colon, bladder, pancreas, stomach, prostate, kidneys, thyroid, and connective tissue.

The second study evaluated both solid and liquid tumors in 29,511 survivors, 65% of whom were included in the same Nordic databases used in the first study, supplemented with patients from Australia, Canada, Scotland, and several other countries.[41] The SIR for all non–germ cell malignancies was 1.65 (95% CI, 1.57–1.73) overall and was not significantly different for seminomas and nonseminomas. In addition to the increased risk of many solid tumors, the study also reported an increased risk of myeloid leukemia (SIR, 3.62; 95% CI, 2.56–4.97) and other nonlymphoid leukemia (SIR, 3.47; 95% CI, 2.20–5.21). The risk of myeloid leukemia was greater for nonseminomas (SIR, 6.77; 95% CI, 4.14–10.5) compared with seminomas (SIR, 2.39; 95% CI, 1.41–3.77). Twenty-year survivors of seminoma had a 9.6% cumulative risk of a second cancer, compared with 6.5% in the age-matched general population. Twenty-year survivors of nonseminoma had a 5.0% risk, compared with 3.1% in the general population (patients with nonseminomas are younger on average and hence the lower expected rate of cancer). Neither of these 2 studies provided strong evidence that men treated with radiotherapy or chemotherapy recently have a lower risk than those treated long ago.

Although the ability of radiotherapy and chemotherapy to cause cancer is clearly established, it is less precisely clear which chemotherapeutic drugs are responsible. Cisplatin, carboplatin, and etoposide have each been linked to a dose-dependent increased risk of nonlymphoid leukemia,[35,45,48,49] but the increased risk of second cancers is documented in patients treated before the use of any of these drugs. The primary implication of the data on second cancers is that unnecessarily aggressive treatment should be avoided when considering and planning treatment with chemotherapy or radiotherapy. Treatment plans that include both chemotherapy and radiotherapy should be avoided whenever possible and are generally only appropriate in patients with seminoma who had disease relapse after radiotherapy for early-stage disease.

Additional screening beyond the standard guidelines for the general population cannot be recommended for patients with testicular cancer at this time because there are no data to support such a recommendation. Indeed, some part of testicular-cancer survivors' increased risk of being diagnosed with a second cancer is likely because of the incidental detection of second cancers on surveillance imaging studies, and the potential risk of overdiagnosis cannot be ignored. Helping patients to identify and change behaviors, such as smoking, that are associated with a higher risk of cancer represents the most promising preventive strategy currently available.

NEUROPATHY

About 15% to 20% of men report sensory peripheral neuropathy manifesting as paresthesias in the fingers and/or toes after 3 or more cycles of cisplatin-based chemotherapy for testicular cancer.[50–52] After 2 cycles of chemotherapy, 8% to 16% of men report neurotoxicity.[53,54] A recent study reported that on clinical examination, 35 of 147 men (24%) who received 3 or 4 cycles of cisplatin-based chemotherapy have detectable peripheral neuropathy, as did 30 of 78 (38%) of those who had received more than 4 cycles. Cisplatin accumulates in and damages dorsal root ganglion cells, and this damage is thought to play a key role in the mechanism of cisplatin neurotoxicity.

No treatment has been convincingly shown to be effective for cisplatin peripheral neuropathy. Proposed neuroprotective agents include acetylcysteine, amifostine, calcium and magnesium, diethyldithiocarbamate, glutathione, Org 2766, oxcarbazepine, and vitamin E, but none has been clearly shown to be of benefit.[55] A recent Cochrane review concluded that none of these agents could be recommended as preventing or limiting neurotoxicity from platinum-based chemotherapy in humans. Nonetheless, there is evidence in support of vitamin E from 2 small randomized controlled trials that studied, respectively, 30 and 41 patients who received more than 300 mg/m^2 of cisplatin. With the trials combined, 31 were randomized to alpha-tocopherol (a daily dose of 600 mg in the first trial and 400 mg in the second trial) and 40 were randomized to the control arms (no treatment in the first trial and placebo in the second trial). In the first trial, neurotoxicity was detected in 21% of those who received vitamin E, compared with 69% of those who did not (RR, 2.51; 95% CI, 1.16–5.47).[56] In the second trial, neurotoxicity was seen in 5.9% of the patients randomized to vitamin E, compared with 42% of those randomized to placebo ($P<.01$).[57] However, a larger trial reported that among 207 subjects receiving neurotoxic chemotherapy who were randomized to 400 mg of vitamin E or placebo twice daily, vitamin E was not associated with a lower rate of grade 2 or higher sensory neuropathy. However, in that trial, the most common neuropathic drugs were taxanes followed by oxaliplatin; so conclusions about cisplatin neurotoxicity in particular could not be drawn.[58]

Cisplatin also causes ototoxicity, which manifests in a dose-dependent fashion as tinnitus and/or loss of high-pitch hearing (3 kHz and more). After cisplatin-based chemotherapy for metastatic disease, 20% to 30% of patients report tinnitus or hearing loss and 20% to 40% have confirmed hearing loss on audiometry.[59,60] Even after 2 cycles of chemotherapy, a 5-dB hearing loss at 8 kHz has been documented as well as transient tinnitus.[61] Cisplatin ototoxicity is often permanent and may worsen over time. No effective treatment or prophylaxis for ototoxicity has been identified.

NEPHROTOXICITY

Cisplatin represents the greatest cause of diminished renal function in the survivors of testicular cancer, but radiotherapy and postchemotherapy RPLND can also affect the kidneys.[62,63] Cisplatin promotes apoptosis of kidney cells and at high doses can cause necrosis. The initial toxic effect is proximal tubular damage, resulting in a reduced capacity for sodium and water reabsorption. Diminished glomerular and distal tubular functions are later effects. Even in patients with no other evidence of renal injury, hyponatremia and hypomagnesemia are common after treatment with cisplatin.[64] Aggressive hydration immediately before and during the administration of cisplatin, with or without the addition of mannitol to enhance diuresis, has long been the standard of care to reduce the risk of renal injury, but no other renal protective measures have been shown to be of benefit.

Studies of men with germ cell tumors receiving at least 3 cycles of cisplatin-based chemotherapy have reported a 10% to 23% decline in the glomerular filtration rate (GFR), and only few patients show subsequent improvement.[65–68] A long-term follow-up study with a median observation time of 14 years reported that 11 of 53 patients (21%) treated with chemotherapy developed below normal GFRs after diagnosis, compared with only 4 of 32 patients (13%) treated without chemotherapy

($P = .02$).[62] There is also evidence that para-aortic radiotherapy results in diminished renal function, whereas patients undergoing surgical treatment alone have not been shown to have reduced renal function.[65] A study of 85 patients who were more than 10 years out from treatment reported that radiotherapy was associated with an 8% decrease in GFR and chemotherapy with a 14% decrease in GFR, whereas those undergoing RPLND had no significant decline.[62] Similar results have been reported by other investigators.[65] However, there is a low risk of undergoing a unilateral nephrectomy during postchemotherapy RPLND to resect the residual masses.[63]

Serum creatinine levels are not sensitive markers of renal injury in patients with germ cell tumors: the studies documenting deteriorated renal function were based on measurements of the GFR rather than estimates of creatinine clearance. A normal serum creatinine level does not equate with the absence of renal injury. However, most patients with cisplatin nephrotoxicity suffer subclinical renal injuries, and the relevance to the patient's health and well-being is not established. There is evidence in other settings that declines in GFR are associated with an increased all-cause cardiovascular mortality, but it is not clear that diminished renal function because of cisplatin carries the same implications as diminished renal function because of hypertension, diabetes, and other more common causes.[69,70]

HYPOGONADISM AND INFERTILITY

The survivors of testicular cancer have an increased incidence of hypogonadism and infertility regardless of the treatment.[18–20,71–76] Hypogonadism is most common after chemotherapy or radiotherapy, with 13% to 25% having low testosterone levels. A Norwegian study of 1235 survivors of testicular cancer with a median follow-up of 11 years reported that compared with healthy controls, the RR of hypogonadism was 4.8 (95% CI, 2.4–9.5) after chemotherapy, 3.5 (95% CI, 1.8–7.0) after radiotherapy, and 2.0 (95% CI, 0.9–4.2) after surgery alone.[20] A UK study of 680 long-term survivors reported that low testosterone levels were seen in 11% of men treated with orchiectomy alone, 13% of those treated with chemotherapy, 15% of those treated with radiotherapy, and 34% of those who received both chemotherapy and radiotherapy.[19] Survivors with low testosterone levels also had an increased body mass index and median systolic and diastolic blood pressures. As noted earlier, there is evidence that hypogonadism leads to insulin resistance and other components of the metabolic syndrome.[23–26]

Those with lower testosterone levels have been found to have lower quality of life regarding sexual function and also in the realms of physical, social, and role functioning.[19,77] An Austrian center found that 34% to 47% of clinical stage I survivors of testicular cancer reported clinical symptoms of androgen deficiency and 25% were hypogonadal.[78] A significant number of survivors of testicular cancer have symptoms of androgen deficiency despite serum testosterone levels above the lower limit of the normal range. This finding is likely due, in part, to the fact that the testosterone threshold below which androgen deficiency symptoms appear varies widely from person to person.[72,78] In men with symptoms of androgen deficiency, administration of supplemental testosterone should be considered if the serum testosterone level is low or in the lower end of the normal range and if the serum luteinizing hormone level is elevated.

Men who develop testicular cancer have reduced fertility both before and after diagnosis. Infertility has been shown to be a risk factor for being diagnosed with testicular cancer.[79–81] At the time of diagnosis, 25% to 75% have abnormally low sperm concentration, and the median preorchiectomy sperm concentration in patients with testicular cancer is 40% lower than that in healthy controls.[82-84] Although sperm counts decrease immediately after orchiectomy, they seem to increase again after successful treatment of the cancer.[85,86] A Viennese study reported that among 22 patients with clinical stage I seminoma, all showed an increase in sperm counts after treatment with carboplatin and the proportion with normospermia increased from 35% to 68%, although a British study failed to confirm these findings in patients treated with cisplatin.[61,86]

Most survivors of testicular cancer are able to father children, but men receiving chemotherapy or radiotherapy have lower success rates than those treated with orchiectomy alone.[19,74,75,87] A study of 451 men in Toulouse reported that 91% of men attempting to father a child succeeded before diagnosis with testicular cancer, compared with 67% after treatment was completed.[75] Norwegian investigators reported that among 544 survivors of testicular cancer attempting to conceive a child, 72% were successful, including 92% of those treated with orchiectomy alone and more than 60% of those who had received no more than 4 cycles of cisplatin-based chemotherapy.[74] Given the decline in fertility after radiotherapy or chemotherapy and the risk of dry ejaculation after RPLND, sperm banking is recommended for all men undergoing any postorchiectomy treatment of testicular cancer.

SUMMARY

Although the extraordinarily high cure rate for testicular cancer represents one of the great achievements of modern oncology, the survivors of testicular cancer face a diverse array of health risks after treatment that can threaten their well-being, quality of life, and ability to father children. The best prophylactic measure available at this time is the avoidance of unnecessary or unnecessarily aggressive treatment. Most survivors of testicular cancer report an undiminished quality of life compared with their peers, but those who suffer complications from treatment often do not. Moreover, late effects of treatment clearly compromise the survival of some men. Effective methods to prevent and/or ameliorate these health problems is needed.

REFERENCES

1. Altekruse SF, Kosary CL, Krapcho M, et al. SEER cancer statistics review, 1975–2007. Bethesda (MD): National Cancer Institute; 2010.
2. Ries LAG, Eisner MP, Kosary CL, et al. SEER cancer statistics review, 1975–2000. Bethesda (MD): National Cancer Institute; 2003.
3. Travis LB, Beard C, Allan JM, et al. Testicular cancer survivorship: research strategies and recommendations. J Natl Cancer Inst 2010;102:1114–30.
4. Fossa SD, Aass N, Harvei S, et al. Increased mortality rates in young and middle-aged patients with malignant germ cell tumours. Br J Cancer 2004;90:607–12.
5. Zagars GK, Ballo MT, Lee AK, et al. Mortality after cure of testicular seminoma. J Clin Oncol 2004;22:640–7.
6. Fossa SD, Gilbert E, Dores GM, et al. Noncancer causes of death in survivors of testicular cancer. J Natl Cancer Inst 2007;99:533–44.
7. Aggarwal N, Parwani AV. Spermatocytic seminoma. Arch Pathol Lab Med 2009; 133:1985–8.
8. Raghavan D, Cox K, Childs A, et al. Hypercholesterolemia after chemotherapy for testis cancer. J Clin Oncol 1992;10:1386–9.
9. Gietema JA, Sleijfer DT, Willemse PH, et al. Long-term follow-up of cardiovascular risk factors in patients given chemotherapy for disseminated nonseminomatous testicular cancer. Ann Intern Med 1992;116:709–15.

10. Sagstuen H, Aass N, Fossa SD, et al. Blood pressure and body mass index in long-term survivors of testicular cancer. J Clin Oncol 2005;23:4980–90.
11. Meinardi MT, Gietema JA, van der Graaf WT, et al. Cardiovascular morbidity in long-term survivors of metastatic testicular cancer. J Clin Oncol 2000;18: 1725–32.
12. Nuver J, Smit AJ, Wolffenbuttel BH, et al. The metabolic syndrome and disturbances in hormone levels in long-term survivors of disseminated testicular cancer. J Clin Oncol 2005;23:3718–25.
13. Wethal T, Kjekshus J, Roislien J, et al. Treatment-related differences in cardiovascular risk factors in long-term survivors of testicular cancer. J Cancer Surviv 2007; 1:8–16.
14. Nuver J, Smit AJ, Sleijfer DT, et al. Microalbuminuria, decreased fibrinolysis, and inflammation as early signs of atherosclerosis in long-term survivors of disseminated testicular cancer. Eur J Cancer 2004;40:701–6.
15. Wethal T, Haugnes HS, Kjekshus J, et al. C-reactive protein; a potential marker of second cancer and cardiovascular disease in testicular cancer survivors? Eur J Cancer 2010;46:3425–33.
16. Nuver J, Smit AJ, van der Meer J, et al. Acute chemotherapy-induced cardiovascular changes in patients with testicular cancer. J Clin Oncol 2005;23:9130–7.
17. Haugnes HS, Wethal T, Aass N, et al. Cardiovascular risk factors and morbidity in long-term survivors of testicular cancer: a 20-year follow-up study. J Clin Oncol 2010;28:4649–57.
18. Eberhard J, Stahl O, Cwikiel M, et al. Risk factors for post-treatment hypogonadism in testicular cancer patients. Eur J Endocrinol 2008;158:561–70.
19. Huddart RA, Norman A, Moynihan C, et al. Fertility, gonadal and sexual function in survivors of testicular cancer. Br J Cancer 2005;93:200–7.
20. Nord C, Bjoro T, Ellingsen D, et al. Gonadal hormones in long-term survivors 10 years after treatment for unilateral testicular cancer. Eur Urol 2003;44:322–8.
21. Huddart RA, Norman A, Shahidi M, et al. Cardiovascular disease as a long-term complication of treatment for testicular cancer. J Clin Oncol 2003;21:1513–23.
22. Siviero-Miachon AA, Spinola-Castro AM, Guerra-Junior G. Detection of metabolic syndrome features among childhood cancer survivors: a target to prevent disease. Vasc Health Risk Manag 2008;4:825–36.
23. Spark RF. Testosterone, diabetes mellitus, and the metabolic syndrome. Curr Urol Rep 2007;8:467–71.
24. Lunenfeld B. Testosterone deficiency and the metabolic syndrome. Aging Male 2007;10:53–6.
25. Haugnes HS, Aass N, Fossa SD, et al. Components of the metabolic syndrome in long-term survivors of testicular cancer. Ann Oncol 2007;18:241–8.
26. Yialamas MA, Dwyer AA, Hanley E, et al. Acute sex steroid withdrawal reduces insulin sensitivity in healthy men with idiopathic hypogonadotropic hypogonadism. J Clin Endocrinol Metab 2007;92:4254–9.
27. van den Belt-Dusebout AW, Nuver J, de Wit R, et al. Long-term risk of cardiovascular disease in 5-year survivors of testicular cancer. J Clin Oncol 2006;24: 467–75.
28. Fossa SD, Chen J, Schonfeld SJ, et al. Risk of contralateral testicular cancer: a population-based study of 29,515 U.S. men. J Natl Cancer Inst 2005;97: 1056–66.
29. Hentrich M, Weber N, Bergsdorf T, et al. Management and outcome of bilateral testicular germ cell tumors: twenty-five year experience in Munich. Acta Oncol 2005;44:529–36.

30. Tabernero J, Paz-Ares L, Salazar R, et al. Incidence of contralateral germ cell testicular tumors in South Europe: report of the experience at 2 Spanish university hospitals and review of the literature. J Urol 2004;171:164–7.
31. Theodore C, Terrier-Lacombe MJ, Laplanche A, et al. Bilateral germ-cell tumours: 22-year experience at the Institut Gustave Roussy. Br J Cancer 2004;90:55–9.
32. Chao CK, Lai PP, Michalski JM, et al. Secondary malignancy among seminoma patients treated with adjuvant radiation therapy. Int J Radiat Oncol Biol Phys 1995;33:831–5.
33. Travis LB, Curtis RE, Hankey BF. Second malignancies after testicular cancer. J Clin Oncol 1995;13:533–4.
34. Travis LB, Curtis RE, Storm H, et al. Risk of second malignant neoplasms among long-term survivors of testicular cancer. J Natl Cancer Inst 1997;89:1429–39.
35. Kollmannsberger C, Beyer J, Droz JP, et al. Secondary leukemia following high cumulative doses of etoposide in patients treated for advanced germ cell tumors. J Clin Oncol 1998;16:3386–91.
36. Bachaud JM, Berthier F, Soulie M, et al. Second non-germ cell malignancies in patients treated for stage I-II testicular seminoma. Radiother Oncol 1999;50: 191–7.
37. Brenner DJ, Curtis RE, Hall EJ, et al. Second malignancies in prostate carcinoma patients after radiotherapy compared with surgery. Cancer 2000;88: 398–406.
38. Houck W, Abonour R, Vance G, et al. Secondary leukemias in refractory germ cell tumor patients undergoing autologous stem-cell transplantation using high-dose etoposide. J Clin Oncol 2004;22:2155–8.
39. Travis LB, Fossa SD, Schonfeld SJ, et al. Second cancers among 40,576 testicular cancer patients: focus on long-term survivors. J Natl Cancer Inst 2005;97: 1354–65.
40. Wierecky J, Kollmannsberger C, Boehlke I, et al. Secondary leukemia after first-line high-dose chemotherapy for patients with advanced germ cell cancer. J Cancer Res Clin Oncol 2005;131:255–60.
41. Richiardi L, Scelo G, Boffetta P, et al. Second malignancies among survivors of germ-cell testicular cancer: a pooled analysis between 13 cancer registries. Int J Cancer 2007;120:623–31.
42. Robinson D, Moller H, Horwich A. Mortality and incidence of second cancers following treatment for testicular cancer. Br J Cancer 2007;96:529–33.
43. van den Belt-Dusebout AW, de Wit R, Gietema JA, et al. Treatment-specific risks of second malignancies and cardiovascular disease in 5-year survivors of testicular cancer. J Clin Oncol 2007;25:4370–8.
44. Hemminki K, Liu H, Sundquist J. Second cancers after testicular cancer diagnosed after 1980 in Sweden. Ann Oncol 2010;21(7):1546–51.
45. Travis LB, Andersson M, Gospodarowicz M, et al. Treatment-associated leukemia following testicular cancer. J Natl Cancer Inst 2000;92:1165–71.
46. Wanderas EH, Fossa SD, Tretli S. Risk of subsequent non-germ cell cancer after treatment of germ cell cancer in 2006 Norwegian male patients. Eur J Cancer 1997;33:253–62.
47. Schairer C, Hisada M, Chen BE, et al. Comparative mortality for 621 second cancers in 29356 testicular cancer survivors and 12420 matched first cancers. J Natl Cancer Inst 2007;99:1248–56.
48. Travis LB, Holowaty EJ, Bergfeldt K, et al. Risk of leukemia after platinum-based chemotherapy for ovarian cancer. N Engl J Med 1999;340:351–7.

49. Smith MA, Rubinstein L, Anderson JR, et al. Secondary leukemia or myelodysplastic syndrome after treatment with epipodophyllotoxins. J Clin Oncol 1999; 17:569–77.

50. Glendenning JL, Barbachano Y, Norman AR, et al. Long-term neurologic and peripheral vascular toxicity after chemotherapy treatment of testicular cancer. Cancer 2010;116:2322–31.

51. Kollmannsberger C, Kuzcyk M, Mayer F, et al. Late toxicity following curative treatment of testicular cancer. Semin Surg Oncol 1999;17:275–81.

52. Mykletun A, Dahl AA, Haaland CF, et al. Side effects and cancer-related stress determine quality of life in long-term survivors of testicular cancer. J Clin Oncol 2005;23:3061–8.

53. Bohlen D, Borner M, Sonntag RW, et al. Long-term results following adjuvant chemotherapy in patients with clinical stage I testicular nonseminomatous malignant germ cell tumors with high risk factors. J Urol 1999;161:1148–52.

54. Kondagunta GV, Motzer RJ. Adjuvant chemotherapy for stage II nonseminomatous germ cell tumors [abstract ix]. Urol Clin North Am 2007;34:179–85.

55. Albers JW, Chaudhry V, Cavaletti G, et al. Interventions for preventing neuropathy caused by cisplatin and related compounds. Cochrane Database Syst Rev 2011; 2:CD005228.

56. Argyriou AA, Chroni E, Koutras A, et al. A randomized controlled trial evaluating the efficacy and safety of vitamin E supplementation for protection against cisplatin-induced peripheral neuropathy: final results. Support Care Cancer 2006;14:1134–40.

57. Pace A, Giannarelli D, Galie E, et al. Vitamin E neuroprotection for cisplatin neuropathy: a randomized, placebo-controlled trial. Neurology 2010;74:762–6.

58. Kottschade LA, Sloan JA, Mazurczak MA, et al. The use of vitamin E for the prevention of chemotherapy-induced peripheral neuropathy: results of a randomized phase III clinical trial. Support Care Cancer 2010. [Epub ahead of print].

59. Bokemeyer C, Berger CC, Hartmann JT, et al. Analysis of risk factors for cisplatin-induced ototoxicity in patients with testicular cancer. Br J Cancer 1998;77: 1355–62.

60. Strumberg D, Brugge S, Korn MW, et al. Evaluation of long-term toxicity in patients after cisplatin-based chemotherapy for non-seminomatous testicular cancer. Ann Oncol 2002;13:229–36.

61. Dearnaley DP, Fossa SD, Kaye SB, et al. Adjuvant bleomycin, vincristine and cisplatin (BOP) for high-risk stage I non-seminomatous germ cell tumours: a prospective trial (MRC TE17). Br J Cancer 2005;92:2107–13.

62. Fossa SD, Aass N, Winderen M, et al. Long-term renal function after treatment for malignant germ-cell tumours. Ann Oncol 2002;13:222–8.

63. Stephenson AJ, Tal R, Sheinfeld J. Adjunctive nephrectomy at post-chemotherapy retroperitoneal lymph node dissection for nonseminomatous germ cell testicular cancer. J Urol 2006;176:1996–9 [discussion: 1999].

64. de Jonge MJ, Verweij J. Renal toxicities of chemotherapy. Semin Oncol 2006;33: 68–73.

65. Aass N, Fossa SD, Aas M, et al. Renal function related to different treatment modalities for malignant germ cell tumours. Br J Cancer 1990;62:842–6.

66. Hamilton CR, Bliss JM, Horwich A. The late effects of cis-platinum on renal function. Eur J Cancer Clin Oncol 1989;25:185–9.

67. MacLeod PM, Tyrell CJ, Keeling DH. The effect of cisplatin on renal function in patients with testicular tumours. Clin Radiol 1988;39:190–2.

68. Fjeldborg P, Sorensen J, Helkjaer PE. The long-term effect of cisplatin on renal function. Cancer 1986;58:2214–7.
69. van der Velde M, Matsushita K, Coresh J, et al. Lower estimated glomerular filtration rate and higher albuminuria are associated with all-cause and cardiovascular mortality. A collaborative meta-analysis of high-risk population cohorts. Kidney Int 2011. [Epub ahead of print].
70. Matsushita K, van der Velde M, Astor BC, et al. Association of estimated glomerular filtration rate and albuminuria with all-cause and cardiovascular mortality in general population cohorts: a collaborative meta-analysis. Lancet 2010;375: 2073–81.
71. Lambert SM, Fisch H. Infertility and testis cancer [abstract xi]. Urol Clin North Am 2007;34:269–77.
72. Lackner JE, Mark I, Schatzl G, et al. Hypogonadism and androgen deficiency symptoms in testicular cancer survivors. Urology 2007;69:754–8.
73. Brydoy M, Fossa SD, Dahl O, et al. Gonadal dysfunction and fertility problems in cancer survivors. Acta Oncol 2007;46:480–9.
74. Brydoy M, Fossa SD, Klepp O, et al. Paternity following treatment for testicular cancer. J Natl Cancer Inst 2005;97:1580–8.
75. Huyghe E, Matsuda T, Daudin M, et al. Fertility after testicular cancer treatments: results of a large multicenter study. Cancer 2004;100:732–7.
76. Spermon JR, Kiemeney LA, Meuleman EJ, et al. Fertility in men with testicular germ cell tumors. Fertil Steril 2003;79:1543–9.
77. Wiechno P, Demkow T, Kubiak K, et al. The quality of life and hormonal disturbances in testicular cancer survivors in Cisplatin era. Eur Urol 2007;52: 1448–54.
78. Lackner JE, Koller A, Schatzl G, et al. Androgen deficiency symptoms in testicular cancer survivors are associated with sexual problems but not with serum testosterone or therapy. Urology 2009;74:825–9.
79. Doria-Rose VP, Biggs ML, Weiss NS. Subfertility and the risk of testicular germ cell tumors (United States). Cancer Causes Control 2005;16:651–6.
80. Jacobsen R, Bostofte E, Engholm G, et al. Risk of testicular cancer in men with abnormal semen characteristics: cohort study. BMJ 2000;321:789–92.
81. Richiardi L, Akre O, Montgomery SM, et al. Fecundity and twinning rates as measures of fertility before diagnosis of germ-cell testicular cancer. J Natl Cancer Inst 2004;96:145–7.
82. van Casteren NJ, Boellaard WP, Romijn JC, et al. Gonadal dysfunction in male cancer patients before cytotoxic treatment. Int J Androl 2010;33(1):73–9.
83. Foster RS, McNulty A, Rubin LR, et al. The fertility of patients with clinical stage I testis cancer managed by nerve sparing retroperitoneal lymph node dissection. J Urol 1994;152:1139–42 [discussion: 1142–3].
84. Petersen PM, Skakkebaek NE, Vistisen K, et al. Semen quality and reproductive hormones before orchiectomy in men with testicular cancer. J Clin Oncol 1999;17: 941–7.
85. Petersen PM, Skakkebaek NE, Rorth M, et al. Semen quality and reproductive hormones before and after orchiectomy in men with testicular cancer. J Urol 1999;161:822–6.
86. Reiter WJ, Kratzik C, Brodowicz T, et al. Sperm analysis and serum follicle-stimulating hormone levels before and after adjuvant single-agent carboplatin therapy for clinical stage I seminoma. Urology 1998;52:117–9.
87. Herr HW, Bar-Chama N, O'Sullivan M, et al. Paternity in men with stage I testis tumors on surveillance. J Clin Oncol 1998;16:733–4.

Index

Note: Page numbers of article titles are in **boldface** type.

A

Adjuvant therapy, chemotherapy, of stage I nonseminomatous germ cell tumors, 521–522
 of stage I testicular seminoma, 509–511
  toxicity of, 511
 radiotherapy of stage I testicular seminoma, 507–509
Apoptosis, in biology of testicular germ cell tumors, 461
 in chemotherapy resistance in testicular germ cell tumors, 463

B

BEP. *See* Bleomycin, etoposide, and cisplatin.
Bevacizumab, for refractory germ cell tumors, 585–587
Biology, of testicular germ cell tumors, **457–471**
 chemosensitivity, 460–462
  apoptosis, 461
  DNA repair pathways, 461–462
  expression of p53, 461
 chemotherapy resistance, 462–464
  cell response to DNA damage, 462–463
  drug metabolism, 462
  epigenetics and cisplatin resistance, 464
  genome-wide studies, 463–464
  transport of cisplatin across cell membrane, 462
 epigenetic changes, 459–460
 gene expression profiling, 460
 genetic changes, 458–459
 preinvasive disease, 457–458
Bleomycin, in first-line chemotherapy of disseminated germ cell tumors, **543–556**
 role in chemotherapy for stage II nonseminoma, 536
Brain metastases, from germ cell tumors, **605–613**
 characteristics of patients with, at first diagnosis of metastatic disease, 605–606
 chemotherapy of patients with, 608–609
 diagnostic procedures for detection of, 607–608
 in patients with relapsed germ cell tumors, 606–607
 multimodal treatment, 610–611
 prognostic impact of, 607
 radiotherapy in patients with, 610
 surgery in patients with, 609–610

C

Carboplatin, role in chemotherapy for stage II nonseminoma, 537
Cardiovascular disease, increased risk in survivors of testicular cancer, 628–631

Hematol Oncol Clin N Am 25 (2011) 641–649
doi:10.1016/S0889-8588(11)00060-8
0889-8588/11/$ – see front matter © 2011 Elsevier Inc. All rights reserved.

hemonc.theclinics.com

Cardiovascular (*continued*)
    events, 630
    prevention, 630–631
    risk factors, 628–629
Cerebral metastases. *See* Brain metastases.
Chemosensitivity, biology of, in testicular germ cell tumors, 460–462
    apoptosis, 461
    DNA repair pathways, 461–462
    expression of p53, 461
Chemotherapy, adjuvant, of stage I nonseminomatous germ cell tumors, 521–522
   adjuvant, of stage I testicular seminoma, 509–511
    toxicity of, 511
   for brain metastases from germ cell tumors, 608–609
   for disseminated germ cell tumors, first-line, **543–556**
    era of delivery (2005 to present), 549–550
    era of development (1985 to 2005), 545–547
    era of discovery (1960s to 1985), 543–545
    intermediate-prognosis and poor-prognosis disease, 547–549
    practical delivery of, 551–553
    work-up of, 550–551
   second-line, **557–576**
    conventional dose, 558–562
    late relapse, 568–569
    prognostic factors, 565–567
    salvage high-dose, 562–565
    seminoma, 567–568
    surgery and, 569
   third-line, **577–591**
    active combination regimens in refractory tumors, 581–583
    active single agents in refractory tumors, 580–581
    for growing teratoma syndrome and teratoma with malignant transformation,
      583–584
    molecular mechanisms of cisplatin resistance, 578–579
    novel agents and refractory tumors, 585–587
    ongoing trials, 587
  for stage II seminoma, residual mass after, 532–533
  primary, duration of for stage II nonseminoma, 536
  role of retroperitoneal lymph node dissection in advanced germ cell tumors after,
    593–604
Chemotherapy resistance, biology of, in testicular germ cell tumors, 462–464
    cell response to DNA damage, 462–463
    drug metabolism, 462
    epigenetics and cisplatin resistance, 464
    genome-wide studies, 463–464
    transport of cisplatin across cell membrane, 462
Chest radiographs, in staging of testicular germ cell tumors, 497
Cisplatin, biology of resistance to, in testicular germ cell tumors, 462–464
    cell response to DNA damage, 462–463
    drug metabolism, 462
    epigenetics and cisplatin resistance, 464
    genome-wide studies, 463–464

transport of cisplatin across cell membrane, 462
in first-line chemotherapy of disseminated germ cell tumors, **543–556**
   practical delivery of BEP regimen, 551–553
in second-line chemotherapy of disseminated germ cell tumors, **557–576**
   conventional dose, 558–560
in third-line chemotherapy of metastatic germ cell tumors, in combination regimens,
   581–583
molecular mechanisms of resistance in metastatic germ cell tumors, 578–579
Computed tomography (CT), in staging of testicular germ cell tumors, 489–495

D

Desperation postchemotherapy retroperitoneal lymph node dissection, 599
Diagnosis, differential, of late relapse of germ cell tumors, 620–621
   of brain metastases of germ cell tumors, 607–608
   of testicular germ cell tumors, imaging studies for, 487–488
DNA repair pathways, in biology of testicular germ cell tumors, 461–462

E

Epidemiologic studies, etiologic differences between seminoma and nonseminoma
   of the testis, **473–486**
Epidermal growth factor receptor, for refractory germ cell tumors, 585–587
Epigenetic changes, in biology of testicular germ cell tumors, 459–460
Epigenetics, and cisplatin resistance in testicular germ cell tumors, 464
Epirubicin, in third-line chemotherapy of metastatic germ cell tumors, in combination
   regimens, 581–583
Etiology, differences between seminoma and nonseminoma of the testis, **473–486**
Etoposide, in first-line chemotherapy of disseminated germ cell tumors, **543–556**
   practical delivery of BEP regimen, 551–553
in second-line chemotherapy of disseminated germ cell tumors, **557–576**
   conventional dose, 558–560
in third-line chemotherapy of metastatic germ cell tumors, **577–591**
   single agent, 580–581

F

First-line chemotherapy. *See* Chemotherapy, first-line.

G

Gemcitabine, in third-line chemotherapy of metastatic germ cell tumors, **577–591**
   in combination regimens, 581–583
   single agent, 580–581
Gene expression profiling, in testicular germ cell tumors, 460
Genetic changes, in biology of testicular germ cell tumors, 458–459
Genome-wide studies, of cisplatin resistance in testicular germ cell tumors, 463–464
Germ cell tumors. *See* Testicular germ cell tumors.
Growing teratoma syndrome, chemotherapy for, 583–584

H

High-dose chemotherapy, of disseminated germ cell tumors in second-line setting,
   562–565

Histopathology, of late relapse of germ cell tumors, 621
Hypogonadism, increased risk in survivors of testicular cancer, 634–635

I

Ifosfamide, in second-line chemotherapy of disseminated germ cell tumors, **557–576**
        conventional dose, 558–560
    in third-line chemotherapy of metastatic germ cell tumors, **577–591**
        single agent, 580–581
Imaging studies, for testicular germ cell tumors, **487–502**
        assessment of tumor response and residual and recurrent disease, 497–500
        diagnosis, 487–488
        staging, 488–497
            chest radiographs, 497
            CT, 489–495
            FDG-PET, 495–496
            MRI, 496
            pattern of spread, 488–489
            ultrasound, 497
Imatinib, for refractory germ cell tumors, 585–587
Infertility, increased risk in survivors of testicular cancer, 634–635
Irinotecan, in third-line chemotherapy of metastatic germ cell tumors, in combination
    regimens, 581–583

L

Late relapse, of germ cell tumors, **615–626**
        detection and differential diagnosis of, 620–621
        histopathology of, 621
        incidence, 615–616
        nonseminoma clinical stage 1, 617–618
        nonseminoma clinical stage greater than 1, 618–620
        seminoma clinical stage 1, 616–617
        seminoma clinical stage greater than 1, 617
        treatment and survival, 621–623
    prognosis of second-line chemotherapy for disseminated germ cell tumors in, 568–569
Life expectancy, in survivors of testicular cancer, 627–628
Lymph node dissection. See Retroperitoneal lymph node dissection.

M

Magnetic resonance imaging (MRI), in staging of testicular germ cell tumors, 496
Malignancies, second, increased risk in survivors of testicular cancer, 631–632
Metastatic germ cell tumors, brain metastases, **605–613**
        characteristics of patients with, at first diagnosis of metastatic disease, 605–606
        chemotherapy of patients with, 608–609
        diagnostic procedures for detection of, 607–608
        in patients with relapsed germ cell tumors, 606–607
        multimodal treatment, 610–611
        prognostic impact of, 607
        radiotherapy in patients with, 610
        surgery in patients with, 609–610
    third-line chemotherapy for, **577–591**

active combination regimens, 581–583

active single agents, 580–581

for growing teratoma syndrome and teratoma with malignant transformation, 583–584

molecular mechanisms of cisplatin resistance, 578–579

novel agents, 585–587

ongoing trials, 587

Mismatch repair pathway, in chemotherapy resistance in testicular germ cell tumors, 462–463

N

Nedaplatin, in combination regimens for third-line chemotherapy of metastatic germ cell tumors, 581–583

Nephrotoxicity, increased risk in survivors of testicular cancer, 633–634

Neuropathy, increased risk in survivors of testicular cancer, 632–633

Nonseminoma. See also Nonseminomatous germ cell tumors.

etiologic differences between seminoma and, **473–486**

late relapse of, 617–620

clinical stage 1, 617–618

clinical stage greater than 1, 618–620

stage II, 533–537

duration of primary chemotherapy, 536

role of bleomycin, 536–537

role of carboplatin, 537

Nonseminomatous germ cell tumors. See also Nonseminoma.

stage I, **517–527**

adjuvant chemotherapy for, 521–522

clinical disease, 518–519

prognostic factors for, 519–520

retroperitoneal lymph node dissection for, 520

stratified approach to management of, 522–523

surveillance for, 520–521

Novel agents, for refractory germ cell tumors, 585–587

O

Oxaliplatin, in third-line chemotherapy of metastatic germ cell tumors, **577–591**

in combination regimens, 581–583

single agent, 580–581

P

p53, expression of, in testicular germ cell tumors, 461

Paclitaxel, in second-line chemotherapy of disseminated germ cell tumors, 560–561

in third-line chemotherapy of metastatic germ cell tumors, **577–591**

in combination regimens, 581–583

single agent, 580–581

Positron emission tomography (PET), FDG-PET in staging of testicular germ cell tumors, 495–496

Profiling, gene expression, in testicular germ cell tumors, 460

Prognostic factors, brain metastases of germ cell tumors, 607
    for nonseminomatous germ cell tumors, 519–520
    with second-line chemotherapy for disseminated germ cell tumors, 565–567

    R

Radiographs, chest, in staging of testicular germ cell tumors, 497
Radiotherapy, adjuvant, of stage I testicular seminoma, 507–509
        dose of radiation, 508
        toxicity, 508–509
        volume of radiation, 507–508
    for stage II seminoma, residual mass after, 532–533
    of brain metastases from germ cell tumors, 610
Recurrent disease, in testicular germ cell tumors, imaging studies for, 497–500
Refractory germ cell tumors, third-line chemotherapy for disseminated, **577–591**
        active combination regimens, 581–583
        active single agents, 580–581
        for growing teratoma syndrome and teratoma with malignant transformation,
            583–584
        molecular mechanisms of cisplatin resistance, 578–579
        novel agents, 585–587
        ongoing trials, 587
Relapsed germ cell tumors, brain metastases in, 606–607
    late relapse, **615–626**
        detection and differential diagnosis of, 620–621
        histopathology of, 621
        incidence, 615–616
        nonseminoma clinical stage 1, 617–618
        nonseminoma clinical stage greater than 1, 618–620
        seminoma clinical stage 1, 616–617
        seminoma clinical stage greater than 1, 617
        treatment and survival, 621–623
    prognosis of second-line chemotherapy for disseminated, 568–569
    stage I testicular seminoma, management of, 512
Residual disease, after radiation or chemotherapy for stage II seminoma, 532–533
    in testicular germ cell tumors, imaging studies for, 497–500
Response, tumor, in testicular germ cell tumors, imaging studies for, 497–500
Retroperitoneal lymph node dissection, in stage I nonseminomatous germ cell tumors, 520
    in stage I testicular seminoma, 511–512
    postchemotherapy, role in advanced germ cell tumors, **593–604**
        classification of, 598–600
            after second-line chemotherapy, 599
            desperation, 599
            for advanced seminoma, 599–600
        patient selection for, in nonseminomatous germ cell tumors, 596–598
        rationale for, in nonseminomatous germ cell tumors, 594–596

    S

Salvage high-dose chemotherapy, of disseminated germ cell tumors, 562–565
        in second-line setting, 563–565
Second malignancies, increased risk in survivors of testicular cancer, 631–632

second primary germ cell tumor, 631
secondary non-germ cell cancers, 631–632
Second-line chemotherapy. See Chemotherapy, second-line.
Seminoma, etiologic differences between nonseminoma and, **473–486**
    late relapse of, 616–617
        clinical stage 1, 616–617
        clinical stage greater than 1, 617
    postchemotherapy retroperitoneal lymph node dissection for advanced, 599
    prognosis of second-line chemotherapy for, 567–566
    stage I testicular, management of, **503–516**
        adjuvant chemotherapy, 509–511
        adjuvant radiotherapy, 507–509
        initial evaluation and management, 503–504
        management of relapse, 512
        retroperitoneal lymph node dissection, 511–512
        surveillance, 504–507
    stage II, 530–533
        residual mass after radiotherapy or chemotherapy, 532–533
Staging, of testicular germ cell tumors, imaging studies for, 488–497
        chest radiographs, 497
        CT, 489–495
        FDG-PET, 495–496
        MRI, 496
        pattern of spread, 488–489
        ultrasound, 497
Sunitinib, for refractory germ cell tumors, 585–587
Surgical management, in the salvage setting for disseminated germ cell tumors, 569
    of brain metastases from germ cell tumors, 609–610
    retroperitoneal lymph node dissection in stage I testicular seminoma, 511–512
Surveillance, of stage I nonseminomatous germ cell tumors, 520–521
    of stage I testicular seminoma, 504–507
        CT screening radiation exposure, 505–507
        predictors of relapse, 504–505
        risk-adapted models, 505
        schedule, 505
Survivors, of testicular cancer, increased risks in, **627–646**
        cardiovascular disease, 628–631
        hypogonadism and infertility, 634–635
        life expectancy, 627–628
        nephrotoxicity, 633–634
        neuropathy, 632–633
        second malignancies, 631–632

T

Teratoma with malignant transformation, chemotherapy for, 583–584
Testicular germ cell tumors, 457–639
    biology of, **457–471**
        chemosensitivity, 460–462
        chemotherapy resistance, 462–464
        epigenetic changes, 459–460
        gene expression profiling, 460

Testicular (*continued*)
    genetic changes, 458–459
    preinvasive disease, 457–458
  brain metastases from, **605–613**
  chemotherapy for disseminated, **543–556, 557–576, 577–591**
    first-line, **543–556**
    second-line, and prognostic models, **557–576**
    third-line, and novel agents for metastatic tumors, **577–591**
  etiologic differences between seminoma and nonseminoma, **473–486**
  imaging studies for, **487–502**
    assessment of tumor response and residual and recurrent disease, 497–500
    diagnosis, 487–488
    staging, 488–497
  late relapse of, **615–626**
  postchemotherapy retroperitoneal lymph node dissection, **593–604**
  stage I nonseminomatous, **517–527**
    adjuvant chemotherapy for, 521–522
    clinical disease, 518–519
    prognostic factors for, 519–520
    retroperitoneal lymph node dissection for, 520
    stratified approach to management of, 522–523
    surveillance for, 520–521
  stage I seminomas, **503–516**
    adjuvant chemotherapy, 509–511
    adjuvant radiotherapy, 507–509
    initial evaluation and management, 503–504
    management of relapse, 512
    retroperitoneal lymph node dissection, 511–512
    surveillance, 504–507
  stage II seminomas and nonseminomas, **529–541**
    nonseminoma, 533–537
      duration of primary chemotherapy, 536
      role of bleomycin, 536–537
      role of carboplatin, 537
    seminoma, residual mass after radiotherapy or chemotherapy, 532–533
      seminoma, 530–533
  survivorship, **627–646**
    cardiovascular disease, 628–631
    hypogonadism and infertility, 634–635
    life expectancy, 627–628
    nephrotoxicity, 633–634
    neuropathy, 632–633
    second malignancies, 631–632
Thalidomide, for refractory germ cell tumors, 585–587
Third-line chemotherapy. *See* Chemotherapy, third-line.
Trastuzumab, for refractory germ cell tumors, 585–587
Tumor response, in testicular germ cell tumors, imaging studies for, 497–500

U

Ultrasound, in staging of testicular germ cell tumors, 497

V

Vascular endothelial growth factor, for refractory germ cell tumors, 585–587
Vinblastine, in second-line chemotherapy of disseminated germ cell tumors, conventional
    dose, 558–560
    second-line chemotherapy of disseminated germ cell tumors, **557–576**

Printed and bound by CPI Group (UK) Ltd, Croydon, CR0 4YY

03/10/2024

01040455-0019